Cystic Tumors of the Pancreas

Marco Del Chiaro
Stephan L. Haas • Richard D. Schulick
Editors

Cystic Tumors of the Pancreas

Diagnosis and Treatment

Springer

Editors
Marco Del Chiaro
Division of Surgery, Department of Clinical Science, Intervention and Technology (CLINTEC)
Karolinska Institute at Center for Digestive Diseases
Karolinska University Hospital
Stockholm
Sweden

Richard D. Schulick
Department of Surgery
University of Colorado at Denver
Aurora, Colorado
USA

Stephan L. Haas
Center for Digestive Diseases
Karolinska University Hospital
Stockholm
Sweden

ISBN 978-3-319-31880-6 ISBN 978-3-319-31882-0 (eBook)
DOI 10.1007/978-3-319-31882-0

Library of Congress Control Number: 2016945764

Printed on acid-free paper

This Springer imprint is published by Springer Nature
The registered company is Springer International Publishing AG Switzerland

Foreword

This publication, entitled *Cystic Tumors of the Pancreas: Diagnosis and Treatment*, is particularly timely. Ten years ago cystic tumors of the pancreas might have made up 5 % of the total pancreatic resections in a large series. Today, cystic tumors comprise 15–20 % of those undergoing pancreatic surgery. This increase is almost entirely made up of intraductal papillary mucinous neoplasms (IPMN). These lesions have changed the face of pancreatic surgery. The three editors, Drs Del Chiaro, Haas, and Schulick, have collected world-class experts on cystic tumors from throughout the world to bring us up to date on how to diagnose and manage these and other cystic lesions of the pancreas. Beginning with Dr Elliot Fishman, who is the recognized leader in diagnosing and defining cystic lesions of the pancreas by computed tomography, to Dr Ralph H. Hruban, who has established many of the pathologic and histologic guidelines for diagnosing and classifying cystic tumors, the contributors are experts from around the world.

This book will undoubtedly go through several editions, because currently the diagnosis, classification, and treatment of cystic neoplasms are still a work in progress. However, for all those currently interested in this topic, which includes primary care physicians, internists, gastroenterologists, surgeons, radiologists, and pathologists, the book is an excellent update.

The cystic tumors that are, of course, of the most interest are IPMNs. These lesions have dramatically changed the face of pancreatic surgery over the past decade. Only infrequently recognized until about 20 years ago, today much of the controversy concerning the diagnosis and management of cystic tumors revolves around IPMNs. The three editors, who themselves are experts in this field, are from different parts of the world—the United States, Europe, and Scandinavia—and are in a unique position to know and recruit experts from around the world to participate in this publication. The resulting book will be of interest to all physicians who see patients with pancreatic diseases and currently set the standard for the diagnosis and management of these lesions.

John L. Cameron, MD
Alfred Blalock Distinguished Service Professor of Surgery
The Johns Hopkins Hospital
Baltimore, MD, USA

Preface

With a prevalence of up to 10 % in the elderly, pancreatic cystic neoplasms (PCNs) represent today the most frequent pancreatic findings in our patients. With the extensive use of high-definition diagnostic modalities for conditions often unrelated to the pancreas, the incidental discovery of a PCN is frequent and represents a challenge not only for the pancreatologist but also for the general practitioner in their daily activity. Some of the PCNs are precursor lesions of pancreas cancer (i.e., intraductal papillary mucinous neoplasm (IPMN)) or can progress to cancer (i.e., mucinous cystic neoplasm (MCN) or solid and pseudopapillary neoplasm (SPN)). In contrast, other neoplasms (i.e., serous cystic neoplasm (SCN)) are benign. Therefore, there are two competing goals. On the one hand, we should aggressively resect lesions that have turned into cancer or are at high risk for doing so. On the other hand, we should not subject patients to the morbidity and mortality of pancreatic resection if they will not be harmed by the PCN. For this reason the correct identification, surveillance, and treatment need careful consideration.

A major issue today is that the preoperative diagnostic accuracy for these neoplasms is very low (inferior to 70 %). For this reason, the management of PCN exposes the patient to the risk of over- or undertreatment of these lesions. Even in patients we decide not to resect, often we subject them to a lifelong regimen of follow-up, because of the low diagnostic accuracy and the impossibility of predicting how individual PCN will evolve. Considering the prevalence of these lesions, this amounts to a tremendous cost for our healthcare systems.

This book was written to be a practical and complete reference for pancreatologists, as well as for gastroenterologists, surgeons, and general practitioners. It will be valuable in the decision-making process in terms of making the correct diagnosis and choosing the correct therapeutic or observational approach for PCNs.

We have been quite successful in collecting and summarizing the experience of some of the most eminent experts in the topic from different disciplines and perspectives. From pathological classification to epidemiology, and from diagnosis to different treatment strategies, the reader has the opportunity to have a complete update on this "burning issue" of the modern pancreatology.

Stockholm, Sweden — Marco Del Chiaro
Stockholm, Sweden — Stephan L. Haas
Aurora, CO, USA — Richard D. Schulick

Contents

Contributors

Peter J. Allen, MD, FACS Department of Surgery, Memorial Sloan Kettering Cancer Center, New York, NY, USA

Unit of Hepatopancreatic Surgery, Memorial Sloan Kettering Cancer Center, New York, NY, USA

Urban Arnelo, MD, PhD Center for Digestive Diseases, Karolinska University Hospital, Stockholm, Sweden

Claudio Bassi, MD, FRCS, FACS Department of Surgery and Oncology, G. B. Rossi Hospital, Verona University Hospital Trust, Verona, Italy

Unit of General and Pancreatic Surgery, University of Verona Hospital Trust, Verona, Italy

Enrico Boninsegna, MD Department of Radiology, Policlinico G. B. Rossi, University of Verona, Verona, Italy

William R. Brugge, MD Department of Gastroenterology, Massachusetts General Hospital, Boston, MA, USA

Marco J. Bruno, MD, PhD Department of Gastroenterology and Hepatology, Erasmus MC, University Medical Center, Rotterdam, The Netherlands

Markus W. Büchler, MD Department of Surgery, University of Heidelberg, Heidelberg, Germany

Djuna L. Cahen, MD, PhD Department of Gastroenterology and Hepatology, Erasmus MC, University Medical Center, Rotterdam, The Netherlands

Güralp O. Ceyhan, MD Department of Surgery, Klinikum Rechts der Isar, Technische Universität München, Munich, Germany

Guido Costamagna, MD, FACG Digestive Endoscopy Unit, Fondazione Policlinico Gemelli – Catholic University, Rome, Italy

Marco Del Chiaro, MD, PhD, FACS Division of Surgery, Department of Clinical Science, Intervention and Technology (CLINTEC), Karolinska Institute at Center for Digestive Diseases, Karolinska University Hospital, Stockholm, Sweden

Ihsan Ekin Demir, MD Department of Surgery, Klinikum Rechts der Isar, Technische Universität München, Munich, Germany

Barish H. Edil, MD, FACS Department of Surgery, University of Colorado Hospital, Aurora, CO, USA

Section of Surgical of Oncology, University of Colorado, Aurora, CO, USA

Elliot K. Fishman, MD Department of Radiology, Johns Hopkins University, Baltimore, MD, USA

Helmut Friess, MD Department of Surgery, Klinikum Rechts der Isar, Technische Universität München, Munich, Germany

Stephan L. Haas, MD, PhD Center for Digestive Diseases, Karolinska University Hospital, Stockholm, Sweden

Thilo Hackert, MD Department of Surgery, University of Heidelberg, Heidelberg, Germany

Ralph H. Hruban, MD Department of Pathology, The Sol Goldman Pancreatic Cancer Research Center, Johns Hopkins University School of Medicine, The Johns Hopkins University, Baltimore, MD, USA

Julio Iglesias-Garcia, MD, PhD Department of Gastroenterology, Foundation for Research in Digestive Diseases, University Hospital of Santiago de Compostela, Santiago de Compostela, Spain

Nirag C. Jhala, MD Department of Pathology and Laboratory Medicine, Professor of Pathology, Temple University School of Medicine, Philadelphia, PA, USA

Ingrid C.A.W. Konings, MD Department of Gastroenterology and Hepatology, Erasmus MC, University Medical Center, Rotterdam, The Netherlands

J. Matthias Löhr, MD Department of Gastrocentrum, Karolinska Institutet, Stockholm, Sweden

Giuseppe Malleo, MD Unit of General and Pancreatic Surgery, G.B. Rossi Hospital, University of Verona Hospital Trust, Verona, Italy

Riccardo Manfredi, MD, MBA Department of Radiology, Policlinico G. B. Rossi, University of Verona, Verona, Italy

Sara Mehrabi, MD Department of Radiology, Policlinico G. B. Rossi, University of Verona, Verona, Italy

Anna Caterina Milanetto, MD Department of Surgery, Oncology and Gastroenterology, Policlinico – University of Padova, Padova, Italy

Unit of Pancreatic and Digestive Endocrine Surgery, Clinica Chirurgica 1, Padova, Italy

Pozzi Mucelli Roberto, MD Department of Radiology, Policlinico G. B. Rossi, University of Verona, Verona, Italy

Takao Ohtsuka, MD, PhD Department of Surgery and Oncology, Graduate School of Medical Sciences, Kyushu University, Fukuoka, Japan

Claudio Pasquali, MD Department of Surgery, Oncology and Gastroenterology, Policlinico – University of Padova, Padova, Italy

Unit of Pancreatic and Digestive Endocrine Surgery, Clinica Chirurgica 1, Padova, Italy

Martha Bishop Pitman, MD Department of Pathology, Massachusetts General Hospital, Professor of Pathology, Harvard Medical School, Boston, MA, USA

Katherine E. Poruk, MD Department of Surgery, The Johns Hopkins Hospital, Baltimore, MD, USA

Siva P. Raman, MD Department of Radiology, Johns Hopkins University, Baltimore, MD, USA

Elena Rangelova, MD Division of Surgery, CLINTEC, Karolinska Institutet at Center for Digestive Diseases, Karolinska University Hospital, Stockholm, Sweden

Roberto Salvia, MD, PhD Department of Surgery, University of Verona – "GB Rossi" Hospital Trust, Verona, Italy

Unit of General and Pancreatic Surgery, University of Verona Hospital Trust, Verona, Italy

Richard D. Schulick, MD, MBA, FACS Department of Surgery, University of Colorado School of Medicine, Aurora, CO, USA

Ralf Segersvärd, MD, PhD Division of Surgery, CLINTEC, Karolinska Institutet at Center for Digestive Diseases, Karolinska University Hospital, Stockholm, Sweden

Camille L. Stewart, MD Department of Surgery, University of Colorado Hospital, Aurora, CO, USA

Section of Surgical of Oncology, University of Colorado, Aurora, CO, USA

Masao Tanaka, MD, PhD, FACS Department of Surgery and Oncology, Graduate School of Medical Sciences, Kyushu University, Fukuoka, Japan

Elke Tieftrunk, MD Department of Surgery, Klinikum Rechts der Isar, Technische Universität München, Munich, Germany

Andrea Tringali, MD, PhD Digestive Endoscopy Unit, Fondazione Policlinico Gemelli – Catholic University, Rome, Italy

Roberto Valente, MD Department of Gastrocentrum, Karolinska University Hospital & Karolinska Institutet, Stockholm, Sweden

Caroline S. Verbeke, MD, PhD, FRCPath Department of Clinical Pathology and Cytology, Karolinska University Hospital, Stockholm, Sweden

Division of Pathology, Department of Laboratory Medicine, Karolinska Institute, Stockholm, Sweden

Christopher L. Wolfgang, MD, PhD Department of Surgery, The Johns Hopkins Hospital, Baltimore, MD, USA

Pathology and Classification of Cystic Tumors of the Pancreas

1

Ralph H. Hruban and Caroline S. Verbeke

1.1 Introduction

A variety of nonneoplastic and neoplastic lesions form cysts in the pancreas (Table 1.1) [1]. The neoplastic lesions range in clinical behavior from entirely benign, to precancerous, to frankly malignant. The management of cystic lesions in the pancreas is therefore complicated, and patients with a pancreatic cyst are best managed by multidisciplinary teams that balance the potential benefits of various treatment options with their risks [2].

An understanding of the pathology of cystic lesions can form a solid foundation for the effective management of patients with a pancreatic cyst. For example, each cyst type has characteristic gross pathology features, and because the radiologic appearance of cystic lesions will be determined by their gross features, an understanding of gross pathology is critical to understanding how imaging can be used to determine cyst type (Tables 1.2 and 1.3) [1]. At the other extreme, the submicroscopic level, each cyst type also has a characteristic pattern of genetic alterations (Table 1.4), and because DNA and other molecules, including miRNAs, proteins, and mucins, shed from the epithelial cells lining a cyst into cyst fluid, an understanding of the genetic and molecular alterations in pancreatic cysts is critical to understanding how analyses of cyst fluid could be used to determine cyst type [3–6].

The major cystic neoplasms of the pancreas include serous cystic neoplasms (SCNs), intraductal papillary mucinous neoplasms (IPMNs), mucinous cystic neoplasms (MCNs), and solid-pseudopapillary neoplasms (SPNs) [1]. In this chapter we will review the gross, microscopic, and immunolabeling characteristics of each of these, with an emphasis on the clinical applications of these pathologic features.

Prepared for "Cystic Tumors of the Pancreas – Diagnosis and Treatment" edited by Marco Del Chiaro, Stephan Haas, and Richard Schulick published by Springer Science+Business Media, New York.

R.H. Hruban, MD (✉)
Department of Pathology, The Sol Goldman Pancreatic Cancer Research Center, Johns Hopkins University School of Medicine, The Johns Hopkins University, 600 N Wolfe Street, Carnegie 415, Baltimore, MD, USA
e-mail: rhruban@jhmi.edu

C.S. Verbeke, MD, PhD, FRCPath
Division of Pathology, Department of Laboratory Medicine, Karolinska Institute, Stockholm 141 86, Sweden

Department of Clinical Pathology and Cytology, Karolinska University Hospital, Stockholm, Sweden
e-mail: caroline.verbeke@ki.se

M. Del Chiaro et al. (eds.), *Cystic Tumors of the Pancreas*, DOI 10.1007/978-3-319-31882-0_1

Table 1.1 Classification of cystic lesions of the pancreas

Epithelial neoplastic	Epithelial nonneoplastic
Acinar cell cystadenoma	Duodenal diverticulum
Acinar cystadenocarcinoma	Endometrial cyst
Intraductal papillary mucinous neoplasm	Hamartoma
Lymphoepithelial cyst[a]	Lymphoepithelial cyst[a]
Mucinous cystic neoplasm	Simple Mucinous cyst
Serous cystadenocarcinoma	Retention cyst
Serous cystic neoplasm (microcystic, oligocystic/macrocystic, solid)	
Solid-pseudopapillary neoplasm	
Teratoma (dermoid cyst)	
Cystic change in a typically solid neoplasm (such as neuroendocrine tumor, ductal adenocarcinoma, etc.)	
Nonepithelial neoplastic	Non epithelial nonneoplastic
Benign nonepithelial neoplasms (e.g., lymphangioma, hemangioma)	Pancreatitis-associated pseudocyst
Malignant nonepithelial neoplasms	Parasitic cyst

[a]It has not been established if these lesions are neoplastic or developmental

Table 1.2 Gross features of serous cystic neoplasms (SCNs), intraductal papillary mucinous neoplasms (IPMNs), mucinous cystic neoplasms (MCNs), and solid-pseudopapillary neoplasms (SPNs)

	SCN	IPMN	MCN	SPN
Localization in the pancreas	Anywhere	Anywhere	Mostly body and tail	Anywhere
Size	Any	Any	Often 5 to >10 cm	1 to >10 cm
Number of locules	Countless (few in oligocystic variant)	1 to many	1 to many	1 to few
Size of cysts	0.1–1 cm (1–5 cm in oligocystic variant)	0.1 to >5 cm	Any	Few mm to few cm
Cyst content	Serous fluid	Thick tenacious mucin	Thick mucin, watery or hemorrhagic fluid possible	Hemorrhagic and necrotic
Cyst lining	Smooth	Velvety – papillary	Smooth – papillary	Irregular
Septa	Thin	Membranous to few mm thick	Membranous to thick (thick pseudocapsule)	Solid tumor tissue of variable thickness
Calcification	Central stellate scar	Uncommon (punctate, eggshell, coarse)	Peripheral (eggshell)	Uncommon
Solid area(s)	Possible (solid variant)	Possible (malignant transformation)	Possible (malignant transformation)	Yes, may predominate
Communication with duct system	No	Yes	No	No
Multifocality	Possible (von Hippel-Lindau syndrome)	Common	No	Extremely rare

Table 1.3 Microscopic features of serous cystic neoplasms (SCNs), intraductal papillary mucinous neoplasms (IPMNs), mucinous cystic neoplasms (MCNs), and solid-pseudopapillary neoplasms (SPNs)

	SCN	IPMN	MCN	SPN
Neoplastic cells	Cuboidal (clear, occasionally eosinophilic cytoplasm)	Columnar (intestinal, gastric foveolar type) or cuboidal (pancreatobiliary type, oncocytic type)	Columnar (mucinous, occasionally goblet or gastric foveolar type)	Polygonal (eosinophilic, occasionally clear cytoplasm)
Growth pattern	Flat with occasional small papillae	Papillae (villiform, fingerlike, or complex) and occasional micropapillae or flat layers	Flat to papillary formations	Pseudopapillae with fibrovascular cores, and solid sheets
Cytological atypia	Absent	Low to high-grade	Low to high-grade	Usually minimal
Mitotic activity	Absent – very low	Low – increased	Low – increased	Very low
Stroma	Acellular collagenous	Delicate fibrovascular stalks of papillae	Ovarian type	Delicate, fibrous, hyaline change or myxoid
Perineural invasion	Unusual	Possible (malignant transformation)	Possible (malignant transformation)	Possible
Hyaline globules	No	No	No	Yes

1.2 Serous Cystic Neoplasm

Serous neoplasms of the pancreas are cystic tumors defined by the morphologic appearance of the neoplastic epithelial cells lining the cysts [1, 7]. These neoplastic cells are cuboidal (and therefore square on cross section) and glycogen rich (and therefore optically clear in most stains), and they produce straw-colored watery fluid [8].

SCNs are virtually always benign, and only a handful of cases that have metastasized have been reported [9–11]. These latter neoplasms are designated serous cystadenocarcinomas. Most serous cystic neoplasms grow slowly, at an average rate of only 0.28–0.56 cm/year, but growth rates vary significantly, and larger SCNs grow faster on average than do smaller SCNs [12–15]. When correctly diagnosed, most small SCNs do not need to be resected. The challenge is that SCNs can grossly, and therefore radiographically, mimic more aggressive neoplasms of the pancreas. For example, oligocystic SCNs can mimic MCNs, and the more solid SCNs can mimic pancreatic neuroendocrine tumors [8, 12, 14, 16, 17].

1.2.1 Gross Appearance

Most SCNs have a distinctive easily recognizable gross appearance. On cross section they are composed of innumerable small (1 mm to 1 cm) cysts that are filled with thin serous fluid [1]. SCNs characteristically have a central stellate scar that can be calcified. The cysts in the center of the lesion are often smaller than those near the periphery of the tumor (Fig. 1.1). There are several gross variants that are important to recognize because, as noted earlier, these variants can mimic other types of tumors in the pancreas. The gross variants include an oligocystic (or macrocystic) variant (Fig. 1.2) and a solid variant (Fig. 1.3) [1]. Recently an "infarcted" variant has been described in which biopsy-induced changes obliterate much of the underlying SCN [18].

Table 1.4 Immunohistochemical and genetic features of serous cystic neoplasms (SCNs), intraductal papillary mucinous neoplasms (IPMNs), mucinous cystic neoplasms (MCNs), and solid-pseudopapillary neoplasms (SPNs)

	SCN	IPMN	MCN	SPN
Immunohistochemistry				
Epithelial markers CK7, 8, 18, 19, EMA	+	+	+	+ in ~ 50 %
Mucins	MUC6 (MUC1) +	MUC2, MUC5AC + (intestinal) MUC1 + (pancreatobiliary) MUC5AC + (gastric foveolar) MUC5AC, MUC6 + (oncocytic)	MUC1 + (invasive) MUC2 + (focal) MUC5AC usually – MUC6 + (rare)	–
Neuroendocrine markers				
NSE	+ (variable)	–	–	+ (diffuse)
Chromogranin	–	–	–	+ (focal)
Synaptophysin	–	–	Scattered cells at base of the epithelium	–
Vimentin	–	–	–	+
Beta-catenin	Membranous	Membranous	Membranous	Nuclear
CD10	–	–	–	+
PR	–	–	+ (stroma)	+
Alpha-1-antichymotrypsin	–	–	–	+
CEA	–	+	+	–
CA 19-9	–	+	+	–
Others				
α-Inhibin	+	–	+ (stroma)	–
Smooth muscle actin	+	–	+ (stroma)	–
Calretinin	+	–	+ (stroma)	–
HIF-1α	+	–	–	–
VEGF	+	–	–	–
E-cadherin	+	+	+	–
Genetics				
VHL	+	wt	wt	wt
GNAS	wt	+	wt	wt
TP53	wt	+ (high-grade dysplasia)	+ (high-grade dysplasia)	wt
SMAD4	wt	+ (invasive)	+ (high-grade dysplasia)	wt
p16/CDKN2A	wt	+	+	wt
KRAS	wt	+	+	wt
CTNB1	wt	wt	wt	+

wt wild type, + mutant or over expressed

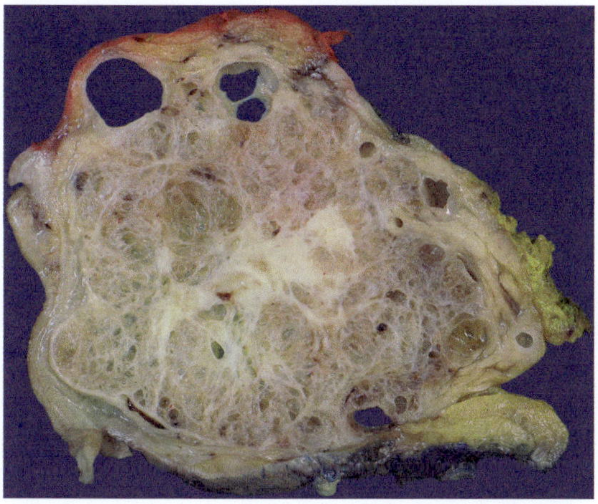

Fig. 1.1 Serous cystic neoplasm (microcystic). This well-circumscribed tumor is composed of innumerable small serous cysts with a central stellate scar

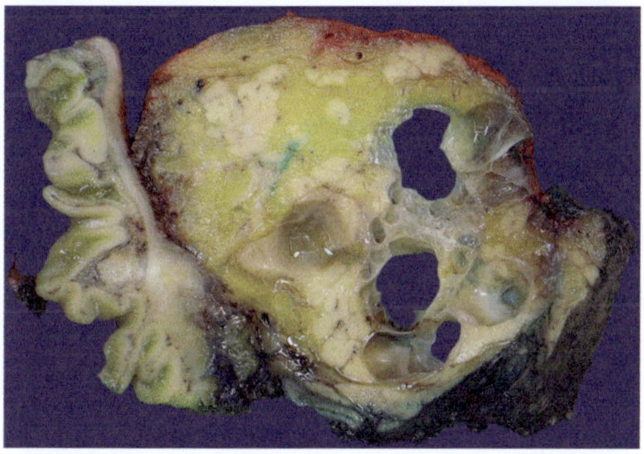

Fig. 1.2 Serous cystic neoplasm (macrocystic variant). The neoplasm consists of a limited number of cysts, most of which measure more than 1 cm in size

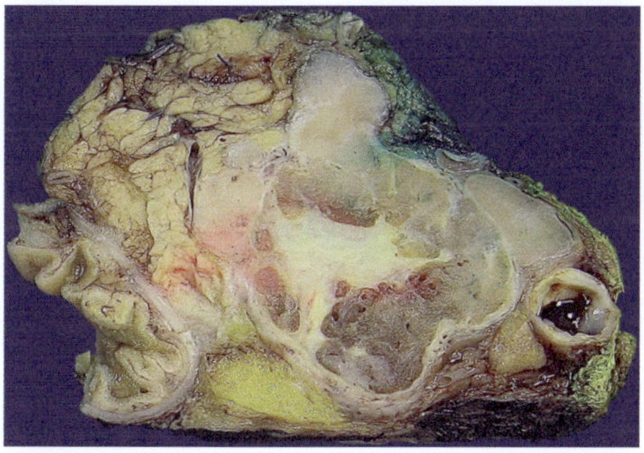

Fig. 1.3 Serous cystic neoplasm (solid variant). The neoplasm is well demarcated and has a central stellate scar. The tumor tissue is mainly solid and focally slightly spongy in appearance

The cysts of SCNs do not grossly communicate with each other, nor do they communicate with the duct system of the pancreas.

1.2.2 Microscopic Appearance

As noted earlier, by definition SCNs are composed of optically clear cuboidal cells with abundant glycogen (Figs. 1.4 and 1.5) [1]. These cells line cysts that are filled with thin serous fluid. Just as was true grossly, the cysts do not communicate microscopically with the pancreatic duct system. The neoplastic cells typically form a single layer, but occasionally are thrown into small papillae. Characteristically, the nuclei of SCNs are extremely uniform, centrally placed in the cell, and round. Nucleoli, when present, are inconspicuous. Mitoses are virtually never seen. The stroma surrounding the cysts is composed of loose acellular collagen and a rich network of small delicate blood vessels. This delicate capillary network lies immediately underneath the epithelial lining of the cysts and is a characteristic feature that can be visualized during endomicroscopic examination. Perineural or vascular invasion is unusual.

Several histologic variants with clinical implications, most of which correspond to the gross variants, should be noted [1, 7]. The oligocystic (or macrocystic) and solid variants are recognized grossly. Microscopically the oligocystic variant is composed of a few larger cysts (>1 cm) with paper thin walls [19–21]. The cysts are lined by cells that are histologically similar to the neoplastic cells of the microcystic SCN. Oligocystic SCNs, however, typically have less stromal collagen, and in some instances the neoplastic cells appear to directly abut pancreatic parenchymal cells. Serous cystic neoplasms with a solid gross appearance are composed of plumper neoplastic cells that form microscopic lumina but not larger cysts [22]. As a result, they appear to be solid masses grossly. Histologically, the “infarcted” variant is characterized by obliteration of much of the neoplasm by hemorrhagic granulation tissue, a sequel of previous biopsy. The cytoplasm of some SCNs is more eosinophilic than clear.

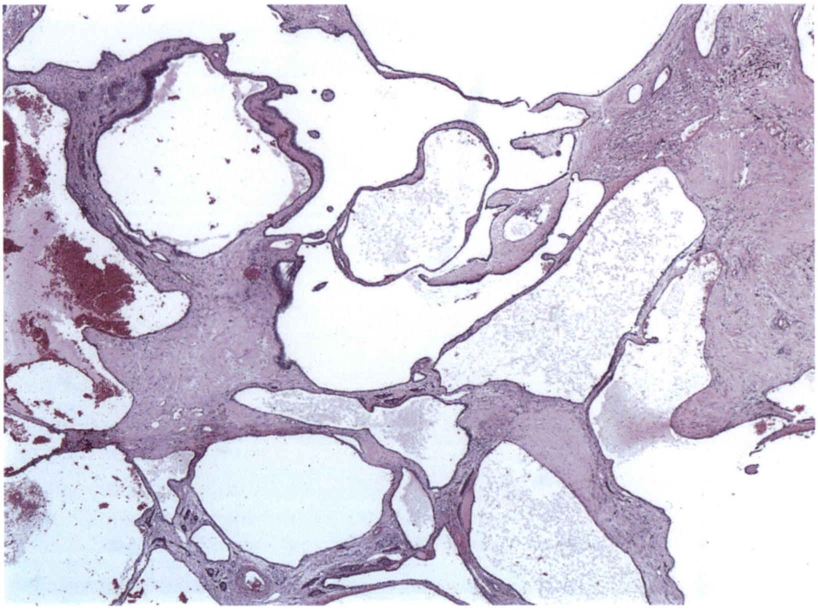

Fig. 1.4 Serous cystic neoplasm. Simple cysts are supported by a bland collagenous stroma with occasional foci of residual pancreatic parenchyma and scattered siderophages

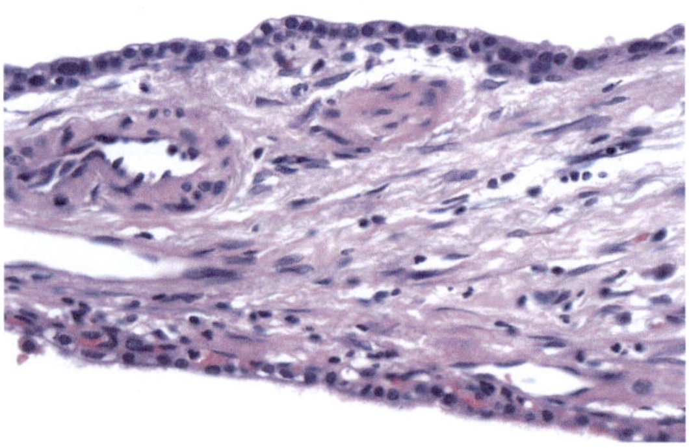

Fig. 1.5 Serous cystic neoplasm. The cysts are lined by a flat layer of cuboidal cells with clear cytoplasm and a uniform, round, centrally placed nucleus

Two microscopic variants of note include the mixed serous-neuroendocrine neoplasms and the von Hippel-Lindau (VHL)-associated SCNs. Mixed serous-neuroendocrine neoplasms are characterized by the presence of two components – a serous cystadenoma intimately admixed with a well-differentiated pancreatic neuroendocrine tumor (PanNET) [1, 7]. VHL-associated SCNs are defined as SCNs that arise in patients with the VHL syndrome [23–25]. Microscopically they are similar to other SCNs, but they are more often of the mixed serous-neuroendocrine neoplasm type and they are more often multifocal. In some cases, the multifocal cysts in patients with VHL involve almost the entire gland.

Several of these variants have clinical significance. The mixed serous-neuroendocrine neoplasm is important to recognize because the PanNET component may be more aggressive than pure SCNs, the VHL-associated variant is important to recognize because of the risk of other neoplasms and the risk to other family members, and the other variants are important to recognize because they can clinically mimic other neoplasms of the pancreas [1]. The variant with eosinophilic cytoplasm has no clinical significance other than that the appearance of the cytoplasm can be diagnostically confusing.

1.2.3 Immunohistochemistry

The immunolabeling pattern of SCNs parallels their morphology and provides insight into the cellular pathways driving these neoplasms [1]. Reflecting their epithelial direction of differentiation, the neoplastic cells of SCNs label with antibodies to keratins 7, 8, 18, and 19, and they express epithelial membrane antigen [1]. The mucins MUC6 (80% of SCNs) and MUC1

(35 % of SCNs) can be expressed, suggesting a centroacinar direction of differentiation [7]. In contrast to mucin-producing cystic neoplasms (MCNs and IPMNs), the epithelial cells of SCNs do not express carcinoembryonic antigen. Finally, the expression of hypoxia-induced factor-1α (HIF-1α) and vascular endothelial growth factor (VEGF) points toward dysregulation of the VHL/HIF-1α pathway [26]. The latter marker, VEGF, is of particular note, because it has been suggested that the presence of VEGFs (VEGF-1, VEGF-2, and VEGF-3) in cyst fluid could be used to support the diagnosis of an SCN [27, 28].

1.2.4 Genetics

Although the genetic changes that characterize SCNs will be discussed in greater detail in the forthcoming chapters, they are worth briefly discussing here as the genes targeted may account for some of the pathologic features of these neoplasms. Targeted sequencing and whole exome sequencing of SCNs have revealed that the *VHL* gene is inactivated in the majority of SCNs [5, 29]. Inactivation of *VHL* would explain some of the dysregulation of the VHL/HIF-1α pathway observed by immunolabeling, and dysregulation of VHL/HIF-1α in turn may explain the clear cell and rich vascularity of these tumors [26]. As is true for overexpressed VEGF (2010), mutant *VHL* genes can be detected in cyst fluid samples, and it too could be used to support the diagnosis of an SCN [28].

1.2.5 Serous Cystadenocarcinoma

Serous cystadenocarcinomas are very rare and should not be overdiagnosed. The single feature that defines malignancy for a serous cystic neoplasm is the presence of distant metastases (noncontiguous spread) [7–11]. While local invasion into organs such as the duodenum certainly suggests a more aggressive pattern of growth, it is not enough to classify a serous neoplasm as malignant [7, 8]. The designation of serous cystadenocarcinoma should therefore be reserved only for cases with documented distant metastases.

Remarkably, other than the fact that the neoplastic cells are located in another organ, serous cystadenocarcinomas are morphologically indistinguishable from benign SCNs. The neoplastic cells lack atypia and other histologic changes typically seen in malignancies.

1.2.6 Clinical Implications of the Pathology

In summary, the vast majority of SCNs are benign, slow-growing neoplasms. Malignancy is rare and is defined by the presence of metastases. While the classic SCNs, microcystic neoplasms with a central calcified star-shaped scar, are usually easily diagnosed clinically, there are a number of variants of SCN that can mimic other neoplasms. Recent advances defining the patterns of gene expression, such as VEGF, and the genetic alterations that drive SCNs, such as *VHL* mutations, suggest a growing opportunity to diagnose SCNs through the analysis of endoscopically obtained cyst fluid. The cysts of SCNs do not communicate with the pancreatic duct system. It is therefore unlikely that analyses of pancreatic "juice" (secretions in the pancreatic duct) will be useful in testing for SCNs.

Finally, it should be noted that in some instances, the pathology can provide a clue that the patient has an underlying genetic syndrome. Multiple cysts and mixed serous-neuroendocrine neoplasms both suggest that the patient may have the von Hippel-Lindau syndrome [23, 30, 31].

1.3 Intraductal Papillary Mucinous Neoplasm

By definition, intraductal papillary mucinous neoplasms (IPMNs) are grossly visible (≥1 cm) epithelial neoplasms that grow within the duct system of the pancreas [1, 7, 32]. The neoplastic cells usually form papillae and they produce sometimes copious amounts of mucin. This mucin and/or papillary tumor tissue can locally distend the duct system, producing a "cystic" lesion. IPMNs are precursor lesions, and if left untreated a minority progress to an invasive adenocarcinoma. Just as adenomas of the colon present an opportunity to cure colonic neoplasia before an invasive cancer develops, so too do IPMNs present the opportunity to cure pancreatic neoplasia before the patient develops an incurable invasive pancreatic cancer [33]. The challenge with IPMNs is that, because of the morbidity and even mortality associated with pancreatic surgery, not all IPMNs can be resected [34]. Instead, clinicians have to carefully balance the risks of surgery with the potential benefits of surgery in individual patients [35]. The malignant potential of IPMNs is often reflected in pathologic features that are detectable clinically. Therefore, as was true for SCNs, a solid understanding of the pathology of IPMNs forms the basis for their clinical management.

1.3.1 Gross Appearance

As noted above, IPMNs, by definition, involve the duct system of the pancreas. Bisecting surgically resected samples along a probe placed in the main pancreatic duct is the best way to detect involvement of the ducts [36]. Alternatively, serial sectioning the tumor along the axial axis (for tumors of the head of the pancreas) or along the sagittal axis (for tumors of the tail of the gland) may provide excellent correlation with preoperative imaging studies. IPMNs that involve the main pancreatic duct are designated "main-duct IPMNs," those that involve a smaller branch of the main pancreatic duct are designated "branch-duct IPMNs," and those that significantly involve the main and branch ducts are designated as "combined main- and branch-duct IPMNs" [1, 7, 32]. This classification is clinically important because main-duct IPMNs, as defined radiographically, are more likely to harbor an associated invasive carcinoma than are branch-duct IPMNs.

IPMNs, as noted above, often form papillary structures and they produce mucin [1, 7, 32]. Both of these features can be appreciated grossly. The papillae look like small fingerlike projections into the lumen of the affected duct (Figs. 1.6 and 1.7). The epithelium in some IPMNs is, however, flat, and the absence of gross papillary structures should therefore not be used to exclude the diagnosis. The mucin produced by IPMNs can be thick, tenacious and viscous, or more watery and thin. IPMNs, in contrast to the other cystic neoplasms of the pancreas, are often multifocal. This multifocality can sometimes be appreciated grossly as two

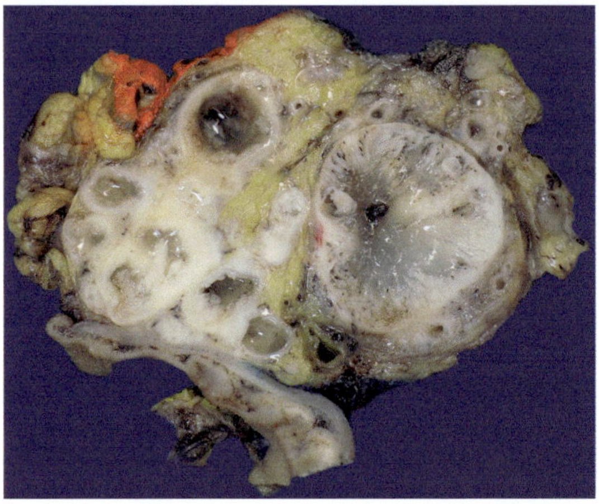

Fig. 1.6 Intraductal papillary mucinous neoplasm. The main pancreatic duct and multiple branch ducts are grossly distended by mucin and villous projections of the neoplastic cells growing along the duct walls

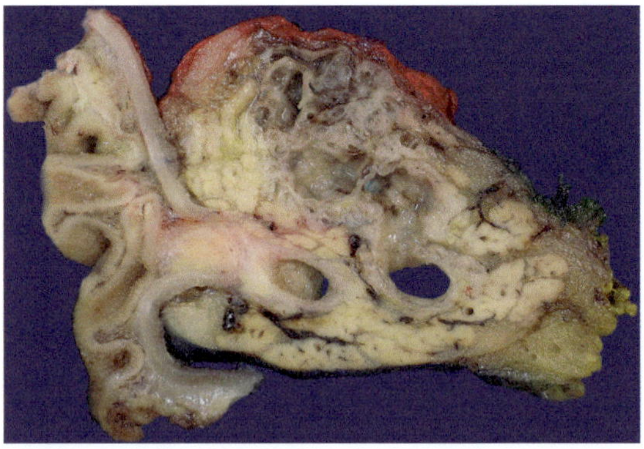

Fig. 1.7 Intraductal papillary mucinous neoplasm. The main pancreatic duct and a cluster of branch ducts are dilated and filled with a small amount of mucin. Focally, intraductal tumor growth is visible as a discreet thickening of the duct wall

distinct lesions separated by grossly normal pancreatic parenchyma [37, 38].

The pancreatic parenchyma upstream from IPMNs often has changes of chronic obstruction including atrophy and fibrosis. The presence of an ill-defined solid mass or of multiple foci of stromal mucin should raise the possibility of an associated invasive carcinoma (Fig. 1.8).

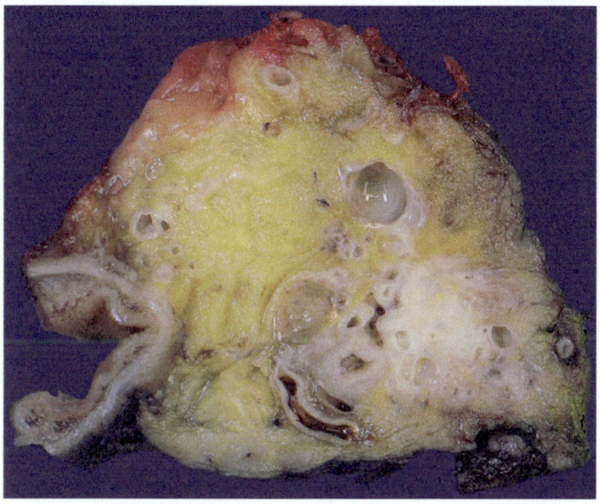

Fig. 1.8 Intraductal papillary mucinous neoplasm. Scattered branch ducts are dilated and contain a small amount of mucin. An area of solid white tissue represents transition into invasive adenocarcinoma

1.3.2 Microscopic Appearance

The microscopic appearance of IPMNs parallels their gross appearance. IPMNs microscopically involve the duct system. This can be appreciated in several ways. The partial involvement of a duct makes it clear that the structure involved is a duct, as does a pattern of growth that conforms to the normal branching pattern of the duct system.

Several directions of differentiation can be appreciated microscopically and the histologic direction of differentiation can be used to classify IPMNs [39]. IPMNs with intestinal differentiation are composed of pseudostratified columnar cells that contain prominent apical mucin. Occasional goblet cells can be appreciated. In many ways, the histologic appearance of an intestinal-type IPMN is similar to that of a villous adenoma of the colon (Fig. 1.9).

The pancreatobiliary-type IPMN is composed of mostly cuboidal cells with scarce mucin [39]. As a result, the cytoplasm of the neoplastic cells is more amphophilic. The papillae tend to be complex and branching in pancreatobiliary-type IPMNs, and they often have high-grade dysplasia with hyperchromatic nuclei and prominent nucleoli.

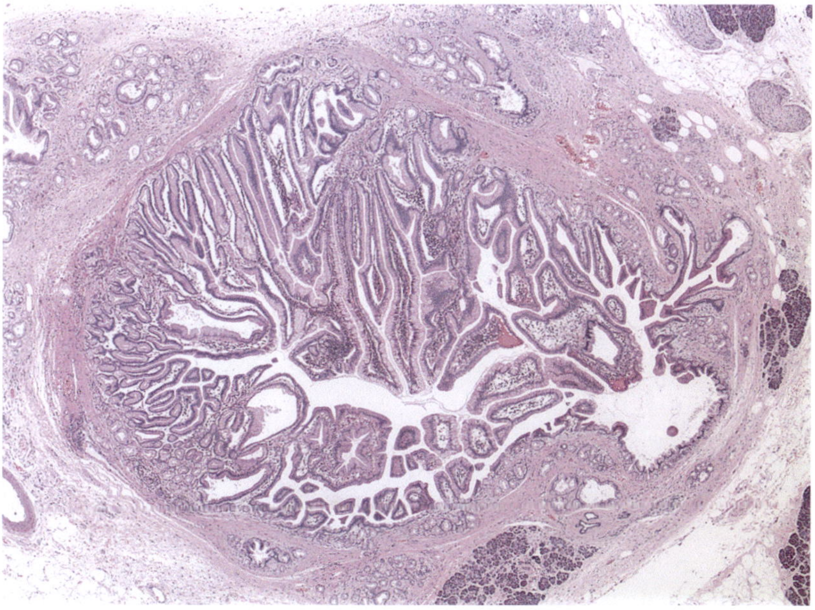

Fig. 1.9 Intraductal papillary mucinous neoplasm. Two dilated branch-duct profiles are lined by tall, partially branched neoplastic papillae

Gastric foveolar-type IPMNs are composed of columnar cells with basally oriented nuclei and apical mucin [39]. The histologic appearance is similar to that of the normal gastric foveolar epithelium. Branch-duct IPMNs often have the gastric foveolar direction of differentiation, and most have low-grade dysplasia.

Oncocytic IPMNs (also known as intraductal oncocytic papillary neoplasms or IOPNs) are easy to recognize because the neoplastic cells have abundant granular eosinophilic cytoplasm [39]. These distinctive neoplasms arise within the duct system, but may have a partially solid appearance, both microscopically and macroscopically. Goblet cells may be scattered among the cells with eosinophilic cytoplasm. The nuclei often contain single prominent nucleoli.

The final histologic variant of the IPMN is the intraductal tubulopapillary neoplasms (ITPNs) [7, 40]. The neoplastic cells of this variant form intraductal tubules and cribriform structures. Focal papillary formation may be present. Comedo-type necrosis is often present, but, in contrast to the other IPMNs, mucin is very scarce.

Much more important than the gross type or the microscopic direction of differentiation is the degree of dysplasia in an IPMN [1, 41]. Low-grade dysplasia, intermediate-grade dysplasia, and high-grade dysplasia are defined histologically. The neoplastic cells of IPMNs with low-grade dysplasia are uniform; they have basally oriented nuclei and minimal pleomorphism. Mitoses are rare. In intermediate-grade dysplasia there is some variability in the nuclei. The nuclei are more stratified than those in low-grade dysplasia, and the nuclei in intermediate-grade dysplasia begin to lose polarity relative to the basement membrane. The nuclei are often a little larger and more pleomorphic than the nuclei of IPMNs with low-grade dysplasia. High-grade dysplasia is characterized by significant architectural and nuclear atypia. Polarity is often lost, the nuclei are pleomorphic and hyperchromatic, and mitoses can be seen.

Dysplasia is important to recognize because invasive carcinomas are most likely to arise from IPMNs with high-grade dysplasia. Because of this, we should spend a moment reflecting on some of the features of high-grade dysplasia that may be detectable clinically before surgery. For example, IPMNs with high-grade dysplasia often have irregular branching papillae. The intraluminal component of these IPMNs is therefore often prominent, and the radiologic correlate of this is a "mural nodule." IPMNs with mural nodules are therefore more likely to be high grade and usually should be surgically resected. Although the correlation is not as strong, larger IPMNs (>3 cm) are more likely to harbor high-grade dysplasia than are smaller IPMNs (<1 cm) [35].

Another histologic feature of IPMNs that has clinical implications is their multifocality [37]. The multifocality of IPMNs that can be appreciated grossly is even more evident microscopically. It is rare to see a single isolated IPMN in an otherwise normal pancreas. Instead, pancreata with an IPMN typically harbor numerous pancreatic intraepithelial neoplasia (PanIN) lesions, small "incipient IPMNs," and in some cases full-blown multifocal IPMNs. This multifocality is clinically very important because it explains why patients who have an IPMN resected are at risk for developing another IPMN or even an invasive carcinoma in their remnant gland [42].

It is very easy to over interpret a separate small innocuous lesion at the margin as part of the larger IPMN that is being resected. When this is done, the risk is that the surgeon will feel obliged to resect additional pancreatic parenchyma with the hope of obtaining a completely negative margin. In our experience this additional surgery is unnecessary. So long as the lesion at the margin is small and lacks high-grade dysplasia, it is unlikely to impact the patient's long-term survival [41]. Removing too much pancreas and creating a brittle diabetic will, however, negatively impact the patient's quality, and perhaps even quantity, of life.

The distinction between an IPMN and a PanIN lesion can be challenging [32]. Three features are helpful. (1) IPMNs are large (≥1 cm) and PanINs are small (<0.5 cm); (2) IPMNs tend to have long fingerlike papillae, and PanINs have short stubby papillae; and (3) IPMNs can produce abundant amounts of thick mucin, and PanINs produce minimal mucin. IPMNs do, however, extend along the duct system, and at their edges, they can involve smaller ducts. In these instances determining the relationship between the lesion in question and the grossly visible IPMN can be helpful. Lesions far from the IPMN are unlikely to be part of the IPMN.

1.3.3 Immunohistochemistry

The immunolabeling pattern of IPMNs reflects the directions of differentiation observed in routine hematoxylin and eosin (H&E)-stained sections [1, 7, 32]. The neoplastic epithelial cells express markers of ductal differentiation such as keratins 7 and 19, CA 19-9, and carcinoembryonic antigen [1]. The pattern of mucin expression relates to the histologic type of IPMN. Intestinal-type IPMNs express MUC2, MUC5AC, and CDX2, pancreatobiliary-type IPMNs express MUC1, gastric foveolar-type IPMNs express MUC5AC, and oncocytic IPMNs express MUC5AC and MUC6 and sometimes HEPAR-1 [39, 43]. ITPNs, as should be expected from the paucity of mucin present in these lesions, usually only weakly label with antibodies to mucins.

1.3.4 Genetics

A number of genes are targeted in IPMNs. These include some, such as *KRAS*, *p16/CDKN2A*, *TP53*, and *SMAD4* (the latter two mostly in invasive cancers that arise from IPMNs), that are also targeted in most infiltrating ductal carcinomas, two (*RNF43* and *PIK3CA*) that are also inactivated in MCNs, and one (*GNAS*) that appears to be specific for the IPMN pathway [5, 6, 44]. The genetic changes correlate with the phenotype of the IPMNs in two ways. First, *GNAS* mutations appear to be more common in intestinal-type IPMNs [5, 6, 44]. Second, the timing of the mutations correlates with histologic grade. *KRAS* and *p16/CDKN2A* are relatively early events (they can be found in low-grade IPMNs), while *TP53* inactivation is a late event, occurring in IPMNs with high-grade dysplasia [1, 7, 32].

1.3.5 Clinical Implications of the Pathology

It is clear from a number of clinical, pathology-based, and molecular studies that noninvasive IPMNs can progress to invasive adenocarcinomas. Histologic grade is one of the best indicators of the likelihood that an IPMN can progress, but grade cannot usually be determined preoperatively. A variety of indirect approaches have therefore been used as surrogates for grade to predict the risk of an IPMN progressing, such as whether or not the IPMN primarily involves the main or branch ducts, its size, and whether or not the cyst contains a mural nodule [35]. Although clinically useful, these features are imperfect markers of dysplasia. Novel molecular-based markers, when integrated with these clinical features, will clearly help determine cyst type and hopefully will help determine grade and therefore likelihood of progression, preoperatively [5, 6, 44]. As noted earlier, IPMNs are often multifocal, and this multifocality suggests that once a patient has one IPMN, they have to be followed clinically as they are at risk for additional IPMNs [38, 45].

Finally, IPMNs, by definition, involve the duct system. This, together with the multifocality of IPMNs, is critical when considering the design of a molecular-based cyst test. Since IPMNs are multifocal, the analysis of cyst fluid obtained by endoscopic ultrasound (EUS)-guided cyst fluid aspiration will provide information only about the single locule aspirated. By contrast, since IPMNs involve the duct system, analyses of pancreatic juice collected at the ampulla of Vater have the potential of more completely sampling the entire duct system and therefore all of the IPMN lesions [46].

1.4 Mucinous Cystic Neoplasm

Mucinous cystic neoplasms are mucin-producing epithelial neoplasms that form cysts and that, by definition, contain a characteristic ovarian type of stroma [1, 7]. MCNs share a number of things in common with IPMNs (both form cysts, both are mucin producing, and both can progress to invasive carcinoma), but there are some key differences in their pathologies that have important clinical ramifications. In contrast to IPMNs, the cysts of the vast majority of MCNs do not communicate with the pancreatic ducts, and, in contrast to IPMNs, most MCNs are unifocal lesions.

1.4.1 Gross Appearance

The vast majority of MCNs arise in the tail of the pancreas, and, as noted above, MCNs do not involve the pancreatic duct system [1, 7]. On cross section, MCNs are composed of multiple cysts, sometimes with a "cyst within a cyst" appearance. The cysts are larger (<1 cm to sometimes as large as 10 cm) than the cysts of SCNs, and the cysts have thick walls. The cysts typically contain thick mucin, but in some instances, the cyst fluid may be more hemorrhagic or turbid (Figs. 1.10, 1.11, and 1.12). This gross pathology is reflected in clinical imaging, as the presence of large thick-walled cysts on imaging should suggest the diagnosis of an MCN [35, 47, 48]. In addition, the variable cyst contents (mucin filled vs. hemorrhagic) can manifest as locules with varying densities on imaging. In some instances the neoplastic epithelium can be seen to project into the lumen of a cyst. Firm, solid foci, the so-called mural nodules, may also be seen (Fig. 1.13). These nodules may contain high-grade dysplasia or even invasive carcinoma and should be sampled carefully.

1.4.2 Microscopic Appearance

Two components are, by definition, present in MCNs [1, 7]. The epithelial component can be flat or papillary and is composed of low columnar to tall columnar mucin-producing cells. These cells will stain with the periodic acid-Schiff (PAS) stain (diastase resistant) and with alcian blue. The stromal component resembles ovarian-type stroma with densely packed plump spindle-shaped cells oriented parallel to the cyst wall (Fig. 1.14) [1, 7]. Luteinized cells may rarely be seen in the stroma. This ovarian stroma often forms a distinct band of nuclei beneath the epithelium. The epithelium of some cysts can be denuded, and when it is the cyst is lined by loose granulation tissue with histiocytes. In these instances the presence of ovarian-type

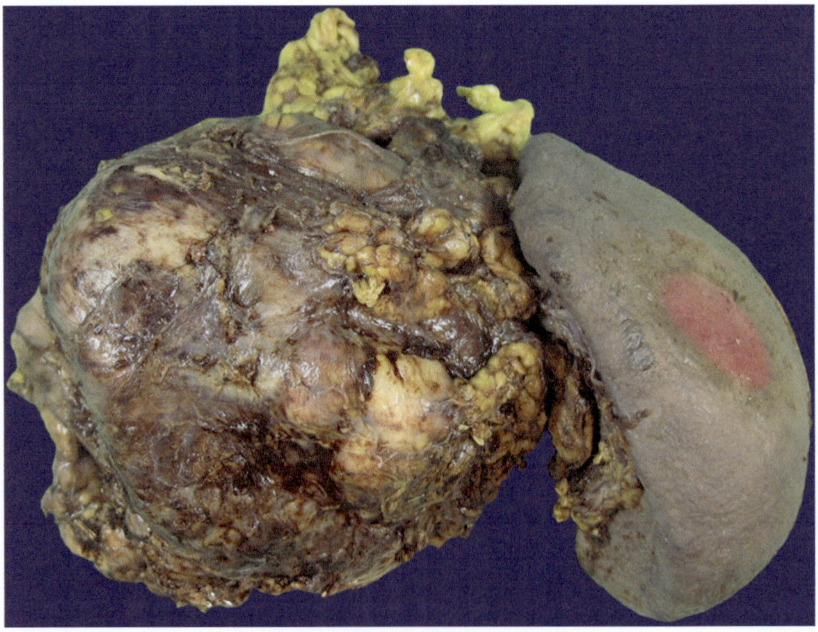

Fig. 1.10 Mucinous cystic neoplasm. A large tumor (12 cm diameter) involves the pancreatic body and tail

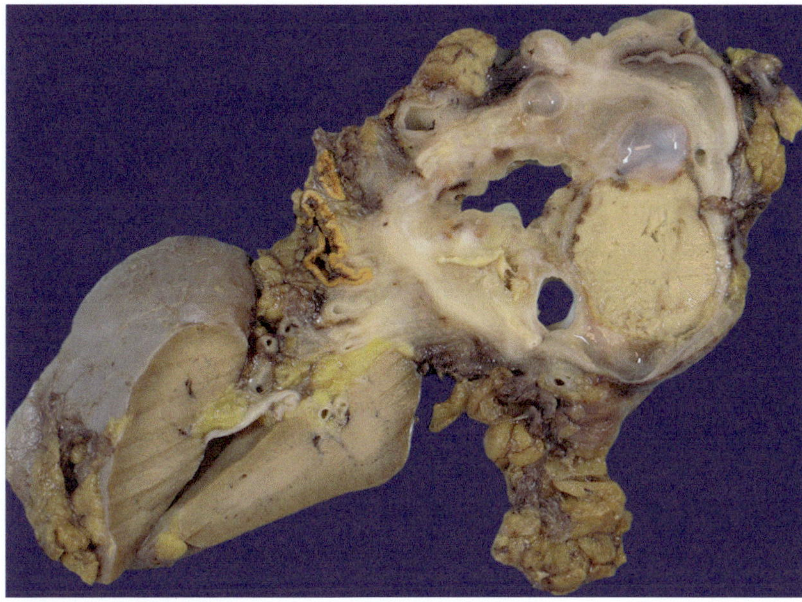

Fig. 1.11 Mucinous cystic neoplasm. Large cysts contain mucin or inflammatory debris. The tumor expands into the gastric wall. Fibrous adhesions extend from the thick pseudocapsule to the adrenal gland and renal hilus

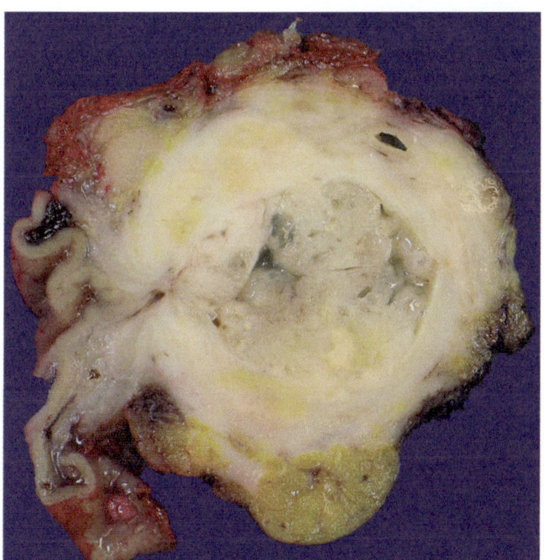

Fig. 1.12 Mucinous cystic neoplasm. A single cyst cavity containing mucin and papillary projections is surrounded by a thick fibrous capsule. The neoplasm had been drained through the stomach following a previous erroneous diagnosis of pseudocyst

stroma can suggest the correct diagnosis even in the absence of an epithelial lining. A variant of MCNs in which the neoplastic cells have a more eosinophilic cytoplasm has been described, but this variant does not have a distinct clinical behavior.

Just as IPMNs can be classified based on the degree of dysplasia, so too are MCNs graded as low, intermediate, and high-grade based on the degree of epithelial architectural and nuclear atypia [1, 7]. In low-grade dysplasia, the neoplastic epithelial cells are well-oriented with uniform, small, and basally located nuclei. Mitoses are, at most, rare. In intermediate-grade dysplasia, the nuclei are slightly enlarged and more crowded (and hence overlapping), they start to lose polarity (and hence one sees pseudostratification), and they exhibit slight pleomorphism. In high-grade dysplasia, there is significant architectural and nuclear atypia. Architecturally, the epithelium can form cribriform structures, sometimes with luminal necrosis. Cytologically, the nuclei are hyperchromatic, enlarged, and poorly oriented. Prominent nucleoli can be appreciated, and mitoses can be seen.

Of note, different locules of a single MCN may have significantly different degrees of dysplasia. For example, the cells lining one locule may have low-grade dysplasia, while the cells lining an adjacent locule in the same neoplasm may have high-grade dysplasia. Therefore, if low-grade dysplasia is identified on fine-needle aspiration, a higher grade component elsewhere in an unsampled locule cannot be excluded.

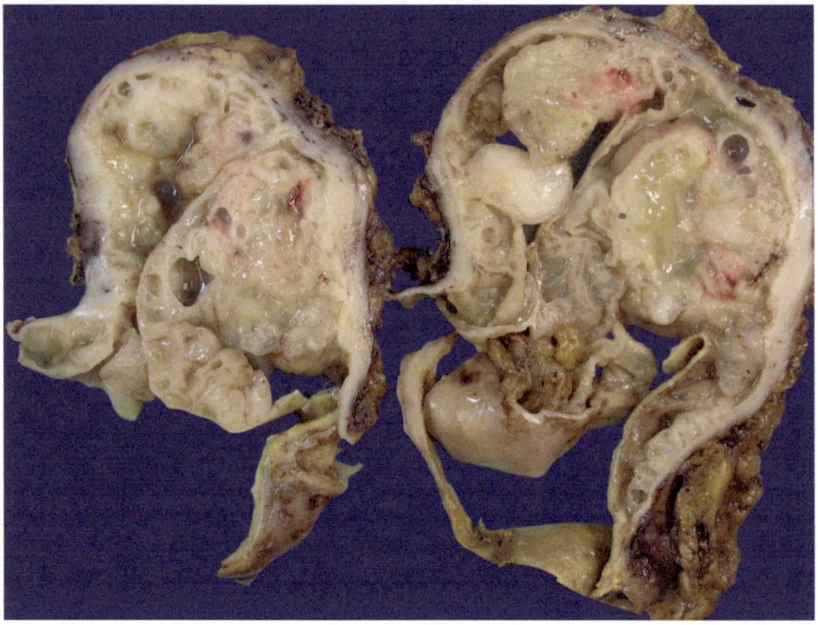

Fig. 1.13 Mucinous cystic neoplasm. Mucin-filled cysts are lined by irregular papillary excrescences and contain several solid mural nodules

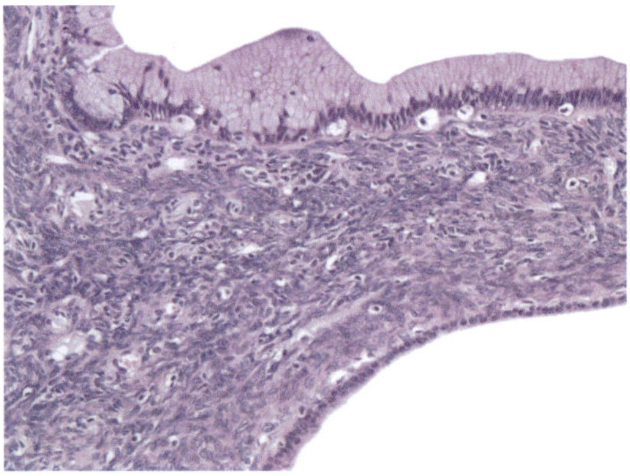

Fig. 1.14 Mucinous cystic neoplasm. The cyst wall is lined by neoplastic mucinous epithelium showing low-grade dysplasia. Cellular ovarian-type stroma characteristically is present

The prognostically most critical determination in evaluating MCNs microscopically is to establish whether or not there is an associated invasive carcinoma. Invasive carcinomas arising in MCNs are defined by the presence of neoplastic epithelial cells crossing the basement membrane and into stromal tissues [49]. This can be difficult to identify in practice, as submucosal glands and trapped atrophic nonneoplastic ducts and acini can mimic invasion. Haphazardly arranged glands, a desmoplastic stromal reaction, and glands where they do not belong (such as around a nerve) are all features that can be used to support the diagnosis of invasive carcinoma arising in association with an MCN. Invasion can be very focal, and therefore sampling that is extensive, if not complete, is needed to rule out focal invasion. It is important to document the grade and size of the invasive carcinoma and to clearly report the invasive component separately from the overall noninvasive MCN [49]. For example, a report could read "2 cm invasive moderately differentiated ductal adenocarcinoma arising in association with a 10 cm mucinous cystic neoplasm with high-grade dysplasia." Reports should not read "12 cm invasive mucinous cystadenocarcinoma," as such reports blur the distinction between the invasive and noninvasive components of the neoplasm. It has recently been suggested that invasive carcinomas limited to the ovarian stroma have a better prognosis than do more deeply invasive carcinomas that extend beyond the ovarian stroma and into adjacent tissues [49].

While the invasive carcinomas that arise in association with MCNs are usually ductal adenocarcinomas, there are several variants that should be noted. In rare cases the associated invasive carcinoma has a sarcomatoid morphology [50]. Genetic analyses have linked these sarcomatoid neoplasms to the epithelial, not the stromal, components of MCNs, helping to establish that they are sarcomatoid carcinomas and not sarcomas derived from the ovarian stroma [50]. Rare cases of undifferentiated carcinomas with osteoclast-like giant cells have also been reported in association with MCNs [51]. Again, genetic analyses link these lesions to the epithelial component of the MCNs, and they too are classified as carcinomas.

1.4.3 Immunohistochemistry

The neoplastic epithelial cells immunolabel with antibodies to keratins 7, 8, 18, and 19, with antibodies to the epithelial membrane antigen (EMA), and with the cancer markers carcinoembryonic antigen (CEA) and CA 19-9 [1, 7]. The neoplastic epithelial cells express the mucin (MUC5AC), and scattered intraepithelial neuroendocrine cells will be synaptophysin and chromogranin A positive [52]. The stromal cells immunolabel with antibodies to smooth muscle actin (SMA) and, belying their "ovarian" phenotype, with antibodies to progesterone receptors (60–90 %) and less commonly estrogen receptors (30 %).

1.4.4 Genetics

The exomes of a series of MCNs have been sequenced, and the genetic landscape of MCNs is now well-characterized. The genes targeted in MCNs include *KRAS*, *p16/CDKN2A*, *PIK3CA*, *RNF43*, *TP53*, and *SMAD4* [5, 53, 54]. Mutations to *KRAS* appear to occur early (they can be seen in low-grade lesions) and are among the most common genetic alterations, while *SMAD4* and *TP53* inactivation occurs late (in high-grade or invasive lesions). Therefore, the abnormal expression of the Smad4 and Tp53 proteins suggests an MCN is high-grade. In contrast to IPMNs, the *GNAS* gene is not commonly altered in MCNs.

1.4.5 Clinical Implications of the Pathology

The gross appearance of MCNs nicely correlates with their appearance on imaging, as the lack of communication of the cysts with the pancreatic duct system, the thick walls of the tumor, and the variable cyst contents (usually mucinous, but sometimes hemorrhagic) can all be appreciated on imaging. Because the cyst walls of MCNs are thick, it can be hard to identify a small invasive carcinoma arising in an MCN on imaging, and, as a result, most MCNs are therefore surgically resected [35]. The unifocality of MCNs seen grossly and microscopically is of note because it suggests that, in contrast to patients with an IPMN who are at risk for synchronous and metachronous disease, most patients are cured after the complete resection of an MCN [55]. The presence of multiple cysts that appear to neither communicate with each other nor with the duct system does present some clinical problems. It suggests that even if a test was developed that could accurately predict the degree of dysplasia in a cyst fluid sample, one could never rule out higher grade dysplasia in an unsampled locule. In addition, the absence of communication between the locules and the pancreatic duct system suggests that tests performed on pancreatic juice samples will not be able to detect changes from MCNs.

1.5 Solid-Pseudopapillary Neoplasm

The neoplastic cells of solid-pseudopapillary neoplasms (SPNs) do not appear to have a nonneoplastic counterpart in the normal pancreas. These neoplasms have therefore been given a name that simply describes their typical gross and microscopic appearance. SPNs are fundamentally solid neoplasms that usually undergo cystic degeneration [1, 7, 56]. The neoplastic cells are uniform, poorly cohesive, and supported by thin branching vessels, giving the neoplasm a pseudopapillary light microscopic appearance. Hyaline globules and foam cells are often present [1, 7]. SPNs are malignant neoplasms, and ~10 % of patients have a metastasis at diagnosis or will develop metastases later in life [1, 7].

1.5.1 Gross Appearance

As noted in the definition of SPNs, they are fundamentally solid neoplasms that frequently undergo cystic degeneration [1, 7]. Most are soft and well-demarcated and on cross section are composed of soft tan-yellow solid areas with admixed foci of necrosis, hemorrhage, and degenerative cystic change. As a result, these neoplasms can range from almost completely solid to almost completely cystic (Fig. 1.15) [57].

1.5.2 Microscopic Appearance

The microscopic appearance of SPNs parallels their gross appearance with solid areas intimately admixed with areas of cystic degeneration [1, 7]. Uniform poorly cohesive cells loosely surround thin delicate vessels, some of which are hyalinized [1, 56]. The pseudopapillae are created when the loosely cohesive cells drop out leaving just a thin layer of neoplastic cells loosely attached to small vessels (Fig. 1.16). This feature of SPNs can be dramatically displayed with smears prepared from the cut surface of the tumor. These smears characteristically reveal delicately branching vessels surrounded by loosely cohesive cells.

The neoplastic cells have eosinophilic, or occasionally clear, cytoplasm. The nuclei are uniform and oval, some with "coffee bean"-style nuclear grooves. Mitoses are usually rare. Eosinophilic periodic acid-Schiff-positive hyaline globules are a characteristic feature [1, 7].

Although most SPNs are grossly well-demarcated, the neoplastic cells at the leading edge of the tumor delicately infiltrate into the non-neoplastic pancreatic parenchyma. They do so very subtly by gently intermingling with nonneoplastic cells [58]. Other histologic features that can be a clue to the diagnosis include foam cells, cells with clear cytoplasm, and cholesterol clefts with associated giant cells. Focal degenerative atypia

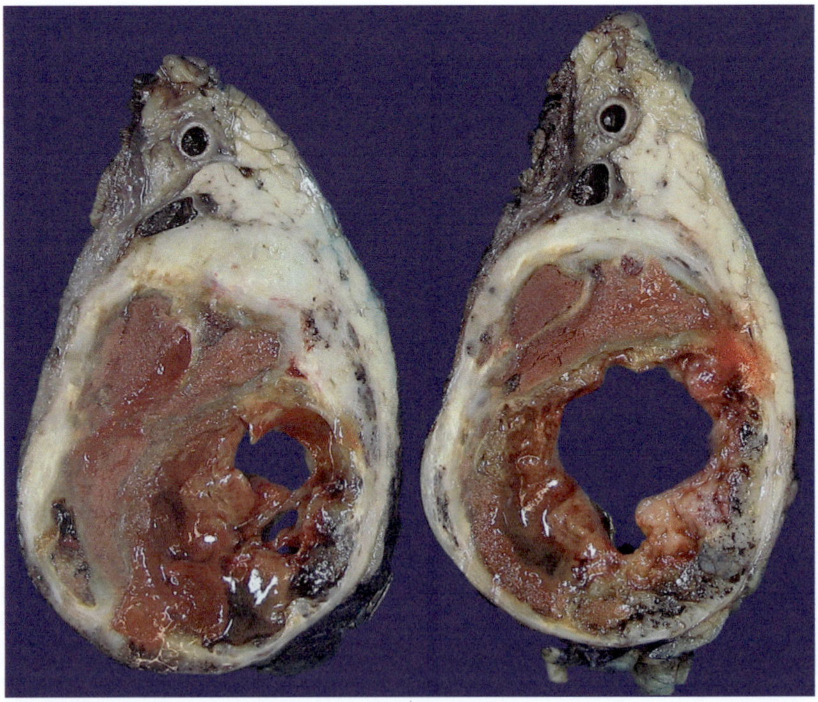

Fig. 1.15 Solid-pseudopapillary neoplasm. The neoplasm is well circumscribed and composed of friable solid tissue with extensive hemorrhage and prominent cystic degeneration

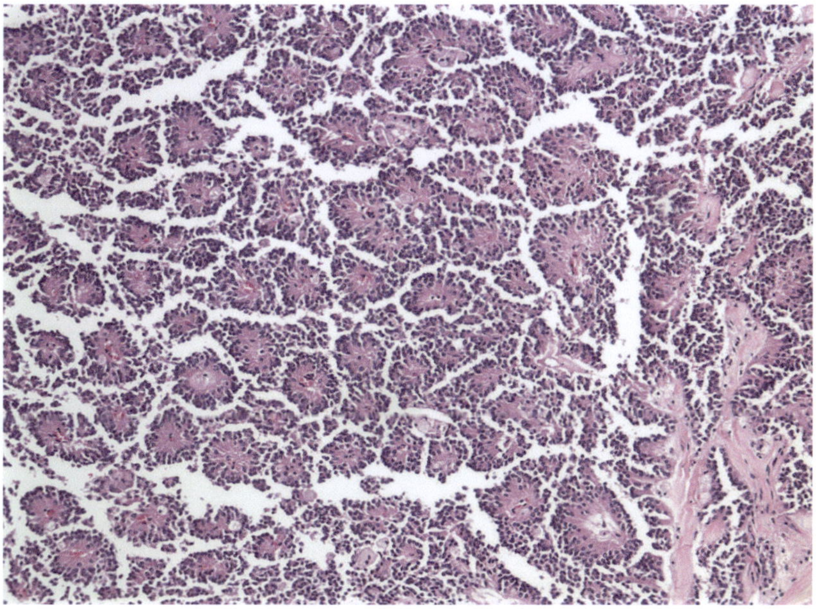

Fig. 1.16 Solid-pseudopapillary neoplasm. The pseudopapillary pattern is characterized by thin layers of neoplastic cells surrounding delicate blood vessels

with enlarged hyperchromatic nuclei is present in approximately 10 % of SPNs, but in most cases this finding has no prognostic significance [59].

Two cases of extremely aggressive SPNs with "sarcomatoid" and undifferentiated areas have been reported [60]. These aggressive SPNs were histologically characterized by a diffuse growth pattern, extensive necrosis, dramatic nuclear atypia, and a very high mitotic rate (35–70 mitoses/50 high-power fields).

1.5.3 Immunohistochemistry

SPNs characteristically express CD10, CD99 (in a dot-like pattern), and nuclear beta-catenin. They also often express α-1-antichymotrypsin, LEF-1, and neuron-specific enolase [1, 7, 61–67]. Interestingly, and perhaps explaining the poorly cohesive nature of the neoplastic cells, the expression of E-cadherin is disrupted in SPNs. The neoplastic cells do not label with antibodies to the extracellular domain of E-cadherin, and an abnormal nuclear pattern is observed when antibodies to the cytoplasmic domain are employed [61–63].

SPNs usually immunostain for vimentin, and only about half of SPNs express keratins at immunohistochemically detectable levels, and these are usually keratins 7, 8, 18, and 19.

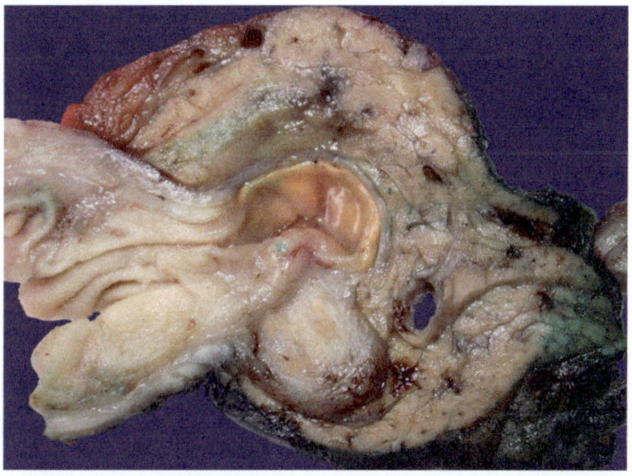

Fig. 1.17 Periampullary diverticulum. A duodenal diverticulum has displaced the ampulla of Vater toward posterior. The diverticular wall shows yellow discoloration due to diverticulitis with accumulation of fatty substances

1.5.4 Genetics

The genetic changes in SPNs are simple. Virtually all SPNs harbor *CTNB1* gene mutations and nothing else [5, 68, 69]. The *CTNB1* gene mutations

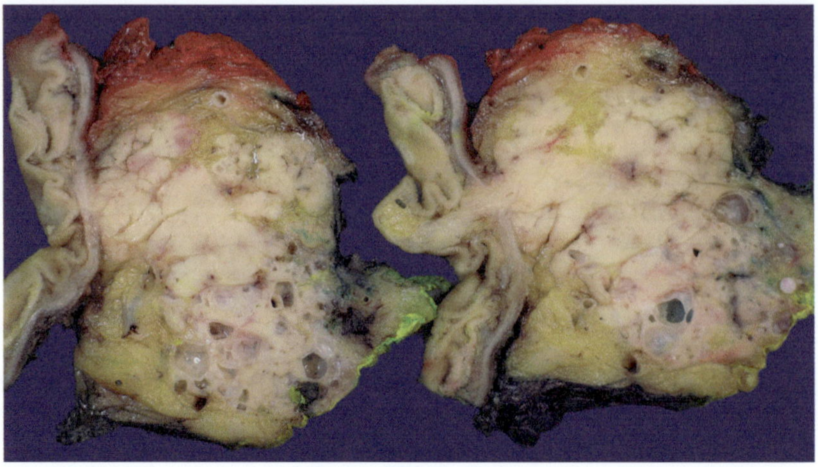

Fig. 1.18 Retention cysts. Dilated pancreatic branch ducts with watery content show smooth membranous walls. On preoperative imaging, the lesion had been diagnosed as side-branch intraductal papillary mucinous neoplasm

explain the nuclear labeling seen with antibodies to the beta-catenin protein as these mutations result in a protein that is longer lived and, as a result, that abnormally accumulates in the nuclei of the neoplastic cells.

1.5.5 Clinical Implications of the Pathology

As is true for the other cystic neoplasms of the pancreas, the gross pathology of SPNs explains their appearance on imaging [57]. SPNs are vascular neoplasms, and they therefore enhance, and they are solid and cystic. With the exception of SPNs with a sarcomatoid appearance, it is difficult to predict the clinical behavior of an SPN. All SPNs are therefore currently classified as malignant.

1.6 Rare Mesenchymal Neoplasms

Several rare mesenchymal neoplasms, such as lymphangiomas and hemangiomas, can be cystic and rarely involve the pancreas [1, 7]. The gross, microscopic, and immunolabeling features of these mesenchymal neoplasms are similar to the gross, microscopic, and immunolabeling features of these neoplasms when they arise in other organs and tissues.

1.7 Other Neoplasms That Can Mimic Truly Cystic Neoplasms

Several neoplasms can mimic the cystic neoplasms of the pancreas. Acinar cell carcinomas can have an extensive intraductal growth pattern and as such can histologically mimic an IPMN, particularly an ITPN [70]. Pancreatic neuroendocrine tumors (PanNETs) can be cystic, and small serotonin-expressing PanNETs can involve the main pancreatic duct producing focal stenosis and secondary upstream dilatation of the pancreatic duct [71, 72]. In addition, just about every variant of solid pancreatic neoplasms can undergo degenerative changes and appear cystic.

1.8 Nonneoplastic Lesions That Can Mimic Cystic Neoplasms

Finally, there are several nonneoplastic lesions that can mimic a cystic neoplasm of the pancreas. The most common of these are pseudocysts. Rarer nonneoplastic cystic lesions include diverticula (Fig. 1.17), retention cysts (Fig. 1.18), endometriosis, parasites, etc.

1.9 Conclusion/Summary

Each cystic neoplasm of the pancreas has characteristic gross, microscopic, immunolabeling, and genetic features. The gross features generally correlate with the appearance of these lesions on imaging, and therefore an understanding of gross pathology is critical to the interpretation of pancreatic imaging [38, 73–75]. The histologic and immunolabeling features of cystic neoplasms of the pancreas are also clinically important. For example, the poorly cohesive nature of the neoplastic cells in SPNs, coupled with the observed loss of expression of E-cadherin, helps explain the mixed solid and cystic appearance of these neoplasms. Finally, mutant DNA is shed from the epithelial cells lining a cyst into cyst fluid. In the near future, we believe that genetic analyses of cyst fluid to determine cyst type will be the standard of care.

References

1. Hruban RH, Pitman MB, Klimstra DS. Tumors of the pancreas. Atlas of tumor pathology, vol. 4, Fascicle 6. Washington, DC: American Registry of Pathology and Armed Forces Institute of Pathology; 2007.
2. Lennon AM, Manos LL, Hruban RH, et al. Role of a multidisciplinary clinic in the management of patients with pancreatic cysts: a single-center cohort study. Ann Surg Oncol. 2014;21(11):3668–74.
3. Jabbar KS, Verbeke C, Hyltander AG, Sjovall H, Hansson GC, Sadik R. Proteomic mucin profiling for the identification of cystic precursors of pancreatic cancer. J Natl Cancer Inst. 2014;106(2):djt439. doi:10.1093/jnci/djt439. djt439 [pii].
4. Siddiqui AA, Kowalski TE, Kedika R, et al. EUS-guided pancreatic fluid aspiration for DNA analysis of KRAS and GNAS mutations for the evaluation of pancreatic cystic neoplasia: a pilot study. Gastrointest Endosc. 2013;77(4):669–70.
5. Wu J, Jiao Y, Dal Molin M, et al. Whole-exome sequencing of neoplastic cysts of the pancreas reveals recurrent mutations in components of ubiquitin-dependent pathways. Proc Natl Acad Sci U S A. 2011;108(52):21188–93.
6. Wu J, Matthaei H, Maitra A, et al. Recurrent GNAS mutations define an unexpected pathway for pancreatic cyst development. Sci Transl Med. 2011;3(92):92ra66.
7. Bosman F, Carneiro F, Hruban RH, Theise N (eds). WHO classification of tumours of the digestive system. 4th ed. Lyon: IARC; 2010.
8. Galanis C, Zamani A, Cameron JL, et al. Resected serous cystic neoplasms of the pancreas: a review of 158 patients with recommendations for treatment. J Gastrointest Surg. 2007;11(7):820–6.
9. Franko J, Cole K, Pezzi CM, Montone KT, Redmond J. Serous cystadenocarcinoma of the pancreas with metachronous hepatic metastasis. Am J Clin Oncol. 2008;31(6):624–5.
10. Le Borgne J, de Calan L, Partensky C. Cystadenomas and cystadenocarcinomas of the pancreas: a multiinstitutional retrospective study of 398 cases. French Surgical Association. Ann Surg. 1999;230(2):152–61.
11. Ohta T, Nagakawa T, Itoh H, Fonseca L, Miyazaki I, Terada T. A case of serous cystadenoma of the pancreas with focal malignant changes. Int J Pancreatol. 1993;14(3):283–9.
12. Chalian H, Tore HG, Rezai P, Bentrem DJ, Yaghmai V. MDCT evaluation of the growth kinetics of serous and benign mucinous cystic neoplasms of the pancreas. Cancer Imaging. 2011;11:116–22.
13. El-Hayek KM, Brown N, O'Rourke C, Falk G, Morris-Stiff G, Walsh RM. Rate of growth of pancreatic serous cystadenoma as an indication for resection. Surgery. 2013;154(4):794–802.
14. Malleo G, Bassi C, Rossini R, et al. Growth pattern of serous cystic neoplasms of the pancreas: observational study with long-term magnetic resonance surveillance and recommendations for treatment. Gut. 2012;61(5):746–51.
15. Menard A, Tomlinson G, Cleary S, Wei A, Gallinger S, Haider MA. Serous cystadenomas of the pancreas: long-term follow-up measurement of growth rate. Can Assoc Radiol J. 2011;62(3):190–6.
16. Chu LC, Singhi AD, Hruban RH, Fishman EK. Characterization of pancreatic serous cystadenoma on dual-phase multidetector computed tomography. J Comput Assist Tomogr. 2014;38(2):258–63.
17. Zaheer A, Pokharel SS, Wolfgang C, Fishman EK, Horton KM. Incidentally detected cystic lesions of the pancreas on CT: review of literature and management suggestions. Abdom Imaging. 2013;38(2):331–41.
18. Panarelli NC, Park KJ, Hruban RH, Klimstra DS. Microcystic serous cystadenoma of the pancreas with subtotal cystic degeneration: another neoplastic mimic of pancreatic pseudocyst. Am J Surg Pathol. 2012;36(5):726–31.
19. Egawa N, Maillet B, Schroder S, Mukai K, Klöppel G. Serous oligocystic and ill-demarcated adenoma of the pancreas: a variant of serous cystic adenoma. Virchows Arch. 1994;424(1):13–7.
20. Goh BK, Tan YM, Yap WM, et al. Pancreatic serous oligocystic adenomas: clinicopathologic features and a comparison with serous microcystic adenomas and mucinous cystic neoplasms. World J Surg. 2006;30(8):1553–9.
21. Santos LD, Chow C, Henderson CJ, et al. Serous oligocystic adenoma of the pancreas: a clinicopathological and immunohistochemical study of three cases with ultrastructural findings. Pathology. 2002;34(2):148–56.
22. Perez-Ordonez B, Naseem A, Lieberman PH, Klimstra DS. Solid serous adenoma of the pancreas. The solid variant of serous cystadenoma? Am J Surg Pathol. 1996;20(11):1401–5.
23. Charlesworth M, Verbeke CS, Falk GA, Walsh M, Smith AM, Morris-Stiff G. Pancreatic lesions in von

Hippel-Lindau disease? A systematic review and meta-synthesis of the literature. J Gastrointest Surg. 2012;16(7):1422–8.
24. Girelli R, Bassi C, Falconi M, et al. Pancreatic cystic manifestations in von Hippel-Lindau disease. Int J Pancreatol. 1997;22(2):101–9.
25. Lee KH, Lee JS, Kim BJ, Lee JK, Kim SH, Lee KT. Pancreatic involvement in Korean patients with von Hippel-Lindau disease. J Gastroenterol. 2009;44 (5):447–52.
26. Thirabanjasak D, Basturk O, Altinel D, Cheng JD, Adsay NV. Is serous cystadenoma of the pancreas a model of clear-cell-associated angiogenesis and tumorigenesis? Pancreatology. 2009;9(1–2):182–8.
27. Yamazaki K, Eyden B. An immunohistochemical and ultrastructural study of pancreatic microcystic serous cyst adenoma with special reference to tumor-associated microvasculature and vascular endothelial growth factor in tumor cells. Ultrastruct Pathol. 2006; 30(1):119–28.
28. Yip-Schneider MT, Wu H, Dumas RP, et al. Vascular endothelial growth factor, a novel and highly accurate pancreatic fluid biomarker for serous pancreatic cysts. J Am Coll Surg. 2014;218(4):608–17.
29. Vortmeyer AO, Lubensky IA, Fogt F, Linehan WM, Khettry U, Zhuang Z. Allelic deletion and mutation of the von Hippel-Lindau (VHL) tumor suppressor gene in pancreatic microcystic adenomas. Am J Pathol. 1997;151:951–6.
30. Mohr VH, Vortmeyer AO, Zhuang Z, et al. Histopathology and molecular genetics of multiple cysts and microcystic (serous) adenomas of the pancreas in von Hippel-Lindau patients. Am J Pathol. 2000;157(5):1615–21.
31. Mukhopadhyay B, Sahdev A, Monson JP, Besser GM, Reznek RH, Chew SL. Pancreatic lesions in von Hippel-Lindau disease. Clin Endocrinol (Oxf). 2002; 57(5):603–8.
32. Hruban RH, Takaori K, Klimstra DS, et al. An illustrated consensus on the classification of pancreatic intraepithelial neoplasia and intraductal papillary mucinous neoplasms. Am J Surg Pathol. 2004;28(8):977–87.
33. Lennon AM, Wolfgang CL, Canto MI, et al. The early detection of pancreatic cancer: what will it take to diagnose and treat curable pancreatic neoplasia? Cancer Res. 2014;74(13):3381–9.
34. Hruban RH, Schulick RD. Is surgery required for patients with intraductal papillary mucinous neoplasms without mural nodules? Nat Clin Pract Gastroenterol Hepatol. 2008;5(11):598–9.
35. Tanaka M, Fernandez-Del Castillo C, Adsay V, et al. International consensus guidelines 2012 for the management of IPMN and MCN of the pancreas. Pancreatology. 2012;12(3):183–97.
36. Westra WH, Hruban RH, Phelps TH, Isacson C. Surgical pathology dissection: an illustrated guide. 2nd ed. New York: Springer; 2003.
37. Matthaei H, Norris AL, Tsiatis AC, et al. Clinicopathological characteristics and molecular analyses of multifocal intraductal papillary mucinous neoplasms of the pancreas. Ann Surg. 2012;255(2):326–33.
38. Raman SP, Kawamoto S, Blackford A, et al. Histopathologic findings of multifocal pancreatic intraductal papillary mucinous neoplasms on CT. AJR Am J Roentgenol. 2013;200(3):563–9.
39. Furukawa T, Klöppel G, Volkan Adsay N, et al. Classification of types of intraductal papillary-mucinous neoplasm of the pancreas: a consensus study. Virchows Arch. 2005;447(5):794–9.
40. Yamaguchi H, Shimizu M, Ban S, et al. Intraductal tubulopapillary neoplasms of the pancreas distinct from pancreatic intraepithelial neoplasia and intraductal papillary mucinous neoplasms. Am J Surg Pathol. 2009;33(8):1164–72.
41. Poultsides GA, Reddy S, Cameron JL, et al. Histopathologic basis for the favorable survival after resection of intraductal papillary mucinous neoplasm-associated invasive adenocarcinoma of the pancreas. Ann Surg. 2010;251(3):470–6.
42. Chari ST, Yadav D, Smyrk TC, et al. Study of recurrence after surgical resection of intraductal papillary mucinous neoplasm of the pancreas. Gastroenterology. 2002;123(5):1500–7.
43. Adsay NV, Merati K, Andea A, et al. The dichotomy in the preinvasive neoplasia to invasive carcinoma sequence in the pancreas: differential expression of MUC1 and MUC2 supports the existence of two separate pathways of carcinogenesis. Mod Pathol. 2002;15(10):1087–95.
44. Amato E, Molin MD, Mafficini A, et al. Targeted next-generation sequencing of cancer genes dissects the molecular profiles of intraductal papillary neoplasms of the pancreas. J Pathol. 2014;233(3):217–27.
45. He J, Cameron JL, Ahuja N, et al. Is it necessary to follow patients after resection of a benign pancreatic intraductal papillary mucinous neoplasm? J Am Coll Surg. 2013;216(4):657–7.
46. Kanda M, Knight S, Topazian M, et al. Mutant GNAS detected in duodenal collections of secretin-stimulated pancreatic juice indicates the presence or emergence of pancreatic cysts. Gut. 2012;62(7):1024–33.
47. Gress F, Gottlieb K, Cummings O, Sherman S, Lehman G. Endoscopic ultrasound characteristics of mucinous cystic neoplasms of the pancreas. Am J Gastroenterol. 2000;95(4):961–5.
48. Procacci C, Carbognin G, Accordini S, et al. CT features of malignant mucinous cystic tumors of the pancreas. Eur Radiol. 2001;11(9):1626–30.
49. Lewis GH, Wang H, Bellizzi AM, et al. Prognosis of minimally invasive carcinoma arising in mucinous cystic neoplasms of the pancreas. Am J Surg Pathol. 2013;37(4):601–5.
50. van den Berg W, Tascilar M, Offerhaus GJ, et al. Pancreatic mucinous cystic neoplasms with sarcomatous stroma: molecular evidence for monoclonal origin with subsequent divergence of the epithelial and sarcomatous components. Mod Pathol. 2000; 13(1):86–91.

51. Westra WH, Sturm PJ, Drillenburg P, et al. K-ras oncogene mutations in osteoclast-like giant cell tumors of the pancreas and liver: genetic evidence to support origin from the duct epithelium. Am J Surg Pathol. 1998;22(10):1247–54.
52. Albores-Saavedra J, Nadji M, Henson DE, Angeles-Angeles A. Entero-endocrine cell differentiation in carcinomas of the gallbladder and mucinous cystadenocarcinomas of the pancreas. Pathol Res Pract. 1988;183(2):169–75.
53. Garcia-Carracedo D, Chen ZM, Qiu W, et al. PIK3CA mutations in mucinous cystic neoplasms of the pancreas. Pancreas. 2014;43(2):245–9.
54. Iacobuzio-Donahue CA, Wilentz RE, Argani P, et al. Dpc4 protein in mucinous cystic neoplasms of the pancreas: frequent loss of expression in invasive carcinomas suggests a role in genetic progression. Am J Surg Pathol. 2000;24(11):1544–8.
55. Wilentz RE, Talamini MA, Albores-Saavedra J, Hruban RH. Pathologic examination accurately predicts prognosis in mucinous cystic neoplasms of the pancreas. Am J Surg Pathol. 1999;23(11):1320–7.
56. Reddy S, Cameron JL, Scudiere J, et al. Surgical management of solid-pseudopapillary neoplasms of the pancreas (Franz or Hamoudi tumors): a large single-institutional series. J Am Coll Surg. 2009;208(5):950–7. discussion 957–9.
57. Raman SP, Kawamoto S, Law JK, et al. Institutional experience with solid pseudopapillary neoplasms: focus on computed tomography, magnetic resonance imaging, conventional ultrasound, endoscopic ultrasound, and predictors of aggressive histology. J Comput Assist Tomogr. 2013;37(5):824–33.
58. Meriden Z, Shi C, Edil BH, et al. Hyaline globules in neuroendocrine and solid-pseudopapillary neoplasms of the pancreas: a clue to the diagnosis. Am J Surg Pathol. 2011;35(7):981–8.
59. Kim SA, Kim MS, Kim SC, Choi J, Yu E, Hong SM. Pleomorphic solid pseudopapillary neoplasm of the pancreas: degenerative change rather than high-grade malignant potential. Hum Pathol. 2014;45(1):166–74.
60. Tang LH, Aydin H, Brennan MF, Klimstra DS. Clinically aggressive solid-pseudopapillary tumors of the pancreas. Am J Surg Pathol. 2005;29:512–9.
61. Audard V, Cavard C, Richa H, et al. Impaired E-cadherin expression and glutamine synthetase overexpression in solid pseudopapillary neoplasm of the pancreas. Pancreas. 2008;36(1):80–3.
62. Burford H, Baloch Z, Liu X, Jhala D, Siegal GP, Jhala N. E-cadherin/{beta}-catenin and CD10: a limited immunohistochemical panel to distinguish pancreatic endocrine neoplasm from solid pseudopapillary neoplasm of the pancreas on endoscopic ultrasound-guided fine-needle aspirates of the pancreas. Am J Clin Pathol. 2009;132(6):831–9.
63. Chetty R, Serra S. Membrane loss and aberrant nuclear localization of E-cadherin are consistent features of solid pseudopapillary tumour of the pancreas. An immunohistochemical study using two antibodies recognizing different domains of the E-cadherin molecule. Histopathology. 2008;52(3):325–30.
64. El Bahrawy MA, Rowan A, Horncastle D, et al. E-cadherin/catenin complex status in solid pseudopapillary tumor of the pancreas. Am J Surg Pathol. 2008;32(1):1–7.
65. Guo Y, Yuan F, Deng H, Wang HF, Jin XL, Xiao JC. Paranuclear dot-like immunostaining for CD99: a unique staining pattern for diagnosing solid-pseudopapillary neoplasm of the pancreas. Am J Surg Pathol. 2011;35(6):799–806.
66. Li L, Li J, Hao C, et al. Immunohistochemical evaluation of solid pseudopapillary tumors of the pancreas: the expression pattern of CD99 is highly unique. Cancer Lett. 2011;310(1):9–14.
67. Singhi AD, Lilo M, Hruban RH, Cressman KL, Fuhrer K, Seethala RR. Overexpression of Lymphoid Enhancer-Binding Factor 1 (LEF1) in solid-pseudopapillary neoplasms of the pancreas. Mod Pathol. 2014;27(10):1355–63.
68. Abraham SC, Klimstra DS, Wilentz RE, et al. Solid-pseudopapillary tumors of the pancreas are genetically distinct from pancreatic ductal adenocarcinomas and almost always harbor beta-catenin mutations. Am J Pathol. 2002;160(4):1361–9.
69. Tanaka Y, Kato K, Notohara K, et al. Frequent beta-catenin mutation and cytoplasmic/nuclear accumulation in pancreatic solid-pseudopapillary neoplasm. Cancer Res. 2001;61(23):8401–4.
70. Toll AD, Mitchell D, Yeo CJ, Hruban RH, Witkiewicz AK. Acinar cell carcinoma with a prominent intraductal growth pattern: case report with review of the literature. Int J Surg Pathol. 2011;19(6):795–9.
71. Kawamoto S, Johnson PT, Shi C, et al. Pancreatic neuroendocrine tumor with cystlike changes: evaluation with MDCT. AJR Am J Roentgenol. 2013;200(3):W283–90.
72. McCall CM, Shi C, Klein AP, et al. Serotonin expression in pancreatic neuroendocrine tumors correlates with a trabecular histologic pattern and large duct involvement. Hum Pathol. 2012;43(8):1169–76.
73. Kawamoto S, Lawler LP, Horton KM, Eng J, Hruban RH, Fishman EK. MDCT of intraductal papillary mucinous neoplasm of the pancreas: evaluation of features predictive of invasive carcinoma. AJR Am J Roentgenol. 2006;186(3):687–95.
74. Kawamoto S, Scudiere J, Hruban RH, Wolfgang CL, Cameron JL, Fishman EK. Solid-pseudopapillary neoplasm of the pancreas: spectrum of findings on multidetector CT. Clin Imaging. 2011;35(1):21–8.
75. Khashab MA, Shin EJ, Amateau S, et al. Tumor size and location correlate with behavior of pancreatic serous cystic neoplasms. Am J Gastroenterol. 2011;106(8):1521–6.

2 Cytology of Cystic Neoplasms of the Pancreas

Martha Bishop Pitman and Nirag C. Jhala

2.1 Introduction

Pancreatic cyst aspirates are often scant specimens with few cells. Cytology alone may not be sufficient for diagnosis. A multimodal approach that utilizes gross cyst fluid characteristics, biochemical testing, and molecular analysis is frequently required to provide sufficient information for patient management [1]. As such optimal cyst fluid triage is necessary to obtain this information. Although a specific diagnosis is always desired, it may not be possible with the limited amount of fluid and cells obtained. Nonetheless, more generic clinical questions that may be answered by the pathologist that directly impact patient management include: (1) Is the cyst a malignant or high-risk cyst that needs to be resected? (2) Is the cyst a low-risk premalignant mucinous cyst that can be closely monitored?

M.B. Pitman, MD (✉)
Department of Pathology, Massachusetts General Hospital, Professor of Pathology, Harvard Medical School, 55 Fruit Street, Boston, MA 01907, USA
e-mail: mpitman@partners.org

N.C. Jhala, MD
Department of Pathology and Laboratory Medicine, Professor of Pathology, Temple University School of Medicine, 3401 N. Broad Street, Philadelphia, PA 19140, USA
e-mail: nirag.jhala@tuhs.temple.edu

2.2 Cyst Fluid Triage and Specimen Processing

Optimal cyst fluid triage will help to answer these questions and potentially make a specific diagnosis [2]. To avoid fluid volume dilution, it is recommended that fresh neat samples of cyst fluid be sent to the cytology laboratory without placing the cyst fluid in any type of transport medium. The clinical question about the cyst coupled with the volume of the cyst fluid will determine which tests should be performed. For example, aspirated cyst fluid that is grossly "thick and mucoid" does not need CEA or molecular testing to confirm its etiology as a mucinous cyst. If the imaging characteristics are diagnostic of a branch-duct intraductal papillary mucinous neoplasm (IPMN), then the only question remaining is the grade, and since cytology is the best test to answer this question, even scant fluid should be processed for cytology only. Any solid nodule or cyst wall mass should be separately aspirated and processed. A proposed triage protocol that maximizes information from the cyst fluid is outlined in Table 2.1.

2.3 Rapid On-Site Interpretation

Rapid on-site evaluation (ROSE) of solid mass lesions provides a benefit of increased accuracy [3]. In fine-needle aspiration (FNA) of pancreatic cysts, however, appropriate triage of cyst fluid for

M. Del Chiaro et al. (eds.), *Cystic Tumors of the Pancreas*, DOI 10.1007/978-3-319-31882-0_2

biochemical analysis or molecular analysis is more important than ROSE. Smearing a cyst fluid for immediate evaluation is not likely to provide information that will influence the yield of the biopsy procedure in contrast to ROSE for endoscopic ultrasound (EUS)-FNA of a solid mass lesion [4, 5].

2.4 Biochemical Testing

Carcinoembryonic antigen (CEA) has been shown to be the most reliable and accurate test for a mucinous cyst compared to mucin stains and cytology [6]. At a level of 192 ng/ml, CEA has an overall accuracy of ~80 % (specificity of 84 % and a sensitivity of 75 %) [7]. At a level of 800 ng/ml, the specificity is 98 % but sensitivity is 48 % [8], so raising the cutoff level this high leaves many mucinous cysts undetected. CEA levels do not correlate with the grade of dysplasia or malignancy [9, 10]. Serous cystadenomas typically have CEA levels <0.5 ng/ml. However, CEA levels may be elevated in pseudocysts and other non-mucinous cysts such as lymphoepithelial cysts [11]. Most importantly, CEA is not always elevated in a mucinous cyst, so a low CEA level should not be interpreted as exclusion of a mucinous cyst. The measured CEA value of a patient's sample can vary depending on the testing procedure used so each laboratory must validate the assay for elevated levels.

The utility of amylase analysis in cyst fluids is to support the clinical and cytological diagnosis of a pseudocyst, serous cystadenoma, or cystic neuroendocrine tumor. Whereas pseudocysts almost always have a markedly elevated amylase level, serous cystadenomas and cystic neuroendocrine tumors consistently have very low amylase levels [8, 12]. Amylase levels are highly variable in mucinous cysts, and elevated levels do not distinguish between IPMN and MCN because MCN can demonstrate high levels despite their lack of connection to the pancreatic ductal system; however, IPMNs should demonstrate an elevated level given their inherent connection to the pancreatic ducts [13] (Table 2.2).

Table 2.1 Pancreatic cyst fluid triage

Fresh, undiluted, unfixed cyst fluid	
Volume (<0.5 cc)	Volume (>0.5 cc)
CEA *or*	Molecular (vortexed, neat; 0.3 cc)
Molecular *or*	Cytology (cell button; cytospin)
Cytology	Amylase (0.3 cc supernatant)
	CEA Amylase (0.3 cc supernatant)
	Bank (residual supernatant)

2.5 Special Stains and Immunohistochemical Stains

Special stains and immunohistochemical stains may be performed on formalin-fixed paraffin-embedded tissue if there is sufficient tissue to make a cellblock. Larger more complex cysts are most likely to produce sufficient tissue for a cellblock. Stains can be performed on destained direct smears if there are proper controls available. When the clinical question is if the cyst is mucinous or non-mucinous, the tissue triage

Table 2.2 Biochemical testing distinguishing mucinous from non-mucinous neoplastic cysts

	IPMN	MCN	SCA	cPanNET
Viscosity	High	High	Low	Low
CEA	High (>192 ng/ml)[a]	High (>192 ng/ml)[a]	Low	Low
Amylase	High	Low/high	Low	Low

IPMN intraductal papillary mucinous neoplasm, *MCN* mucinous cystic neoplasm, *SCA* serous cystadenoma, *cPanNET* cystic pancreatic neuroendocrine tumor, *CEA* carcinoembryonic antigen

[a]Accuracy ~80 % at this level; lower CEA values have been noted without affecting accuracy. Each laboratory may use their cutoff values following a validation of the protocol that they use

should follow the algorithm as stated above with the extra cyst fluid processed as a cellblock. If the cyst is more complex or solid and cystic, then effort should be made to obtain sufficient tissue for a cellblock since high in the differential diagnosis are secondarily cystic solid neoplasms that greatly benefit from ancillary testing with immunohistochemical stains. Ancillary testing is discussed in more detail with each neoplasm.

2.6 Molecular Analysis

The molecular characteristics of pancreatic cystic neoplasms are covered in detail in Chap. 4. Clinically useful molecular tests in the preoperative assessment of cyst fluid are rather limited with respect to their value-added benefit over less expensive biochemical tests and cytology. While the assessment of CEA is certainly a more cost-effective test to determine the mucinous nature of a cyst, not all mucinous cysts have an elevated CEA, and an elevated CEA is not 100 % specific for a mucinous neoplasm. When CEA is not elevated, detection of *KRAS*, *GNAS*, and/or *RNF43* mutations supports the diagnosis of a mucinous cyst [14–18]. *RNF43* is not as frequently mutated as *KRAS* and *GNAS* and adds no additional clinically useful information, so analysis of just *KRAS* and *GNAS* is sufficient [17]. The detection of a *KRAS or GNAS* mutation supports the presence of a neoplastic mucinous cyst, and the detection of a *GNAS* mutation appears to distinguish an IPMN from an MCN. Unfortunately, these molecular markers are present in all grades of dysplasia, so the detection of neither mutant gene distinguishes a low-grade from high-grade mucinous cyst. In addition, the absence of both markers does not exclude a mucinous neoplasm. *TP53* mutation and loss of *SMAD4* are late mutations in the progression to carcinoma, and detection with next-generation sequencing is advantage over single-gene mutational analysis [17].

Other helpful mutations include 3p25 (the von Hippel-Lindau gene) seen in some serous cystadenomas [19] and the beta-catenin gene, which is mutated in virtually all solid pseudopapillary neoplasms [20] (Table 2.3).

Table 2.3 Molecular studies that help distinguish a mucinous cyst from non-mucinous neoplastic cyst

	IPMN	MCN	SCA
KRAS mutation	Present	Present	Absent
GNAS mutation	Present	Absent	Absent
RNF43 mutation	Present	Present	Absent
VHL gene	Absent	Absent	Present

2.7 Cytological Analysis and Test Integration

One of the major challenges that pathologists face in the diagnosis of pancreatic cysts is the distinction between mucinous and non-mucinous cysts. Once this distinction has occurred via observation of sufficiently thick extracellular mucin grossly or microscopically, via CEA elevation or via detection of *KRAS/GNAS/RFN43* mutation, the second challenge is to determine the degree of cytological atypia, especially in a mucinous cyst. Secondarily cystic neoplasms such as neuroendocrine tumors can demonstrate diagnostic epithelial atypia [12].

While reviewing morphology it is very important to have knowledge of the location of the cyst, imaging characteristics of the cyst, and access utilized by the gastroenterologist to obtain the FNA sample. For example, a highly cellular specimen of abundant mucinous glandular epithelium from a small (<2 cm), simple unilocular cyst obtained using a transgastric approach should raise suspicion of gastric contamination. Recognition of multiple types of glandular cells and their morphologic characteristics helps to distinguish neoplastic epithelium from contaminating glandular cells from the gastrointestinal tract such as duodenal surface epithelium (Fig. 2.1) and gastric foveolar epithelium from the stomach (Fig. 2.2). Correlating demographic information and imaging characteristics, such as multiplicity, status of the main pancreatic duct, and communication with the main pancreatic duct, aid in making a specific diagnosis of an IPMN.

Malignancy or high-grade epithelial atypia is assessed by cytological analysis. In a mucinous cyst, less than overt malignancy is best interpreted

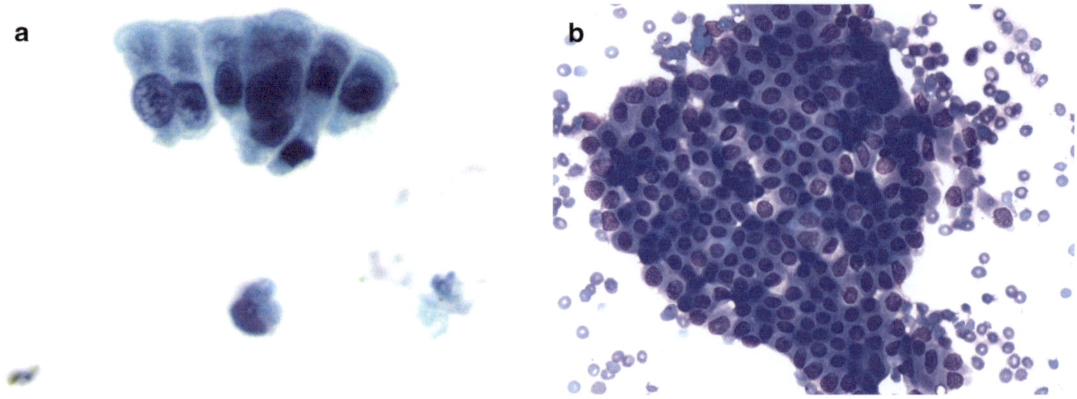

Fig. 2.1 Duodenal epithelium. Contaminating duodenal enterocytes are non-mucinous columnar glandular cells in a strip with a brush border (**a**) or a flat honeycombed sheet punctuated by goblet cells and lymphocytes (b) (**a**. Papanicoloua; **b**. Diff-quik)

Fig. 2.2 Gastric epithelium. Foveolar-type epithelium from the stomach is mucinous and is virtually identical to the low-grade dysplastic gastric-type cyst-lining cells of the typical branch-duct IPMN (Papanicolaou)

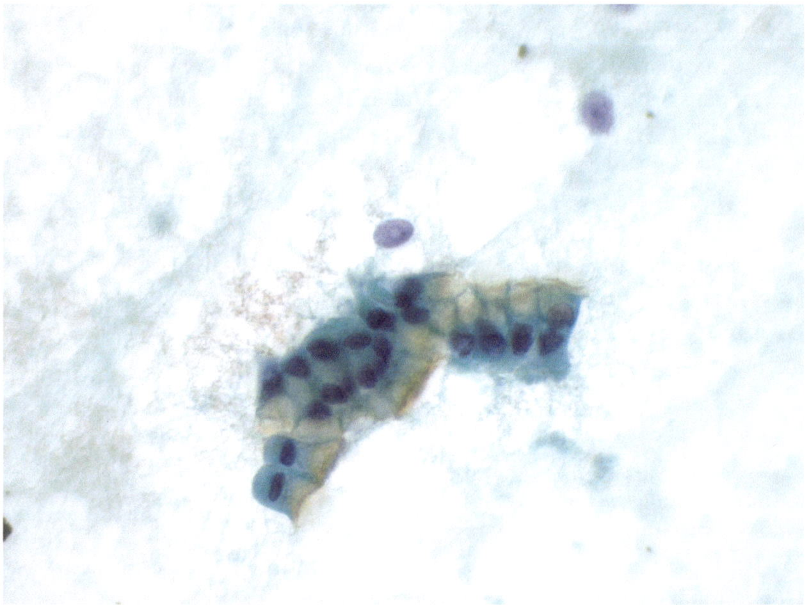

as either low-grade or high-grade atypia as the accuracy in distinguishing intermediate-grade (moderate) dysplasia from high-grade dysplasia is difficult if not impossible [21]. Cytological criteria distinguishing high-grade atypia from low-grade atypia have recently been described [22]. Cells smaller than a 12 μm duodenal enterocyte showing an increased nuclear to cytoplasmic ratio, an abnormal chromatin pattern, and background necrosis represent high-grade epithelial atypia (high-grade dysplasia or adenocarcinoma) placing the cyst in a high-risk category. Cytology is also the best test for accurate diagnosis of a cystic neuroendocrine tumor [12]. The cytological features are illustrated below with each neoplasm.

2.8 Standardized Reporting of Pancreaticobiliary Cytology

The Papanicolaou Society of Cytopathology has proposed a unified, standardized method of reporting pancreaticobiliary cytology [23]. Per these guidelines, pancreatic aspirates are placed into one of six general groups (Table 2.4). Having a clear understanding of the current histological

Table 2.4 Papanicolaou Society of Cytopathology System for Reporting Pancreaticobiliary Cytology

I. Nondiagnostic
II. Negative (for malignancy)
(a) Benign pancreatic tissue (in appropriate clinical setting)
(b) Acute pancreatitis
(c) Chronic pancreatitis
(d) Autoimmune pancreatitis
(e) Pseudocyst
(f) Lymphoepithelial cyst
(g) Splenule/accessory spleen
III. Atypical
IV. Neoplastic
(a) Benign
(i) Serous cystadenoma
(ii) Neuroendocrine microadenoma
(iii) Lymphangioma
(b) Other
(i) Well-differentiated neuroendocrine tumor
(ii) Intraductal papillary mucinous neoplasm, all grades of dysplasia
(iii) Mucinous cystic neoplasm, all grades of dysplasia
(iv) Solid pseudopapillary neoplasm
V. Suspicious (for malignancy)
VI. Positive/malignant
(a) Ductal adenocarcinoma of the pancreas and its variants
(b) Cholangiocarcinoma
(c) Acinar cell carcinoma
(d) Poorly differentiated (small- and large-cell) neuroendocrine carcinoma
(e) Pancreatoblastoma
(g) Lymphoma
(g) Metastatic malignancy

terminology and nomenclature as well as the management algorithms used to treat patients with cystic neoplasms is essential in order for the pathologist to render a diagnosis that is understood by the clinician and useful for patient management.

2.9 Cytology of Neoplastic Cysts

2.9.1 Serous Cystadenoma

Aspirates of serous cystadenoma (SCA) produce scant specimens when cysts are small, but when cysts are large (macrocystic variant), aspirates may procure abundant thin fluid that may be bloody or clear. Smears from SCA are paucicellular, and, as such, most FNAs are nondiagnostic. The background is devoid of thick, colloid-like mucin, although contaminating mucin from the gastrointestinal tract can be a pitfall. Bloody fluids produce bloody backgrounds and clear fluids yield clean backgrounds on direct smears. Placing an aliquot of fluid into a liquid-based preservative may increase the yield of diagnostic material. Fresh cyst fluid, however, is required for biochemical testing.

Neoplastic cells are small cuboidal cells with round regular nuclear membranes and inconspicuous nucleoli [24] (Fig. 2.3a). Cytoplasm is scant, pale, foamy, and vacuolated but non-mucinous [24, 25]. The cells are fragile, so direct smears often destroy the cells leaving fibrosis tissue fragments from the stripped cyst septa. Given the high vascularity of the septa which bleed, hemosiderin-laden macrophages may be noted (Fig. 2.3b), and these cells may serve as a surrogate marker for the diagnosis [24].

2.9.1.1 Ancillary Studies

The absence of thick mucin, mucinous epithelial cells, and high-grade cytological atypia, coupled with low amylase and CEA levels are characteristic findings that support the diagnosis. If there is a cellblock or core biopsy with neoplastic cells, the use of periodic acid-Schiff (PAS) stain with and without diastase digestion confirms the glycogen in the cytoplasm (Fig. 2.4). Use of cytokeratin and CD68 stain may help distinguish macrophages from neoplastic epithelial cells. It is important to recognize contaminating gastrointestinal glandular cells to avoid a false diagnosis of a neoplastic mucinous cyst [25, 26]. If sufficient cyst fluid is available, molecular analysis may detect the *VHL* gene mutation, which would support the diagnosis. Due to the high vascularity of SCA, analysis of the cyst fluid for VEGF has been proposed as an accurate test for SCA [27]; however, this remains to be validated. A recent study of clinical cyst fluids did not show sufficient sensitivity or specificity for clinical utility [28].

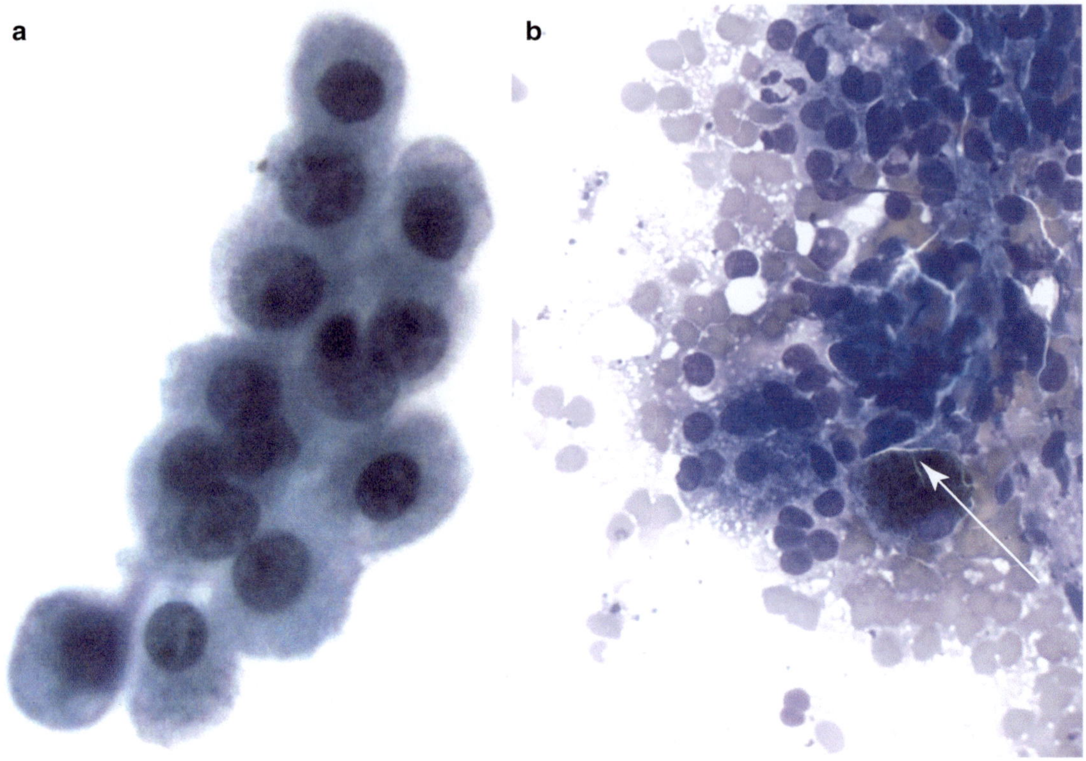

Fig. 2.3 Serous cystadenoma. Cyst-lining cells are nonmucinous cuboidal cells with benign round nuclei and finely vacuolated cytoplasm rich in glycogen (**a**). Hemosiderin-laden macrophages (*arrow*) are not uncommon and act as a surrogate marker of the highly vascular septa of this neoplasm (**b**) (**a.** Papanicoloua; **b.** Diff-Quik)

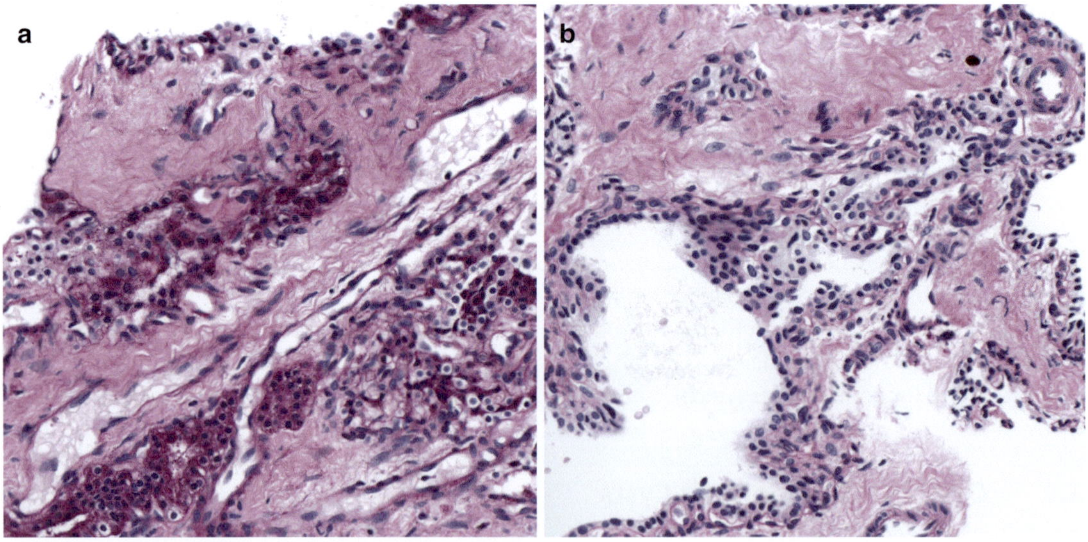

Fig. 2.4 Serous cystadenoma. Cellblock or core biopsy provides tissue for ancillary tests. The glycogen-rich cytoplasm is demonstrated by PAS stain (**a**), which, in contrast to mucin, is removed with diastase (**b**) (**a**. Periodic acid-Schiff; **b**. periodic acid-Schiff with diastase)

2.9.2 Mucinous Cysts

IPMNs and MCN are biologically distinct neoplastic mucinous cysts of the pancreas that share common cytomorphological features. The distinction between these entities is often not possible on cytology alone as a specific diagnosis typically requires correlation with clinical and imaging findings as well as ancillary tests. The distinction is important for clinical management, however, since all MCN are resected regardless of grade, and most branch-duct IPMNs, which are usually low risk by imaging, are observed [29].

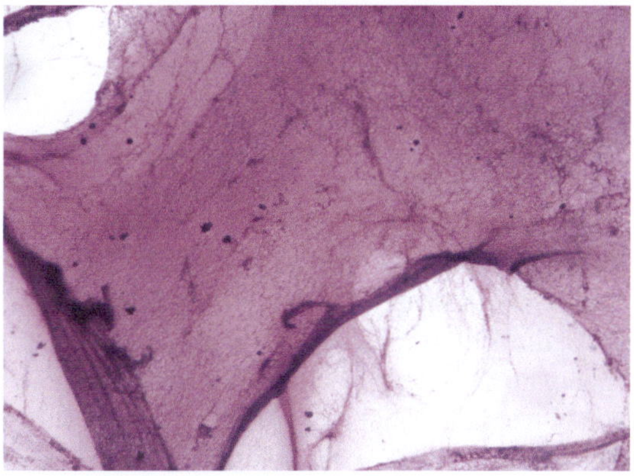

Fig. 2.5 Mucinous cyst. Thick, colloid-like extracellular mucin is not consistent with gastrointestinal contamination and supports the diagnosis of a mucinous cyst, regardless of the presence of an epithelial component (hematoxylin and eosin)

2.9.3 Cytological Features Associated with IPMN and MCN

The volume of fluid aspirated from mucinous cysts is highly variable, obviously dependent on the size of the cyst(s) accessible to the needle. The gross characteristics of the cyst fluid can be very informative and these features should be recorded in the endoscopy note and relayed to the pathologist. A gross description such as "thick and viscous fluid" indicates a mucinous cyst fluid. These descriptions act as a surrogate marker for viscosity. In lieu of viscosity, a "string test" performed by placing the fluid between the thumb and index finger and pulling apart to form a "string" can roughly assess viscosity; fluid that "strings" to 3.5 mm is considered mucinous [30]. The volume of cyst fluid is also important to record. The pathologist will note an obvious noncorrelation when only a "drop" of fluid is obtained during aspiration, and the slide is very cellular or covered with extracellular mucin or tissue. Such discordance should prompt the pathologist to consider gastrointestinal contamination or normal pancreatic tissue as the source of the tissue.

Smears of grossly thick, viscous mucin correlate with colloid-like, thick extracellular mucin, which is not consistent with gastrointestinal contamination and supports the diagnosis of a mucinous cyst (Fig. 2.5). Another clue that the mucin is from the cyst includes the presence of degenerated cells and debris floating in the mucin. The absence of an epithelial component in such mucin should not lead to a nondiagnostic report, but instead a report of a neoplastic mucinous cyst. Thin mucin may be difficult to appreciate on smears and especially in fluids which are processed by placing the fluid in liquid preservatives such as PreservCyt® and CytoRich Red™. Liquid-based processing dilutes and attenuates the extracellular mucin, which may be mistaken for fibrin. Special stains for mucin such as mucicarmine and alcian blue pH 2.5 may be helpful if positive, but contaminating gastrointestinal tract mucin may give a false-positive result in some cases and a negative mucin stain does not exclude a mucinous etiology.

Evaluation of the cells in the cyst fluid is the best test for establishing the cyst grade since neither CEA nor the presence of *KRAS/GNAS* mutations correlate with grade. Many cysts are paucicellular, especially when they are small (<3 cm) and unilocular. The more complex the cyst, the more likely the cyst is to be cellular. When cyst-lining cells become denuded, the cyst fluids are dominated by inflammation, histiocytes, and cell debris mimicking a pseudocyst. This finding is more frequently noted with MCN. Adjacent epithelial cells may also demonstrate changes associated with cell injury. Such epithelial cells may demonstrate nuclear and nucleolar enlargement mimicking high-grade dysplasia.

IPMNs are associated with four distinct types of lining epithelium. Gastric (null)-type epithelium is the most common lining epithelium of branch-duct IPMN. These cells are consistent with low-grade dysplasia and are virtually identical to the gastric foveolar epithelial cells of the stomach. Intestinal-type epithelial cells are more commonly associated with main-duct IPMN and by definition are intermediate-grade dysplasia. Pancreaticobiliary-type lining cells are by definition high-grade dysplasia as are oncocytic epithelial cells. Gastric-type epithelial cells can progress from low-grade to high-grade dysplasia, and these higher grade gastric-type cells can be impossible to distinguish from the other cell types. It is not necessary to make such a specific diagnosis of cell type on cytology. The most important distinction is between low-grade cells and high-grade cells since it is the high-grade cells that will represent a high-risk feature for malignancy. MCN are lined by mucinous epithelial cells similar to gastric-type epithelial cells. The progression from low-grade to high-grade cyst-lining cells of an MCN is similar to that of the low-grade dysplastic gastric-type cyst-lining cells of IPMN.

Cytological features associated with various grades of dysplasia (low, intermediate, and high) have been described for IPMN [22, 31–35]. These findings are similar for MCN. Interobserver variability among pathologists in diagnosing and grading mucinous lesions of the pancreas is a real issue, not only for cytology but for histology as well [21, 36]. For this reason, the two-tiered cytological grading is recommended with low- and intermediate-grade dysplasia grouped as low-grade atypia and high-grade dysplasia and invasive carcinoma grouped as high-grade atypia [21]. Of course, if the features on cytology are unequivocally diagnostic of malignancy, then the diagnosis should be positive for adenocarcinoma.

Cytological features associated with grades of dysplasia are as follows.

2.9.3.1 Low-Grade Atypia

Low-Grade Dysplasia (Fig. 2.6) Mucinous epithelium shows two-dimensional cell groups and sheets of mucinous cells with preserved nuclear to cytoplasmic ratio and cytoplasmic mucin. In cases where distinction between neoplastic and gastric contaminating epithelium cannot be made, then the cells are best characterized as low-grade epithelial atypia.

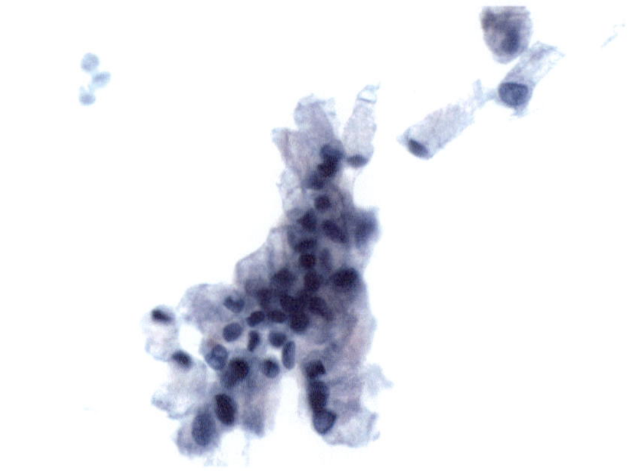

Fig. 2.6 IPMN with low-grade dysplasia. Columnar mucinous epithelial cells show abundant mucinous cytoplasm and minimal nuclear atypia (Papanicolaou)

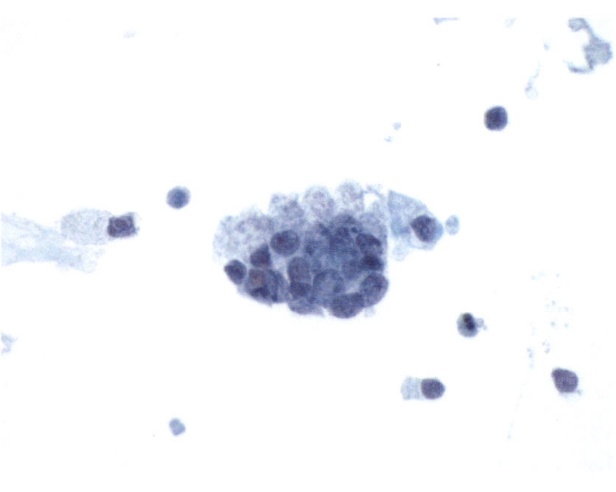

Fig. 2.7 IPMN with intermediate-grade dysplasia. Cells show stratification of the nuclei and moderate cytological atypia with mild anisonucleosis and slight loss of polarity (Papanicolaou)

Intermediate-Grade Dysplasia (Fig. 2.7) Mucinous epithelial cells are usually in cohesive cell clusters of various sizes and the nuclei show crowding and some loss of polarity. Stratification of the nuclei recapitulates the increasing complexity of the lining epithelium noted on histology. The cells demonstrate increased nuclear to cytoplasmic ratio and may also demonstrate mild nuclear atypia including inconspicuous nucleoli and membrane irregularity.

2.9.3.2 High-Grade Atypia

High-Grade Dysplasia (Fig. 2.8) Atypical epithelial cells are noted in small bud-like clusters and single cells. These cells are usually smaller than a 12 μm duodenal enterocyte. They will have increased nuclear to cytoplasmic ratio and abnormal chromatin (hypochromasia or hyperchromasia), some have irregular nuclear membranes, and the cytoplasm is variably vacuolated. In addition, background necrosis is usually present.

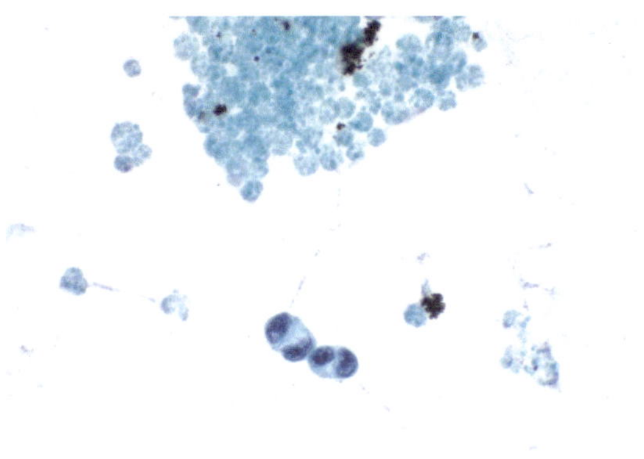

Fig. 2.8 IPMN with high-grade dysplasia. Cells are small (<12 μm duodenal enterocyte), often in small clusters, and singly, with abnormal chromatin and typically associated with background necrosis (Papanicolaou)

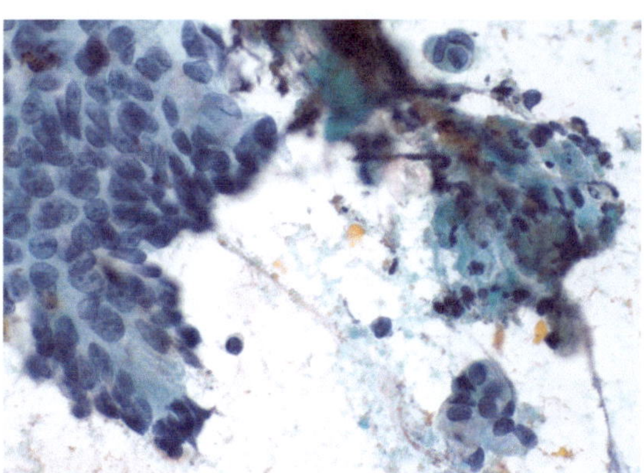

Fig. 2.9 MCN with invasive carcinoma (adenocarcinoma). Cells show irregular spacing in a sheet with nuclear crowing and overlap, anisonucleosis of 4:1, and irregular nuclear membranes. Note the smaller clusters of high-grade epithelial cells and degenerated collagen (Papanicolaou)

Adenocarcinoma (Fig. 2.9) Three-dimensional groups and single cells show variable anisonucleosis of at least 1:4 in a single sheet, irregular nuclear membranes, prominent nucleoli, and variably vacuolated cytoplasm, present in a background of necrosis in most cases.

2.9.3.3 Ancillary Studies

Establishing that the cyst is mucinous is accomplished either by gross inspection of the cyst fluid, special stains for mucin such as mucicarmine or alcian blue pH 2.5, documentation of cyst fluid CEA elevation, or molecular analysis documenting *KRAS*, *GNAS*, or *RNF43* mutation (see above). Grading atypia requires cytological analysis of the cells. Detection of mutations known to occur late in progression to malignancy such as *TP53* or deletion of *SMAD4* supports malignancy [17, 18].

2.9.4 Secondarily Cystic Solid Neoplasms

Secondarily cystic neoplasms include solid pseudopapillary neoplasm, neuroendocrine tumor, acinar cell carcinoma, and conventional ductal adenocarcinoma. These cystic neoplasms are complex cysts usually with more solid than cystic components. Rarely do typically solid neoplasms mimic primary cysts of the pancreas, but this does occur. EUS-FNA targeting of the solid component produces cellular aspirates and should provide sufficient tissue for cellblocks, which should be a goal of the FNA to ensure tissue for ancillary testing. The cytomorphological characteristics are identical to those of their solid counterparts and are outlined in Table 2.5. The ancillary studies used to distinguish these neoplasms are outlined in Table 2.6.

2.9.5 Solid Pseudopapillary Neoplasm

Solid pseudopapillary neoplasms (SPNs) demonstrate characteristic cytological findings [37–41]. Smears from this tumor are usually cellular with

Table 2.5 Cytomorphology of secondarily cystic solid masses

Feature	SPN	PanNET	ACC	PDAC
Cellularity	Moderate to high	Variable	Variable	Moderate to high
Architecture	Papillary groups and single cells	Single cells	Single cells	Clusters and single cells
Cells	Epithelioid	Plasmacytoid	Round to polygonal	Glandular
Nuclei	Round to oval	Usually round	Usually round	Pleomorphic
Membrane irregularity	Yes "coffee bean"	No	Usually no	Yes
Nucleoli	Inconspicuous	May be present	Often prominent centrally placed	Variable
Cytoplasm	Scant tags, ill-defined	Moderate and defined; eccentric	Well-defined circumferential	Variable
Cytoplasmic character	Focal cytoplasmic vacuoles, hyaline globules	Dense, non-mucinous Neurosecretory granules	Eosinophilic and granular, zymogen granules	Mucinous
Background	Metachromatic matrix and cyst debris	Cyst debris	Cyst debris	Mucin and cyst debris

Table 2.6 Ancillary studies differentiating secondarily cystic neoplasms

Stain	SPN	PanNET	ACC
Chromogranin	Negative	Positive	Negative
CD56	Positive	Positive	Negative
Synaptophysin	Negative	Positive	Negative
E-cadherin	Membrane negative	Membrane positive	Positive
Beta-catenin	Positive (nuclear)	Positive (membrane and cytoplasmic)	Positive (membrane and cytoplasmic)
CD10	Positive	Positive (10 %)	Negative
Progesterone receptor	Positive	Positive	Negative

SPN solid pseudopapillary neoplasm, *PanNET* pancreatic neuroendocrine tumor, *ACC* acinar cell carcinoma

many dyscohesive single cells as well as branching and papillary cell groups (Fig. 2.10a). Papillary cell clusters show a central fibromyxoid stromal core, which stains a bright magenta on air-dried Romanowsky stain (Fig. 2.10b). The cells from SPN reveal a high nuclear to cytoplasmic ratio, but the nuclei are bland with round to oval shape, even chromatin, and frequent nuclear grooves or indentations, which yields a "coffee bean" appearance (Fig. 2.10c). They do not demonstrate mitotic activity. The cytoplasm of these cells is typically scant and ill-defined and may show large clear cytoplasmic vacuoles or well-defined hyaline globules which are PAS positive (Fig. 2.10d) (both best highlighted on air-dried Romanowsky stain) [41, 42]. The smear background may be clean or filled with hemorrhagic cyst debris, foamy histiocytes, and multinucleated giant cells.

2.9.5.1 Ancillary Studies

These tumors are usually straightforward to diagnosis since most present in the characteristic young female with solid and cystic imaging features or a cellblock demonstrates the classic papillary architecture of the neoplasm (Fig. 2.11a). Some, however, pose significant challenges to diagnosis [39, 43]. The primary differential diagnosis of SPN is with PanNET. Most SPNs show no or weak staining for cytokeratin (AE1/AE3, CAM5.2), which is generally strongly positive in PanNETs and other epithelial-rich tumors in the pancreas. SPN tumor cells also demonstrate nuclear staining for beta-catenin (Fig. 2.11b) in contrast to the cytoplasmic staining of PanNET tumor cells. In addition, staining for E-cadherin, the cell-anchoring protein, shows no staining in SPN, whereas membrane positivity is noted in

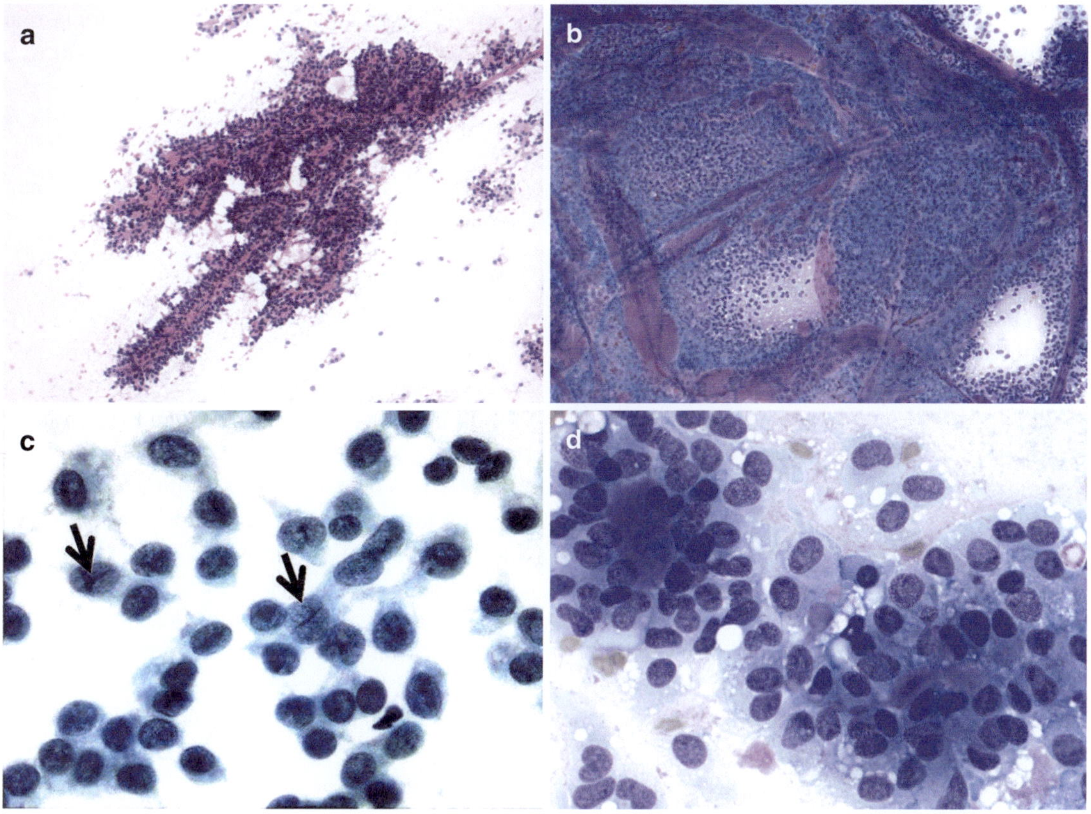

Fig. 2.10 Solid pseudopapillary neoplasm. Smears from SPN are cellular with many dyscohesive single cells and branching, papillary groups (**a**). Papillary cell clusters show bright magenta central fibromyxoid stromal core on Romanowsky stain (**b**). The cells are bland with a high nuclear to cytoplasmic ratio and commonly a "coffee bean" appearance (arrows) (**c**). The typically scant cytoplasm may show large clear cytoplasmic vacuoles or hyaline globules (**d**) (**a**. Hematoxylin and eosin; **b**. Diff-Quik; **c**. Papanicolaou; **d**. Diff-Quik)

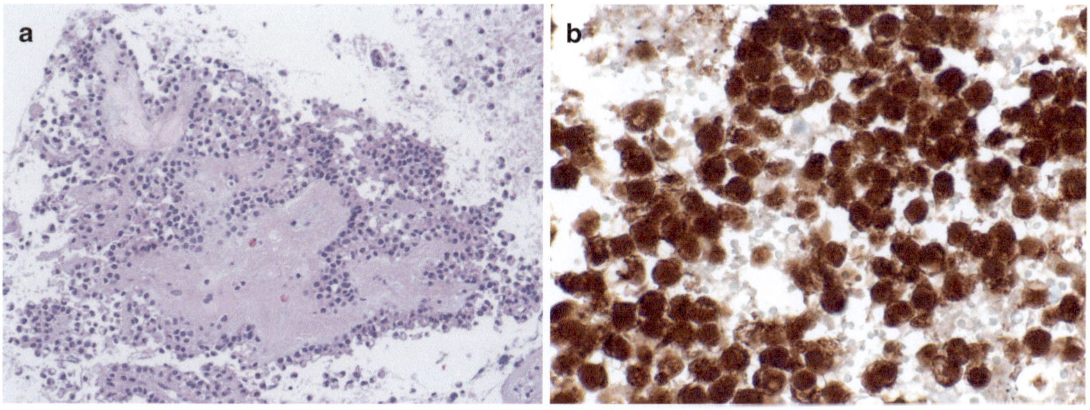

Fig. 2.11 Mxyoid stromal of the papillary cores is diagnostic (**a**). An immunohistochemical stain for beta-catenin shows strong nuclear staining (**b**) (peroxidase-antiperoxidase) (**a.** Cellblock, hematoxlin and eosin; **b.** Solid pseudopapillary neoplasm)

PanNET and other epithelial tumors [44]. SPN is positive for alpha-1 antitrypsin, CD10, CD56, and vimentin. Variable expression is seen with synaptophysin and chromogranin A, endocrine markers which are usually strongly positive in PanNET [45]. The majority of SPNs show a point mutation in exon 3 of the beta-catenin gene, but molecular testing is not needed in most instances since the vast majority of tumors are either morphologically diagnostic or confirmed by immunohistochemistry [44, 46].

2.9.6 Cystic Neuroendocrine Tumors

The cytological features of PanNET are similar whether the aspirate is from a solid tumor or a cystic lesion [12, 47–49]. In contrast to the smears from solid PanNET, which are usually very cellular, aspirates of cystic PanNET can be quite limited. A clue to the diagnosis from EUS-FNA is the presence of thick cyst walls and yellow cyst fluid [12]. Compared to imaging, cytology is the best test for making an accurate diagnosis [12, 50]. The neoplastic cells are usually individual cells with coarse, stippled chromatin and a plasmacytoid appearance caused by the eccentrically located nucleus (Fig. 2.12a). These characteristic features may be diminished in specimens processed by liquid-based means and nucleoli may be prominent (Fig. 2.12b). That being said, the cells are relatively small with a high nuclear to cytoplasmic ratio with coarse chromatin, consistent with the "high-grade" atypia of a high-risk mucinous cyst, so even if the neuroendocrine nature of the cells is not appreciated on cytology, the cells should be recognized as neoplastic and "high-grade" leading to surgical resection.

2.9.6.1 Ancillary Studies

Immunohistochemical stains supporting endocrine differentiation is typically all that is needed to support the diagnosis of PanNET. Synaptophysin is more sensitive than chromogranin and usually provides diffuse strong staining, whereas chromogranin A produces a patchier staining pattern and may not be positive in scant samples (Fig. 2.13). Specific markers for insulin, glucagon, somatostatin, and pancreatic polypeptide are variably positive; gastrin, vasoactive intestinal polypeptide, cholecystokinin, and adrenocorticotropic hormone are generally not necessary unless the patient is syndromic and labeling is requested for clinical correlation. Cystic PanNETs may not provide sufficient cellularity for such testing. Grading of cystic PanNETs is also not necessary for any tumor that will be resected. PanNETs are, by definition, "tumors" that are well differentiated. If the cytology shows a small-cell neuroendocrine carcinoma or large-cell neuroendocrine carcinoma, then that is the diagnosis, not a neuroendocrine "tumor." Accurate grading of PanNET requires evaluation of the most mitotically active area as determined

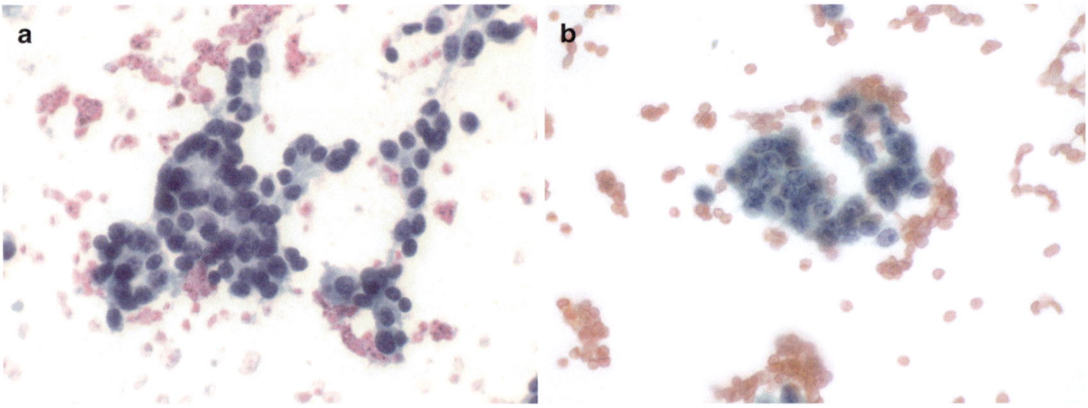

Fig. 2.12 Cystic neuroendocrine tumor. The neoplastic cells are usually individual cells with coarse, stippled chromatin and a plasmacytoid appearance typical of solid tumors (**a**). These characteristic features may be diminished in specimens processed by liquid-based means (**b**) (**a**, **b**. Papanicolaou)

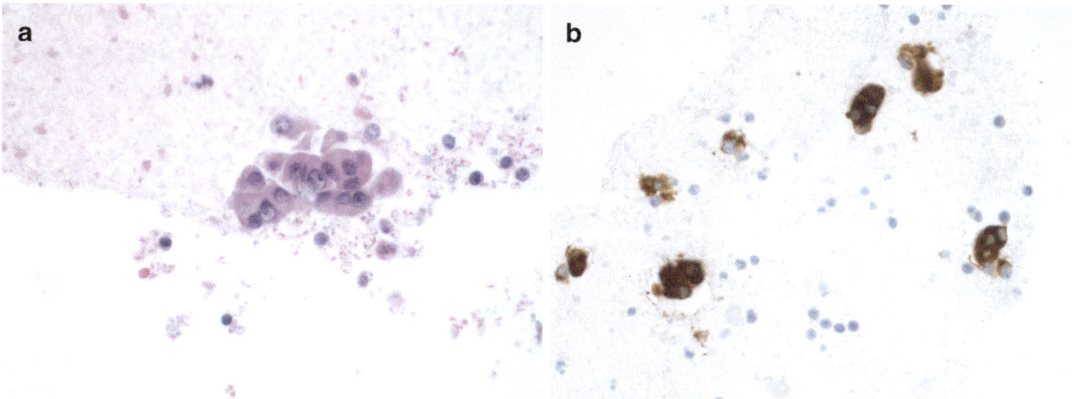

Fig. 2.13 Cystic neuroendocrine tumor. Cellblock preparations (**a**) provide cells for immunohistochemical staining that can confirm the neuroendocrine nature of the cells, such as synaptophysin (**b**) (**a**. Hematoxylin and eosin; **b**. peroxidase-anti-peroxidase)

from complete histological evaluation. That being said, if the tumor is unresectable, then ki-67 proliferation marker may be able to separate a grade 1 or 2 tumor from a grade 3 carcinoma if all or most of the cells show nuclear staining [51].

Cyst fluid analysis shows low CEA and amylase levels with rare exception of an elevated CEA [12, 50].

2.9.7 Cystic Acinar Cell Carcinoma

Cystic acinar cell carcinoma is rare. Cellular clusters of various sizes and single cells may be noted. Cells from the solid counterpart of this tumor may be very bland with a polygonal cell shape, granular cytoplasm, and low nuclear to cytoplasmic ratio, but in a cyst, the cells round up and the characteristic cytoplasmic features are not well appreciated (Fig. 2.14). Tumor cells also demonstrate coarse chromatin and usually prominent nucleoli. Cytoplasm is fragile and frequently stripped from the tumor cells leaving bare tumor nuclei [52, 53].

2.9.7.1 Ancillary Studies

The primary ancillary tests include those that highlight the exocrine nature of the cells: periodic acid-Schiff (PAS)/dPAS histochemical stains and immunohistochemical stains such as trypsin, chymotrypsin, and lipase. Trypsin is the most sensitive maker of acinar origin. Positivity for this marker should be strong and diffuse and all that is necessary to distinguish acinar cell carcinoma from PanNET. High background staining is common, but the labeling of the cells should still stand out. Markers for chymotrypsin and lipase are also usually positive. Epithelial cell markers for keratins Cam5.2 and AE1:3 are positive and so is membranous staining for E-cadherin and beta-catenin. EMA is positive in about 50 % of cases [54].

2.10 Cystic Ductal Adenocarcinoma

Secondarily cystic conventional ductal carcinomas are relatively rare and typically high-grade. Aspirates of these tumors show variably cellular samples, but since the solid component of these tumors is what is targeted on FNA, the cells present are similar to those aspirated from solid tumors. FNA smears generally show cohesive sheets as well as single obviously malignant epithelial cells. Cells in groups and sheets show loss of polarity and cellular and nuclear pleomorphism often giving the appearance of a "drunken honeycomb" (Fig. 2.15). Individual cells have enlarged nuclei that are about 2–3 times the size of the red blood cells. The nuclei demonstrate marked membrane irregularity, coarse chromatin clumping, conspicuous nucleoli, and abnormal mitoses. The cytological diagnosis is straightforward and ancillary studies are not necessary.

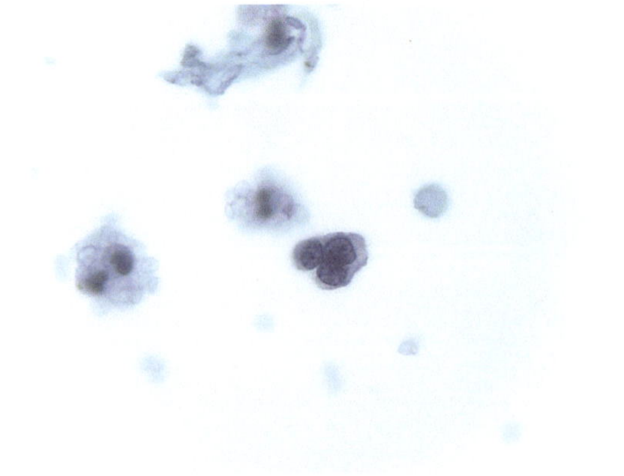

Fig. 2.14 Cystic acinar cell carcinoma. The tumor cells round up in cyst fluid and the polygonal cell shape, granular cytoplasm, and low nuclear to cytoplasmic ratio of the solid tumor counterpart are not well (Papanicolaou)

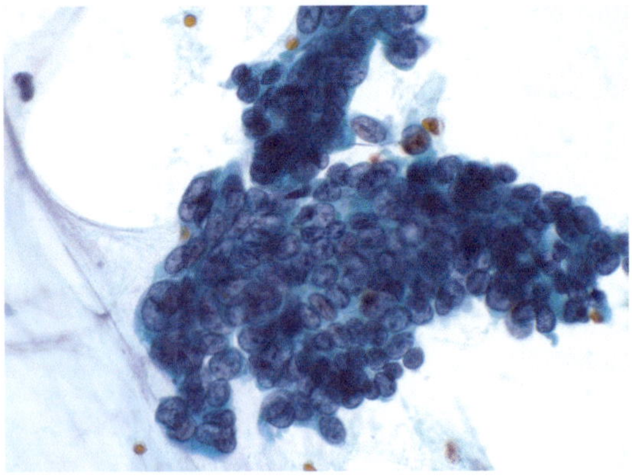

Fig. 2.15 Cystic ductal adenocarcinoma. Cellular groups of cells with nuclear crowding and overlapping of nuclei with irregular nuclear membranes, anisonucleosis of 4:1, and abnormal chromatin pattern meet the criteria for malignancy (adenocarcinoma) (Papanicolaou)

2.11 Summary

The cytopathologist plays a pivotal role in the management of patients with pancreatic lesions. Management options for patients are broad and increasingly conservative. It cannot be overemphasized that the accurate diagnosis of pancreatic cysts depends upon a multimodal team approach that combines the clinical and radiological patient information with the cytological impression and the results of ancillary studies. The gastroenterologist must understand the optimal methods of tissue handling and processing and the pathologist must be familiar with pancreatic histopathology and the nomenclature of pancreatic cytology for accurate diagnosis.

References

1. Pitman MB, Deshpande V. Endoscopic ultrasound-guided fine needle aspiration cytology of the pancreas: a morphological and multimodal approach to the diagnosis of solid and cystic mass lesions. Cytopathology. 2007;18(6):331–47.
2. Pitman MB. Pancreatic cyst fluid triage: a critical component of the preoperative evaluation of pancreatic cysts. Cancer Cytopathol. 2013;121(2):57–60.
3. Hebert-Magee S, et al. The presence of a cytopathologist increases the diagnostic accuracy of endoscopic ultrasound-guided fine needle aspiration cytology for pancreatic adenocarcinoma: a meta-analysis. Cytopathology. 2013;24(3):159–71.
4. da Cunha Santos G, et al. "The petals and thorns" of ROSE (rapid on-site evaluation). Cancer Cytopathol. 2013;121(1):4–8.
5. Collins BT, et al. Rapid on-site evaluation for endoscopic ultrasound-guided fine-needle biopsy of the pancreas decreases the incidence of repeat biopsy procedures. Cancer Cytopathol. 2013;121(9):518–24.
6. Cizginer S, et al. Cyst fluid carcinoembryonic antigen is an accurate diagnostic marker of pancreatic mucinous cysts. Pancreas. 2011;40(7):1024–8.
7. Brugge WR, et al. Diagnosis of pancreatic cystic neoplasms: a report of the cooperative pancreatic cyst study. Gastroenterology. 2004;126(5):1330–6.
8. van der Waaij LA, van Dullemen HM, Porte RJ. Cyst fluid analysis in the differential diagnosis of pancreatic cystic lesions: a pooled analysis. Gastrointest Endosc. 2005;62(3):383–9.
9. Nagula S, et al. Evaluation of cyst fluid CEA analysis in the diagnosis of mucinous cysts of the pancreas. J Gastrointest Surg. 2010;14(12):1997–2003.
10. Kucera S, et al. Cyst fluid carcinoembryonic antigen level is not predictive of invasive cancer in patients with intraductal papillary mucinous neoplasm of the pancreas. JOP. 2012;13(4):409–13.
11. Raval JS, et al. Pancreatic lymphoepithelial cysts express CEA and can contain mucous cells: potential pitfalls in the preoperative diagnosis. Mod Pathol. 2010;23(11):1467–76.
12. Morales-Oyarvide V, et al. Cystic pancreatic neuroendocrine tumors: the value of cytology in preoperative diagnosis. Cancer Cytopathol. 2014;122(6):435–44.
13. Moparty B, Pitman MB, Brugge WR. Pancreatic cyst fluid amylase is not a marker to differentiate IPMN from MCN. Gastrointest Endosc. 2007;65(5):AB303.
14. Shen J, et al. Molecular analysis of pancreatic cyst fluid: a comparative analysis with current practice of diagnosis. Cancer Cytopathol. 2009;117(3):217–27.

15. Nikiforova MN, et al. Integration of KRAS testing in the diagnosis of pancreatic cystic lesions: a clinical experience of 618 pancreatic cysts. Mod Pathol. 2013; 26(11):1478–87.
16. Wu J, et al. Recurrent GNAS mutations define an unexpected pathway for pancreatic cyst development. Sci Transl Med. 2011;3(92):92ra66.
17. Amato E, et al. Targeted next-generation sequencing of cancer genes dissects the molecular profiles of intraductal papillary neoplasms of the pancreas. J Pathol. 2014;233(3):217–27.
18. Layfield LJ, et al. Utilization of ancillary studies in the cytologic diagnosis of biliary and pancreatic lesions: the Papanicolaou Society of Cytopathology guidelines. Cytojournal. 2014;11 Suppl 1:4.
19. van Asselt SJ, et al. Pancreatic cyst development: insights from von Hippel-Lindau disease. Cilia. 2013; 2(1):3.
20. Abraham SC, et al. Solid-pseudopapillary tumors of the pancreas are genetically distinct from pancreatic ductal adenocarcinomas and almost always harbor beta-catenin mutations. Am J Pathol. 2002;160 (4):1361–9.
21. Pitman MB, et al. Grading epithelial atypia in endoscopic ultrasound-guided fine-needle aspiration of intraductal papillary mucinous neoplasms: an international interobserver concordance study. Cancer Cytopathol. 2013;121(12):729–36.
22. Pitman MB, et al. Cytological criteria of high-grade epithelial atypia in the cyst fluid of pancreatic intraductal papillary mucinous neoplasms. Cancer Cytopathol. 2014;122(1):40–7.
23. Pitman MB, et al. Standardized terminology and nomenclature for pancreatobiliary cytology: the Papanicolaou Society of Cytopathology guidelines. Diagn Cytopathol. 2014;42(4):338–50.
24. Belsley NA, et al. Serous cystadenoma of the pancreas: limitations and pitfalls of endoscopic ultrasound-guided fine-needle aspiration biopsy. Cancer. 2008; 114(2):102–10.
25. Lal A, et al. Microcystic adenoma of the pancreas: clinical, radiologic, and cytologic features. Cancer. 2004;102(5):288–94.
26. Collins BT. Serous cystadenoma of the pancreas with endoscopic ultrasound fine needle aspiration biopsy and surgical correlation. Acta Cytol. 2013;57(3):241–51.
27. Yip-Schneider MT, et al. Vascular endothelial growth factor, a novel and highly accurate pancreatic fluid biomarker for serous pancreatic cysts. J Am Coll Surg. 2014;218(4):608–17.
28. Wu R, et al. Analysis of VEGF/PlGF heterodimer level in pancreatic cyst fluid as a biomarker for serous cystadenoma. J Am Soc Cytopathol. 2015;4:79–83.
29. Tanaka M, et al. International consensus guidelines 2012 for the management of IPMN and MCN of the pancreas. Pancreatology. 2012;12(3):183–97.
30. Leung KK, et al. Pancreatic cystic neoplasm: the role of cyst morphology, cyst fluid analysis, and expectant management. Ann Surg Oncol. 2009;16(10): 2818–24.
31. Emerson RE, Randolph ML, Cramer HM. Endoscopic ultrasound-guided fine-needle aspiration cytology diagnosis of intraductal papillary mucinous neoplasm of the pancreas is highly predictive of pancreatic neoplasia. Diagn Cytopathol. 2006;34(7):457–62.
32. Zhai J, Sarkar R, Ylagan L. Pancreatic mucinous lesions: a retrospective analysis with cytohistological correlation. Diagn Cytopathol. 2006;34(11):724–30.
33. Michaels PJ, et al. Intraductal papillary mucinous neoplasm (IPMN) of the pancreas: cytohistologic analysis and correlation with histologic grade. Cancer Cytopathol. 2006;108(3):163–73.
34. Pitman MB, et al. Cytological and cyst fluid analysis of small (< or =3 cm) branch duct intraductal papillary mucinous neoplasms adds value to patient management decisions. Pancreatology. 2008;8(3). 277–84.
35. Genevay M, et al. Cytology adds value to imaging studies for risk assessment of malignancy in pancreatic mucinous cysts. Ann Surg. 2011;254(6):977–83.
36. Sigel CS, et al. Low interobserver agreement in cytology grading of mucinous pancreatic neoplasms. Cancer Cytopathol. 2014;123(1):40–50.
37. Pettinato G, et al. Solid-pseudopapillary tumor of the pancreas: a neoplasm with distinct and highly characteristic cytological features. Diagn Cytopathol. 2002; 27(6):325–34.
38. Pelosi G, et al. Solid and cystic papillary neoplasm of the pancreas: a clinico-cytopathologic and immunocytochemical study of five new cases diagnosed by fine-needle aspiration cytology and a review of the literature. [Review] [106 refs]. Diagn Cytopathol. 1995;13(3):233–46.
39. Bardales RH, et al. Endoscopic ultrasound-guided fine-needle aspiration cytology diagnosis of solid-pseudopapillary tumor of the pancreas: a rare neoplasm of elusive origin but characteristic cytomorphologic features. Am J Clin Pathol. 2004;121(5):654–62.
40. Jhala N, Siegal GP, Jhala D. Large, clear cytoplasmic vacuolation: an under-recognized cytologic clue to distinguish solid pseudopapillary neoplasms of the pancreas from pancreatic endocrine neoplasms on fine-needle aspiration. Cancer. 2008;114(4):249–54.
41. Samad A, et al. Cercariform cells: another cytologic feature distinguishing solid pseudopapillary neoplasms from pancreatic endocrine neoplasms and acinar cell carcinomas in endoscopic ultrasound-guided fine-needle aspirates. Cancer Cytopathol. 2013;121 (6):298–310.
42. Adams AL, Siegal GP, Jhala NC. Solid pseudopapillary tumor of the pancreas: a review of salient clinical and pathologic features. Adv Anat Pathol. 2008;15(1): 39–45.
43. Hooper K, et al. Diagnostic error assessment and associated harm of endoscopic ultrasound-guided fine-needle aspiration of neuroendocrine neoplasms of the pancreas. Cancer Cytopathol. 2013;121(11): 653–60.
44. Burford H, et al. E-cadherin/beta-catenin and CD10: a limited immunohistochemical panel to distinguish

pancreatic endocrine neoplasm from solid pseudopapillary neoplasm of the pancreas on endoscopic ultrasound-guided fine-needle aspirates of the pancreas. Am J Clin Pathol. 2009;132(6):831–9.
45. Liu X, et al. Solid-pseudopapillary neoplasm of the pancreas: three cases with a literature review. Appl Immunohistochem Mol Morphol. 2006;14(4): 445–53.
46. Layfield L, et al. Utilization of ancillary studies in the cytologic diagnosis of biliary and pancreatic lesions: the papanicolaou society of cytology guidelines of pancreatobiliary cytology. Diagn Cytopathol. 2014;42 (4):351–62.
47. Jhala D, et al. Fine needle aspiration biopsy of the islet cell tumor of pancreas: a comparison between computerized axial tomography and endoscopic ultrasound-guided fine needle aspiration biopsy. Ann Diagn Pathol. 2002;6(2):106–12.
48. Levy GH, et al. Cytoplasmic vacuolization: an under-recognized cytomorphologic feature in endocrine tumors of the pancreas. Diagn Cytopathol. 2013;41 (7):623–8.
49. Gu M, et al. Cytological diagnosis of endocrine tumors of the pancreas by endoscopic ultrasound-guided fine-needle aspiration biopsy. Diagn Cytopathol. 2005;32(4):204–10.
50. Yoon WJ, et al. Cystic pancreatic neuroendocrine tumors: endoscopic ultrasound and fine-needle aspiration characteristics. Endoscopy. 2013;45(3):189–94.
51. Weynand B, et al. Pancreatic neuroendocrine tumour grading on endoscopic ultrasound-guided fine needle aspiration: high reproducibility and inter-observer agreement of the Ki-67 labelling index. Cytopathology. 2014;25(6):389–95.
52. Stelow EB, et al. Cytology of pancreatic acinar cell carcinoma. Diagn Cytopathol. 2006;34(5):367–72.
53. Sigel CS, Klimstra DS. Cytomorphologic and immunophenotypical features of acinar cell neoplasms of the pancreas. Cancer Cytopathol. 2013;121(8): 459–70.
54. Hruban RH, Pitman MB, Klimstra DS. Tumors of the pancreas. Atlas of tumor pathology, vol. 4, fascicle 6. Washington, D.C.: American Registry of Pathology; Armed Forces Institutes of Pathology; 2007.

Pathology and Classification of Cystic Tumors of the Pancreas: Epidemiology

3

Elke Tieftrunk, Güralp O. Ceyhan, Ihsan Ekin Demir, and Helmut Friess

3.1 Introduction

Cystic tumors of the pancreas are rare, but attract increasing interest as their prognosis is good and the disease is very often curable. One of the most interesting questions dealing with pancreatic cystic tumors remains, whether they appear more frequently in the last decades or the diagnostic tools improved in such a way that they are more frequently diagnosed and classified. As cystic tumors were diagnosed earlier, their resection rate also increased accordingly, allowing a detailed histopathological classification of the tumors. This led to a more precise pathomorphological description and a better classification of cystic pancreatic tumors. In this book chapter, we will give an overview of epidemiological data for the most common cystic pancreatic tumors.

3.2 Intraductal Papillary Mucinous Neoplasm (IPMN)

The first description of intraductal papillary mucinous neoplasm (IPMN) dates back to the 1980s. Three subtypes can be differentiated: main-duct IPMN, side-branch IPMN, and mixed-type IPMN. Current data show an increasing incidence estimated to be approximately 2.04 per 100,000 person-years (95 % confidence interval: 1.28–2.80) [1]. IPMN is a disease primarily of the elder patient, as the mean age is reported to lie between 65 and 68 years [2, 3]. Noninvasive IPMN patients are on average 6.4 years younger than patients with invasive/malignant IPMN [2]. IPMN is often diagnosed as an incidental finding, when imaging (ultrasound, CT, MRI) is used for other reasons. In a study of 1064 patients with pancreatic cystic lesions from South Korea, 436 patients were diagnosed with IPMN, in which the sex distribution between men and women was comparable [4]. In Europe, Marchegiani et al. showed a slight tendency toward women being more often affected (55 versus 45 %) by main-duct IPMN than men [3]. In a large Californian pancreatic cancer study with 15,296 pancreatic cancer cases, Le et al. verified the good prognosis even of malignant IPMN compared with ductal adenocarcinomas. In general, the prognosis of malignant IPMNs especially in early tumor stage is better than for pancreatic adenocarcinomas. In the Californian register, malignant IPMNs have the best prognosis (5-year overall survival 60–65 %) compared with pancreatic ductal adenocarcinoma (5-year overall survival 2 %) and mucinous tumors (5-year overall survival 5 %) but also in comparison with neuroendocrine pancreatic tumors (5-year overall survival 30 %) [2, 5]. The 5-year overall survival rate for patients with

E. Tieftrunk, MD • G.O. Ceyhan, MD
I.E. Demir, MD • H. Friess, MD (✉)
Department of Surgery, Klinikum rechts der Isar, Technische Universität München, Munich, Germany
e-mail: elke.tieftrunk@tum.de; gueralp.ceyhan@tum.de; ekin.demir@tum.de; helmut.friess@tum.de

M. Del Chiaro et al. (eds.), *Cystic Tumors of the Pancreas*, DOI 10.1007/978-3-319-31882-0_3

resected main-duct IPMN is 69 %; the disease-specific survival rate within this patient cohort even reaches 83 %. The recurrence rate for resected main-duct IPMNs at 10 years is stated with 25 % [3]. Salvia et al. split up the survival rates in benign and malignant IPMN in a cohort of 137 resected IPMN patients and could show that the survival rate for benign/noninvasive IPMN (adenoma, borderline tumors, carcinoma in situ) was 100 % even after 10 years. In contrast, for invasive IPMN, the 5- and 10-year survival rate was 60 % and 50 %, respectively [2].

3.2.1 Risk Factors for the Development of IPMN

There are a number of investigations analyzing risk factors for the development of IPMN in the medical literature; however, no relevant risk factors have been clearly defined so far. Most studies revealed that there is no correlation between common risk factors and IPMN. In a retrospective analysis of 446 patients, 47 % of the patients were smokers. There was a correlation to smoking history, as smokers were more likely to have a main-duct IPMN in comparison with nonsmokers. However, there was no correlation between smoking and grade of dysplasia or invasiveness of IPMN [6].

Pancreatitis was proposed as a risk factor for the development of IPMN. However, a current retrospective single-center study could not prove that patients with pancreatitis have a higher risk of malignancy or invasiveness. Interestingly, patients with IPMN without a history of pancreatitis, who revealed elevated or decreased serum pancreatic enzyme levels, had a higher malignancy rate [7]. There is also a positive correlation between elevated serum pancreatic enzyme levels and the invasiveness of IPMN [7].

Although obesity is a common and known risk factor for pancreatic adenocarcinoma, there was no correlation between the BMI and invasive main-duct IPMN in a single-center prospective study [8]. However, patients with malignant branch-duct IPMN were found to be more often obese [8].

In addition to pancreatitis, a multicenter case-control study identified a positive family history of pancreatic adenocarcinoma and previous history of diabetes as independent risk factors for the development of IPMN [9]. Patients with diabetes that required insulin supplementation revealed an even higher risk of developing IPMN [9].

3.2.2 Extrapancreatic Malignancies in Patients with IPMN

In recent years, there have been several reports on the potential association of IPMN with extrapancreatic malignancies (EPM; Table 3.1). These reports mainly represent retrospective case series in which a large spectrum of EPM have been considered to be in potential association with IPMN. Although the genetic basis of this clinical suspicion has not yet been subject to study, several studies provided retrospective data with a positive relationship. Concerning the association of EPM incidence in patients with pancreatic ductal adenocarcinoma (PDAC) versus IPMN, Riall et al. reported high rates of EPM both in patients with PDAC and with IPMN. In their cohort of 19,647 patients, 95 % had sporadic PDAC and 5 % invasive IPMN. In the cohort of patients with sporadic PDAC, 10.3 % had one or more EPM, and this rate was comparable to 10.1 % within the invasive IPMN cases. The most common sites of EPM were the breast (19.9 %), prostate (16.6 %), urinary system (11.1 %), and lung (9.8 %). Interestingly, among the 2017 patients with EPM, 86 % were primarily detected before and 14 % after the diagnosis of PDAC. The authors concluded that although the rates of EPM were not different between sporadic and IPMN-associated PDAC cases, the relatively high prevalence of EPM in the IPMN cohort may warrant surveillance of these patients for common malignancies [13]. However, there are also several studies reporting higher EPM rates in IPMN patients. Sugiyama et al. reported a high rate of 36 % EPM in a small cohort of 42 IPMN patients. The malignancies included mainly colorectal and gastric carcinomas. The comparison of EPM between PDAC and IPMN patients revealed a

Table 3.1 Incidence and subtypes of extrapancreatic neoplasms (EPN) among patients with IPMN

Investigator	Year	Cohorts	No. of patients	EPN prevalence	EPN subtypes
Sugiyama et al. [10]	1999	IPMN	42	48 %	21 % colorectal adenoma 12 % colorectal carcinoma 10 % gastric carcinoma
Kamisawa et al. [11]	2005	IPMN	79	35 % (28)	Gastric cancer (12 cases) Colonic cancer (7 cases) Esophageal cancer (4 cases) Pulmonary cancer (4 cases)
Choi et al. [12]	2006	IPMN	61	39 % (24) EPN 30 % (18) EPM	33 % gastric adenocarcinoma 17 % colorectal adenocarcinoma
Riall et al. [13]	2007	PDAC	18,655	10.3 % (1917)	19.9 % colorectal 20 % breast 16.7 % prostate 11 % urinary tract
		IPMN	992	10.1 % (100)	25 % colorectal 18 % breast 14 % prostate 13 % urinary tract
Baumgaertner et al. [14]	2008	IPMN Matched controls	178 356	16.8 % 8.4 %	30 % breast 10 % prostate 10 % colorectal
Reid-Lombardo et al. [15]	2010	IPMN	471	52 % ($p=0.002$) PDAC: 36 % General population: 43 %	24 % colon polyps 7 % nonmelanoma skin cancer 5 % prostate 4 % colorectal cancer
Marchegiani et al. [16]	2014	IPMN	1340	21.6 %	12 % kidney 19 % colorectal 9 % prostate 21 % breast

Overview of epidemiological data on cystic pancreatic neoplasms
IPMN intraductal papillary mucinous neoplasm, *PDAC* pancreatic ductal adenocarcinoma, *EPM* extrapancreatic malignancy

higher frequency of EPM among IPMN (11 %) versus PDAC patients (7 %) [10]. In a similar study with 79 patients, 35 % of the IPMN patients were diagnosed with EPM, particularly gastric, colonic, esophageal, pulmonary, and independent PDAC [11]. Similar rates of EPM reaching up to 30 % within their cohort of 61 IPMN patients were reported. Also in this study, the main sites of EPM were identified as colonic and gastric carcinomas. Different from other studies, the authors also compared the frequency of EPM in IPMN patients to those with mucinous cystic neoplasm (MCN) and found clearly higher rates of EPM in IPMN patients than in MCN patients (39 % versus 8 %) [12].

In a population study on the incidence of IPMN, Reid-Lombardo et al. identified nonmelanoma skin (7 %), breast (5 %), prostate (5 %), and colorectal (4 %) cancer and carcinoid (1 %) tumors among a small cohort of 28 IPMN patients [17].

A common denominator for these initial studies on the high rates of EPM in IPMN patients is the lack of demographically matched control cohorts. This deficiency was addressed in the case-control study by Baumgaertner et al.

comparing 178 patients with resected IPMN (hyperplasia/low-grade dysplasia, $n=91$; high-grade dysplasia/invasive cancer, $n=87$) versus 356 age- and gender-matched controls. In this analysis, EPM were diagnosed in 16.8 % patients with IPMN (70 % of which preceding IPMN) and in 8.4 % controls ($p=0.003$). The most frequent sites of cancer in patients with IPMN and controls were the breast (30 % in each group), prostate (10 % and 13 %, respectively), and colon/rectum (10 and 6 %, respectively). The authors found no correlation between the prevalence of EPM and the grade of dysplasia in IPMN. Importantly, the vast majority of IPMNs were detected after the diagnosis of EPM. For this reason, the authors postulated that this observation, despite the high rate of co-occurrence of EPM with IPMN, does not sufficiently justify extension of the current screening recommendations [14].

An important study that addressed the incidence of extrapancreatic neoplasia (EPN) after the diagnosis of mainly branch-duct IPMN was performed by Marchegiani and colleges who followed up 816 patients with IPMN over a period of 4 years for EPN incidence. Fifty patients developed an EPN after a median surveillance time of 46 months after study enrollment. When compared to the sex-specific, age-standardized general cancer incidence estimates on the incidence of cancer in Italy, Sweden, Germany, and Turkey (obtained from national registries), the incidence of any EPN was not greater in patients with or without IPMN (IR of 1.48 in men and of 1.39 in women). Furthermore, the 5- and 10-year cumulative incidence rates for EPN in patients with IPMN were 7.9 and 16.6 % in men and 3.4 and 23.1 % in women. Based on this observational study, the authors concluded that an additional screening procedure beyond the routine screening for the general population is not necessary for IPMN patients [16].

In a large case-control study from the Mayo Clinic, Reid-Lombardo et al. compared the prevalence of EPN, i.e., including benign lesions such as colonic polyps and Barrett's neoplasia, among IPMN patients with two gender- and age-matched control groups consisting of patients with a diagnosis of ductal pancreatic adenocarcinoma (group 1) and a general referral population (group 2). The proportion of IPMN patients having any EPN diagnosed before or coincident to the index date was 52 % compared with 36 % in group 1 ($p<0.001$) and 43 % in group 2 ($p=0.002$). The most common neoplasms were colonic polyps; Barrett's neoplasia; nonmelanoma skin, breast, prostate, and colorectal cancers; and carcinoid neoplasms. As colonic polyps were the most common neoplasia of IPMN patients, the authors recommended that screening colonoscopy should be considered in all patients with IPMN [15]. However, screening colonoscopy is recommended in men and women above the age of 50 years, independent on an additive IPMN diagnosis.

Comparison of the characteristics of all these studies reveals that these observed differences regarding the incidence of EPM/EPN in IPMN patients may be due to the geographic (Asian versus European cohorts) differences or due to the lack of appropriate control groups. Even in the study by Marchegiani et al., a major question that arises is whether the IPMN population was subject to the same intensity and frequency of cancer screening as the general population of the four countries. Ideally, to effectively address this question, a prospective case-control study with subjects exposed to the same extent of post-diagnosis screening examinations is necessary. Nonetheless, current evidence does not convincingly justify intensified screening of IPMN patients for EPM/EPN.

3.3 Mucinous Cystic Neoplasm (MCN)

MCNs are a mucin-producing, septated, cystic epithelial neoplasia of the pancreas that are characterized by the presence of an ovarian stroma [18]. One distinguishing feature between IPMN and MCN is that MCNs do not have a communication with the ductal system. They are usually solitary; their size at diagnosis ranges between 0.3 and 35 cm with a thick fibrotic or calcifying wall [19, 20]. Epidemiologically, a characteristic feature of

MCN is the absolute predominance in women (with a reported female to male ratio around 20:1) [21], and the mean age at diagnosis is around 40–50 years (age range 14–95 years) [19]. The overwhelming majority of MCNs are located in the pancreatic body and tail. MCNs are less common than IPMN (e.g., 91 % of cystic tumors representing IPMN versus only 9 % MCN [22]).

Based on the degree of dysplasia, MCNs are classified as mucinous cystic adenoma (mild dysplasia), borderline MCN (moderate dysplasia), and MCN carcinoma in situ (severe dysplasia). Histopathological signs of malignancy include a thickened wall with peripheral calcification, papillary proliferations with mural nodules, size greater than 5 cm, vascular involvement, and hypervascular pattern. The incidence of invasive MCN was reported to be 6–36 %, reaching up to 51 % when carcinoma in situ is included [19].

In case of no histological evidence for invasive carcinoma within the MCN at time of resection, the overall survival probability is not altered. But once invasive cancer is detected, the 5-year survival rate drops down to 20–60 %. In case of anaplastic pancreatic carcinoma in conjunction with MCN, the 3-year survival rate is reported to be lower than 3 % [19].

There seems to be no geographic difference with regard to the epidemiological characteristics of MCN. In a multicentric, retrospective series of 156 MCN patients, Yamao et al. detected 129 mucinous cystic adenomas (82.7 %) and 21 noninvasive (13.4 %) and 6 invasive carcinomas (3.9 %). Nearly all patients were exclusively women (98.1 %) with a mean age of 48.1 years. In accordance with other studies, in 155 patients (99.4 %), the tumors were located in the pancreatic body/tail region with a mean size of 65.3 mm. Interestingly, the authors detected communication between the cyst and the pancreatic duct in 18.1 %. The 3-, 5-, and 10-year survival rates were 97.6 %, 96.6 %, and 96.6 %, respectively. In this analysis, cyst diameter and presence of mural nodules were predictive parameters of malignant MCN [23].

In a study on invasive MCN, Kargozaran et al. compared the characteristics of 185 patients with MCN and 641 patients with invasive IPMN in the *S*urveillance, *E*pidemiology, and *E*nd *R*esults (*SEER*) database (1996–2006). MCNs were more common (73 %) among women when compared to invasive IPMN (48 %, $p<0.0001$) [24]. Importantly, lymph node metastases were more frequently encountered in IPMN than in MCN (46 % versus 24 %, $p<0.0001$). In the early stages of disease (i.e., stage I), overall survival after resection was better for patients with MCN compared to IPMN patients ($p=0.0005$). No difference could be detected in stages equal or greater to stage II or in the comparison of node-positive MCN with node-positive IPMN ($p=0.2263$). Therefore, in the presence of node-negative early-stage disease, invasive MCN seems to be associated with a better outcome than invasive node-negative IPMN [24].

In a comprehensive comparative analysis of all mucin-producing cystic tumors (MPT) of the pancreas (i.e., IPMN, main duct IPMN/MD-IPMN, branch-duct IPMN/BD-IPMN), Crippa et al. analyzed the clinicopathological features of 557 cases. They found that 168 patients (30 %) had MCN, 159 (28.5 %) BD-IPMN, 149 (27 %) combined IPMN, and 81 (14.5 %) MD-IPMN. In the demographic analysis, patients with MCN were almost exclusively women (95 %), and the few male patients were significantly older (63 versus 44 years). In contrast, only 44 % of patients with main- or mixed-duct IPMN and 57 % of those with branch-duct IPMN were women. In accordance with previous studies, MCNs were single lesions located in the distal pancreas (95 %), with malignant transformation in 11 % of the cases. In comparison, IPMNs are commonly located in the proximal pancreas, and invasive cancer is present in 11 %, 42 %, and 48 % of BD-, combined, and MD-IPMNs, respectively. Importantly, the mean age of patients with invasive MCN was greater than for those with noninvasive tumors (55 versus 44 years) [21]. The 5-year disease-specific survival rate is 100 % for patients with noninvasive tumors and 58 % for invasive MCN when compared to 56 %, 51 %, and 64 % for BD-IPMN, MD-IPMN, and combined-type IPMN, respectively. Based on these characteristics, MCN possesses distinct epidemiological and morphological characteristics. Regarding prognosis, MCN seem to largely resemble other cystic tumors of the pancreas [25].

3.4 Serous Cystic Neoplasm (SCN)

Serous cystic neoplasm (SCN) of the pancreas is commonly termed serous cystadenoma and represents over 32 % of all cystic tumors of the pancreas in a study with 522 patients performed by Le Borgne et al. [26]. SCN are mostly encountered among women (75 % of cases) with a median age of ca. 60 years [27], and the cysts do not seem to have a predominant site of origin in the pancreas. They can be either microcystic or macrocystic, although the microcystic form was reported to be more frequent (app. 93 % microcystic versus 7 % macrocystic). Therefore, a classical SCN is microcystic, has a central area of calcification, and contains a watery, nonviscous fluid. Macroscopically, macrocystic SCN can appear to be very similar to pseudocysts or MCNs. SCN is widely believed to have no malignant potential, although a small number of cases of malignant serous cystadenocarcinomas have been reported.

In one of the first retrospective studies on macrocystic SCN, Chatelain et al. detected seven women and one man with macrocystic SCN, with a mean age of 48 years and a mean cyst size of 3 cm (range: 1.5–5 cm) [28]. In a simultaneous comparison of SCN with other cystic pancreatic neoplasms among 851 cases from the Massachusetts General Hospital, SCN comprised 16 % of all cystic pancreatic neoplasms when compared to IPMN (38 %), MCN (23 %), and cystic neuroendocrine neoplasm (7 %) [29]. In a similar retrospective study from Korea, Yoon et al. compared the clinicopathological data and risk factors for malignancy among 1064 patients with pancreatic cystic tumors from 30 university hospitals throughout Korea. In this large cohort, 436 (41 %) were IPMN, 268 (25 %) MCN, 195 (18 %) solid pseudopapillary neoplasm (SPN), and 162 (15 %) SCN [4]. Therefore, SCN account for 15–32 % of all cystic tumors in the pancreas.

3.5 Solid Pseudopapillary Neoplasm (SPN)

SPNs are the rarest cystic tumors of the pancreas. They occur in approximately 0.5 % of all solid pancreatic lessons [30]. Mainly women are affected, and the female frequency in the literature lies between 85 and 100 % [31, 32]. A literature review of 1014 patients with SPN showed male patients only in 137 cases (13.5 %). The incidence of SPN metastasis in males is twofold, and the death rate is three times higher than in females [33]. The mean age of affected patients is 27 years, and 5-year survival rates are over 96 % [34, 35]. However, SPNs do have malignant potential, since about 23 % of the resected SPNs are pseudopapillary carcinomas [36]. Most SPNs are diagnosed due to symptoms, such as abdominal pain (58–100 %) [32, 33, 37].

In a case series from the Johns Hopkins University with 37 patients, 33 (89 %) were women, and the median age at diagnosis was 32 years. The most common symptom was abdominal pain (81 %). Median tumor size was 4.5 cm. From these 37 patients, 34 patients underwent an R0 resection (92 %), 1 had an R1 resection, and 1 had an R2 resection, and after resection 34 (94 %) patients remained alive after a remarkable observation period of 38 years [20]. In a retrospective review of 181 pancreatic resections, Cecka et al. reported on SPN in four cases (2.2 %). All these patients were females, and the average age was 34 years [38]. In a pediatric patient series, Speer et al. identified SPN in 11 cases, 64 % of them were female with a median age of 14 years (9–17 years). The median tumor diameter in these children was 5 cm (3.5–12 cm) [39]. In another larger series presented by Guo et al., 23 of 24 patients were women, and the mean age of all patients was 31 years [40]. Overall, SPN has an excellent prognosis. In the case study by Brecht et al., the authors analyzed the SEER database regarding the prognosis of malignant pancreatic tumors in children. Here, even malignant SPNs demonstrated an excellent 5-year survival rate of 88 % [41]. In a similar series by Kim et al., 86.9 % of the resected 114 patients were female, and the median age was 36 years (range: 11–75). Twenty-six patients (22.8 %) revealed solid pseudopapillary carcinoma (SPC). Although the authors detected no difference in symptoms (e.g., abdominal/back pain, indigestion, jaundice) among the SPN versus SPC patients, recurrence was only detected among the SPC cases (4 out of 26 patients). Patients with recurrence were young patients (mean age of patients with no recurrence, 36, versus of those with recurrence, 23 years) with metastasis at first operation, invasion of an adjacent organ, and a large tumor (≥13 cm) [36]. Therefore, overall, SPN can be regarded as a tumor of young female patients that has a low malignancy potential and an excellent prognosis after curative resection.

3.6 Pseudocysts

Pancreatic pseudocysts are encapsulated fluid collections without an epithelial lining (hence "pseudo"cyst) and can be attributed to the leakage of the pancreatic fluid after damage to the ductal system during acute or chronic pancreatitis or subsequent to abdominal trauma. Acute pancreatitis was reported to be associated with pseudocysts in 5.1–16 %, and reaches up to 20–40 % in patients with chronic pancreatitis [42–44]. They are usually single cystic lesions without septations or solid parts. The cyst fluid contains high levels of amylase and has low viscosity. The main indications for intervention are associated symptoms (such as pain or feeling of abdominal pressure). In their prospective multicenter study, Cui et al. detected a pseudocyst incidence of 6.3 % and a higher frequency of pseudocysts with decreasing age, with alcoholic acute pancreatitis and higher serum LDH levels. Furthermore, they detected that approximately 84 % of the pseudocysts disappeared or decreased in size during follow-up [30].

3.7 Summary

In summary, from an epidemiological point of view, cystic tumors of the pancreas still represent a rare entity. However, there are a number of indicators for the increasing incidence or at least increased detection rate of these lesions in routine imaging diagnostics. The key epidemiological features of pancreatic cystic tumors and a comprehensive list of the studies that provided epidemiological data on pancreatic cystic tumors were presented on Tables 3.2 and 3.3. Knowledge on the typical epidemiological characteristics of cystic pancreatic tumors, particularly related to the peak of their occurrence, gender, and age predilection, may help in the diagnosis and clinical decision-making process. Since cystic pancreatic tumors are relatively recently recognized disorders, there is ongoing need for large-scale major epidemiological studies. Such studies necessitate a close collaboration between gastroenterologists, radiologists, and surgeons within large centers and establishment of "cystic pancreatic tumor referral centers" which may enable the performance of such studies.

Table 3.2 Overview of the most common cystic pancreatic tumors

Investigator	Year	Entity	No. of patients	Male/female ratio	Age (years)	Prognosis
Sugiyama et al. [10]	1999	IPMN	42	27/15	65 (median)	100 % 5-Y survival: for noninvasive 82 % IPM-C
Le Borgne et al. [26]	1999	Cystadenoma SCA MCA MCAC	398 144 150 78	14/86 13/87 39/61	58.5 50.5 65	100 % mean follow-up 38 months 91 % mean follow-up 47 months 63 % 5-Y survival
Chatelain et al. [28]	2002	Macrocystic SCA	8	1/7	48	100 % mean follow-up 6 years
Salvia et al. [2]	2004	MD-IPMN	140 (83 malignant, 57 benign)	40/43 for malignant 31/26 for benign	60.9 for benign (median) 67.3 for malignant (median)	5-Y survival: Benign/CIS: 100 % Malignant: 60 %
Kamisawa et al. [11]	2005	IPMN	79	8/20	71.9 for pts with EPN 66.8 for pts w/o EPN	N/A
Tseng et al. [27]	2005	SCA	106	26/80	61.5	N/A
Choi et al. [12]	2006	IPMN	61	38/23	62.4 (mean)	100 % for noninvasive 68.2 % for IPM-C
Murakami et al. [22]	2006	IPMN	70	53/17	66 (mean)	84 %
		MCN	7	0/7	55 (mean)	100 %
Riall et al. [13]	2007	IPM-C	992	48/52	67.7 (mean)	5 % 5-Y survival for IPM-C
Yoon et al. [4]	2008	IPMN	436	167/115 for benign 88/47 for malignant	60.7 for benign 62.4 for malignant (both mean age)	N/A
		MCN	268	34/157 for benign 21/56 malignant	50.2 for benign 56.3 for malignant (both mean age)	N/A
		SPN	195	28/167	34.9 (mean)	N/A
		SCN	162	52/110	52.6 (mean)	N/A
Reid-Lombardo et al. [17]	2008	IPMN	28	N/A	73.1 (median)	59.6 % 5-Y survival rate
Baumgaertner et al. [14]	2008	IPMN Matched controls	178 356	86/92 86/92	66 (median) 66 (median)	N/A

Crippa et al. [21]	2008	MCN	163	8/155	40–50 (mean)	Noninvasive MCN: 100 % 5-Y survival Invasive MCN (mucinous cystadenocarcinoma: 57 % 5-Y survival)
Reddy et al. [20]	2009	SPN	37	4/33	32	36 disease-free after median follow-up 4.8 years
Khan et al. [1]	2010	IPMN	28	N/A	73.1 (median)	N/A
Testini et al. [19]	2010	Invasive MCN		1/20		Noninvasive MCN: 100 % OS Invasive MCN (mucinous cystadenocarcinoma: 20–60 % 5-Y survival)
Crippa et al. [25]	2010	MD-IPMN	81	45/36	67 (median)	65 % 5-Y survival
		BD-IPMN	159	68/91	66 (median)	91 % 5-Y survival
		Mixed-type IPMN	149			77 % 5-Y survival
		MCN	168	8/160		94 % 5-Y survival
Lin et al. [33]	2010	SPN SPN literature review	11 1014	2/9 137/877		100 % mean follow-up 63.4 months (women) 0 % (men)
Yamao et al. [23]	2011	MCN (with ovarian-type stroma)	156			96.6 % 5-Y survival
Kargozaran et al. [24]	2011	MCN (invasive)	185			46.7 % 5-Y survival
		IPMN (invasive)	41			26 % 5-Y survival
Yu et al. [35]	2011	SPT	11	0/11	29.5	100 % median follow-up 45.5 months
Kim et al. [36]	2011	SPT	114	16/98	36	100 % follow-up 11–177 months
Guo et al. [40]	2011	SPN	24	1/23	31	91 % median follow-up 68 months (curative resection) 50 % (R1 resection, 2 patients)
Brecht et al. [41]	2011	Malignant pancreatic tumors Carcinoma Endocrine tumors SPN Pancreatoblastoma	228 100 85 8 11	N/A	<30	37 % OS (males), 55 % OS (females) 33 % 58 % 88 % 66 %

(continued)

Table 3.2 (continued)

Investigator	Year	Entity	No. of patients	Male/female ratio	Median age	Prognosis
Valsangkar et al. [29]	2012	Cystic pancreatic neoplasm IPMN MCN SCA Cystic NET SPT	851 326 (38 %) 199 (23 %) 137 (16 %) 63 (7 %) 29 (3.4 %)	323/519 43–50/50–57 % 16/84 % 32/68 % 53/47 % 12/88 %	60 68–69 51 61 54 33	87 % 5-Y survival 83–88 % 5-Y survival N/A 97 % N/A 100 %
Speer et al. [39]	2012	SPT	11		14	100 % median follow-up 1.4 years
Sturm et al. [8]	2013	IPMN	274	137/137	67 (mean)	9 % recurrence rate of all types of IPMN
Capurso et al. [9]	2013	IPMN	390	166/224	65 (mean)	N/A
Gil et al. [18]	2013	MCN with ovarian stroma	47	4/43	48.5 (mean)	Invasive type: 2 out of 5 had recurrence Noninvasive type: no recurrence
		MCN without ovarian stroma	23	4/19	53.8 (mean)	Invasive type: 4 out of 5 had recurrence Noninvasive type: no recurrence
Park et al. [31]	2013	SPT	60	5/55	34	100 % mean follow-up of 143 months
Cai et al. [32]	2013	SPN	33	3/30	29.2	97 % follow-up 4–118 months
Rezaee et al. [6]	2014	IPMN	446	51/49 55/45	68.0 (mean)	Median OS 70 months (smokers) 88 months (nonsmokers)
Roch et al. [7]	2014	IPMN	364	100/103	67 (mean)	N/A
Marchegiani et al. [16]	2014	IPMN	1340	545/795	67 (median)	N/A
Estrella et al. [34]	2014	SPN	64	10/54	33	10-Y disease-specific survival rate 96 %
Manuballa et al. [37]	2014	SPN	6	0/6	27.7	
Cecka et al. [38]	2014	Pancreatic tumor SPT	181 4	0/4	34	N/A

IPMN intraductal papillary mucinous neoplasm, *CIS* carcinoma in situ, *MCN* mucinous cystic neoplasm, *SCN* serous cystic neoplasm, *SPN* solid pseudopapillary neoplasm, *SPT* solid papillary tumor, *Y* year, *OS* overall survival

Table 3.3 Overview of epidemiological data on cystic pancreatic neoplasms

Entity	Gender ratio (male/female)	Age	Localization	Prognosis (5-Y survival rate)
IPMN	1:1.2	65–68	Head	56 % for invasive branch-duct IPMN 51 % for invasive main-duct IPMN
MCN	1:20	40–50	Body-tail	100 % for noninvasive, 58 % for invasive MCN
SCN	1:7	60		
Microcystic	1:9	71	Body-tail (75 %)	Near 100 %
Macrocystic	1:1	48–63	Head (60 %)	Near 100 %
SPN	1:9	27	No preference	>90 %
Pseudocysts	3:1	No preference	No preference	

IPMN intraductal papillary mucinous neoplasm, *IPM-C* intraductal papillary mucinous carcinoma, *SCN* serous cystic neoplasm, *MCN* mucinous cystic neoplasm, *SPN* solid pseudopapillary neoplasm, *MD* main duct, *BD* branch duct, *Y* year, *N/A* not available

References

1. Khan S, Sclabas G, Reid-Lombardo KM. Population-based epidemiology, risk factors and screening of intraductal papillary mucinous neoplasm patients. World J Gastrointest Surg. 2010;2(10):314–8.
2. Salvia R, et al. Main-duct intraductal papillary mucinous neoplasms of the pancreas: clinical predictors of malignancy and long-term survival following resection. Ann Surg. 2004;239(5):678–85; discussion 685–7.
3. Marchegiani G, et al. IPMN involving the main pancreatic duct: biology, epidemiology, and long-term outcomes following resection. Ann Surg. 2015;261:976–83.
4. Yoon WJ, et al. Cystic neoplasms of the exocrine pancreas: an update of a nationwide survey in Korea. Pancreas. 2008;37(3):254–8.
5. Le H, et al. A population-based, descriptive analysis of malignant intraductal papillary mucinous neoplasms of the pancreas. Cancer Epidemiol Biomarkers Prev. 2008;17(10):2737–41.
6. Rezaee N, et al. Smoking is not associated with severe dysplasia or invasive carcinoma in resected intraductal papillary mucinous neoplasms. J Gastrointest Surg. 2015;19:656–65.
7. Roch AM, et al. Abnormal serum pancreatic enzymes, but not pancreatitis, are associated with an increased risk of malignancy in patients with intraductal papillary mucinous neoplasms. Surgery. 2014;156(4):923–9.
8. Sturm EC, et al. Obesity increases malignant risk in patients with branch-duct intraductal papillary mucinous neoplasm. Surgery. 2013;154(4):803–8; discussion 808–9.
9. Capurso G, et al. Risk factors for intraductal papillary mucinous neoplasm (IPMN) of the pancreas: a multicentre case-control study. Am J Gastroenterol. 2013;108(6):1003–9.
10. Sugiyama M, Atomi Y. Extrapancreatic neoplasms occur with unusual frequency in patients with intraductal papillary mucinous tumors of the pancreas. Am J Gastroenterol. 1999;94(2):470–3.
11. Kamisawa T, et al. Malignancies associated with intraductal papillary mucinous neoplasm of the pancreas. World J Gastroenterol. 2005;11(36):5688–90.
12. Choi MG, et al. High incidence of extrapancreatic neoplasms in patients with intraductal papillary mucinous neoplasms. Arch Surg. 2006;141(1):51–6; discussion 56.
13. Riall TS, et al. Incidence of additional primary cancers in patients with invasive intraductal papillary mucinous neoplasms and sporadic pancreatic adenocarcinomas. J Am Coll Surg. 2007;204(5):803–13; discussion 813–4.
14. Baumgaertner I, et al. Prevalence of extrapancreatic cancers in patients with histologically proven intraductal papillary mucinous neoplasms of the pancreas: a case-control study. Am J Gastroenterol. 2008;103(11):2878–82.
15. Reid-Lombardo KM, et al. Frequency of extrapancreatic neoplasms in intraductal papillary mucinous neoplasm of the pancreas: implications for management. Ann Surg. 2010;251(1):64–9.
16. Marchegiani G, et al. Association between pancreatic IPMNs and extra-pancreatic malignancies. Clin Gastroenterol Hepatol. 2015;13(6):1162–9.
17. Reid-Lombardo KM, et al. Incidence, prevalence, and management of intraductal papillary mucinous neoplasm in Olmsted County, Minnesota, 1984–2005: a population study. Pancreas. 2008;37(2):139–44.
18. Gil E, et al. Mucinous cystic neoplasms of the pancreas with ovarian stroma. ANZ J Surg. 2013;83(12):985–90.

19. Testini M, et al. Management of mucinous cystic neoplasms of the pancreas. World J Gastroenterol. 2010;16(45):5682–92.
20. Reddy S, et al. Surgical management of solid-pseudopapillary neoplasms of the pancreas (Franz or Hamoudi tumors): a large single-institutional series. J Am Coll Surg. 2009;208(5):950–7; discussion 957–9.
21. Crippa S, et al. Mucinous cystic neoplasm of the pancreas is not an aggressive entity: lessons from 163 resected patients. Ann Surg. 2008;247(4):571–9.
22. Murakami Y, et al. Intraductal papillary-mucinous neoplasms and mucinous cystic neoplasms of the pancreas differentiated by ovarian-type stroma. Surgery. 2006;140(3):448–53.
23. Yamao K, et al. Clinicopathological features and prognosis of mucinous cystic neoplasm with ovarian-type stroma: a multi-institutional study of the Japan pancreas society. Pancreas. 2011;40(1):67–71.
24. Kargozaran H, et al. Invasive IPMN and MCN: same organ, different outcomes? Ann Surg Oncol. 2011;18(2):345–51.
25. Crippa S, et al. Mucin-producing neoplasms of the pancreas: an analysis of distinguishing clinical and epidemiologic characteristics. Clin Gastroenterol Hepatol. 2010;8(2):213–9.
26. Le Borgne J, de Calan L, Partensky C. Cystadenomas and cystadenocarcinomas of the pancreas: a multiinstitutional retrospective study of 398 cases. French Surgical Association. Ann Surg. 1999;230(2):152–61.
27. Tseng JF, et al. Serous cystadenoma of the pancreas: tumor growth rates and recommendations for treatment. Ann Surg. 2005;242(3):413–9; discussion 419–21.
28. Chatelain D, et al. Macrocystic form of serous pancreatic cystadenoma. Am J Gastroenterol. 2002;97(10):2566–71.
29. Valsangkar NP, et al. 851 resected cystic tumors of the pancreas: a 33-year experience at the Massachusetts General Hospital. Surgery. 2012;152(3 Suppl 1):S4–12.
30. Cui ML, et al. Incidence, risk factors and clinical course of pancreatic fluid collections in acute pancreatitis. Dig Dis Sci. 2014;59(5):1055–62.
31. Park JK, et al. Natural history and malignant risk factors of solid pseudopapillary tumors of the pancreas. Postgrad Med. 2013;125(2):92–9.
32. Cai H, et al. Solid-pseudopapillary neoplasms of the pancreas: clinical and pathological features of 33 cases. Surg Today. 2013;43(2):148–54.
33. Lin MY, Stabile BE. Solid pseudopapillary neoplasm of the pancreas: a rare and atypically aggressive disease among male patients. Am Surg. 2010;76(10):1075–8.
34. Estrella JS, et al. Solid pseudopapillary neoplasm of the pancreas: clinicopathologic and survival analyses of 64 cases from a single institution. Am J Surg Pathol. 2014;38(2):147–57.
35. Yu PF, et al. Solid pseudopapillary tumor of the pancreas: a review of 553 cases in Chinese literature. World J Gastroenterol. 2010;16(10):1209–14.
36. Kim CW, et al. Solid pseudopapillary tumor of the pancreas: can malignancy be predicted? Surgery. 2011;149(5):625–34.
37. Manuballa V, Amin M, Cappell MS. Clinical presentation and comparison of surgical outcome for segmental resection vs. Whipple's procedure for solid pseudopapillary tumor: report of six new cases & literature review of 321 cases. Pancreatology. 2014;14(1):71–80.
38. Cecka F, et al. Solid pseudopapillary tumour of the pancreas: diagnosis, treatment, and prognosis. Acta Chir Belg. 2014;114(1):58–62.
39. Speer AL, et al. Solid pseudopapillary tumor of the pancreas: a single-institution 20-year series of pediatric patients. J Pediatr Surg. 2012;47(6):1217–22.
40. Guo N, et al. Diagnosis and surgical treatment of solid pseudopapillary neoplasm of the pancreas: analysis of 24 cases. Can J Surg. 2011;54(6):368–74.
41. Brecht IB, et al. Malignant pancreatic tumors in children and young adults: evaluation of 228 patients identified through the Surveillance, Epidemiology, and End Result (SEER) database. Klin Padiatr. 2011;223(6):341–5.
42. Barthet M, et al. Management of cysts and pseudocysts complicating chronic pancreatitis. A retrospective study of 143 patients. Gastroenterol Clin Biol. 1993;17(4):270–6.
43. Ammann RW, et al. Course and outcome of chronic pancreatitis. Longitudinal study of a mixed medical-surgical series of 245 patients. Gastroenterology. 1984;86(5 Pt 1):820–8.
44. Elliott DW. Pancreatic pseudocysts. Surg Clin North Am. 1975;55(2):339–62.

4 Multidetector Computed Tomography in the Evaluation of Cystic Tumors of the Pancreas

Siva P. Raman and Elliot K. Fishman

4.1 Introduction

Over the course of the last two decades, dramatic improvements in the spatial and temporal resolution of multidetector computed tomography (MDCT), as well as the routine utilization of multiplanar reformations and three-dimensional reconstruction tools, have had a significant impact on our ability to evaluate a variety of pancreatic diseases with increasing accuracy and sophistication. Nowhere is this more evident than in the assessment of pancreatic cystic neoplasms, which are increasingly being identified incidentally as a result of improvements in the spatial resolution of both MDCT and magnetic resonance imaging (MRI). Given that roughly 1 % of all hospitalized patients in the United States and 25 % of all cadavers are found to harbor pancreatic cysts, it is not surprising that pancreatic cysts are frequently being identified on studies being performed for completely unrelated reasons and this has consequently created a vital role for imaging in the diagnosis and risk stratification of these cystic lesions [1].

While it is undoubtedly true that there are some lesions (particularly when small) for which MDCT cannot provide a specific diagnosis, many cystic pancreatic neoplasms do have imaging features that may allow a radiologist either to provide a specific and accurate diagnosis or, alternatively, to narrow the differential diagnosis to a few salient entities. Moreover, imaging now serves as the primary tool to risk stratify cysts and determine which lesions can be safely managed conservatively with serial follow-up imaging examinations and which lesions need to be more aggressively managed with either endoscopic ultrasound or surgical resection [2].

This chapter will provide a brief overview of the standard MDCT imaging techniques and protocols utilized in the evaluation of pancreatic cysts, followed by a detailed description of the imaging features of a number of common pancreatic cystic neoplasms, including intraductal papillary mucinous neoplasms (IPMN), serous cystadenomas, mucinous cystic neoplasms, cystic neuroendocrine tumors, solid pseudopapillary neoplasms, and lymphoepithelial cysts.

4.2 Imaging Technique

Whenever a disorder of the pancreas is suspected (either based on clinical symptomatology or the result of a prior imaging study), the imaging acquisition should be specifically tailored for a focused evaluation of the pancreas. These patients are typically not given positive oral contrast agents, as dense contrast pooling in the stomach or duodenum can result in beam hardening and

S.P. Raman, MD (✉) • E.K. Fishman, MD
Department of Radiology, Johns Hopkins University, JHOC 3251, 601N. Caroline Street, Baltimore, MD 21287, USA
e-mail: srsraman3@gmail.com; efishman@jhmi.edu

M. Del Chiaro et al. (eds.), *Cystic Tumors of the Pancreas*, DOI 10.1007/978-3-319-31882-0_4

streak artifacts that can obscure subtle lesions in the adjacent pancreas and, moreover, interfere with standard 3-D post-processing techniques. Rather, patients are typically given roughly 1500 cc of water immediately prior to the scan in order to distend the stomach and duodenum and consequently improve our ability to differentiate primary pancreatic pathology from a duodenal or gastric lesion. The administration of intravenous contrast is absolutely vital in the evaluation of pancreatic cysts, as many lesions cannot even be visualized without intravenous contrast (especially when small), while the internal architecture and morphology of larger cysts cannot be adequately assessed without intravenous contrast. Typically, 100–120 cc of nonionic intravenous contrast is administered in a rapid bolus (3–5 cc/s) in order to maximize enhancement. It is now routinely accepted that the evaluation of pancreatic lesions requires a dual-phase acquisition, with arterial phase images typically acquired at roughly 30–40 s after the injection of intravenous contrast, while venous phase images are acquired roughly 60–70 s after contrast injection. As we will discuss later, each of these two phases has their own strengths in terms of lesion assessment, and different lesions might be more readily evaluated on one of the two phases.

On most modern scanners, images are acquired with extremely thin collimation, usually with a slice thickness of only 0.625–0.75 mm, with these source images being then reconstructed into 3–5 mm axial sections for routine review. Moreover, the source images are used to create coronal and sagittal reformations directly at the scanner soon after image acquisition, as well as to create 3-D reconstructions at an independent workstation using dedicated software packages. In addition, at our institution, we also routinely create "coned-down," magnified reconstructions centered on the pancreas itself, which we have found very helpful in the identification of tiny lesions.

3-D reconstruction has now proven to be an extremely valuable adjunct technique for the evaluation of pancreatic cystic lesions, in many cases providing insight into cysts that may not be appreciable on the routine axial image review. While a variety of 3-D techniques have been developed, the two most commonly utilized include (1) maximum intensity projection (MIP) imaging and (2) volume rendering (VR). MIP images highlight the highest-attenuation voxels in a dataset and project these voxels into a three-dimensional display. MIP images are very helpful for evaluating the vasculature and illustrating the vascularity associated with lesions, including feeding vessels. Moreover, subtle peripheral hyperenhancement (as seen with serous cystadenomas and cystic neuroendocrine tumors) may be increased in conspicuity with MIP technique, as will subtle sites of hypervascular mural nodularity. Volume rendering is a much more mathematically and computationally intensive process that entails assigning a specific color and transparency to different voxels based on their attenuation values and then presenting this data as an interactive 3-D display. We have found this technique to be very helpful for lesion identification, assessing the internal architecture of pancreatic cystic lesions and demonstrating the relationship of a cystic lesion to the adjacent pancreatic duct.

Overall, given these advancements, multiple studies in the literature have shown MDCT to be very accurate in the characterization of pancreatic cystic lesions, with accuracy rates not dissimilar to MRI. Several studies have shown accuracy rates ranging from 56 to 85 %, with accuracies as high as 79 % for differentiating benign and malignant lesions and as high as 85 % for distinguishing mucinous and non-mucinous lesions [1–4].

4.3 Serous Cystadenoma

Serous cystadenomas are benign pancreatic tumors composed of glycogen-rich cuboidal epithelium arising from acinar cells that account for roughly 20 % of all pancreatic cystic neoplasms [5]. 80 % of lesions are found in women and are mostly diagnosed in patients over the age of 60, therefore leading these tumors to be classically described as "grandmother" tumors. These lesions are almost always benign (with only a few isolated reports describing extraordinarily rare malignant or locally aggressive variants), and in most cases, lesions (particularly when small) typically demonstrate very indolent growth rates and are unlikely to cause symptoms due to mass effect. It is important, however, to note that larger lesions can sometimes grow quite rapidly, particularly when they reach a threshold of roughly 4 cm in size (growing as fast as 2 cm/year), sometimes necessitating surgical resection to avoid symptoms due to mass effect or local growth [6, 7]. Given that these lesions can grow slowly over several years before reaching clinical attention, serous cystadenomas are not infrequently quite large at presentation, since smaller lesions may not cause symptoms and thus not reach clinical attention. Given their typically indolent growth pattern, serous cystadenomas are frequently diagnosed incidentally on imaging (~50 % of cases) [8]. The vast majority of cases are sporadic, although serous cystadenomas are found with increasing frequency in patients with von Hippel-Lindau syndrome (VHL), with VHL patients frequently demonstrating multiple lesions [6].

Serous cystadenomas typically demonstrate three common morphologic patterns (Figs. 4.1, 4.2, and 4.3) which can be seen on MDCT: (1) microcystic pattern, (2) macrocystic or oligocystic pattern, and (3) solid pattern. The microcystic pattern (i.e., microcystic serous cystadenoma) is the appearance most classically associated with serous cystadenomas and is the most likely to allow a specific imaging diagnosis. Microcystic serous cystadenomas typically demonstrate a "honeycomb" or "sponge" pattern with innumerable (classically > 6 cysts) tiny (<2 cm) cysts comprising a larger cystic mass (Figs. 4.2 and 4.3). Innumerable avidly enhancing septations are often seen within the mass, and a central stellate enhancing scar (seen in roughly 30 %) with calcification may be present. If multiphase imaging is performed, the septations and periphery of the mass show avid enhancement on the arterial phase images, while the central scar may demonstrate delayed enhancement [9]. While this pattern allows a specific diagnosis (which may allow the lesion to be followed conservatively without the need for further tests or surgical resection), it is unfortunately seen in less than ¼ of all cases [5].

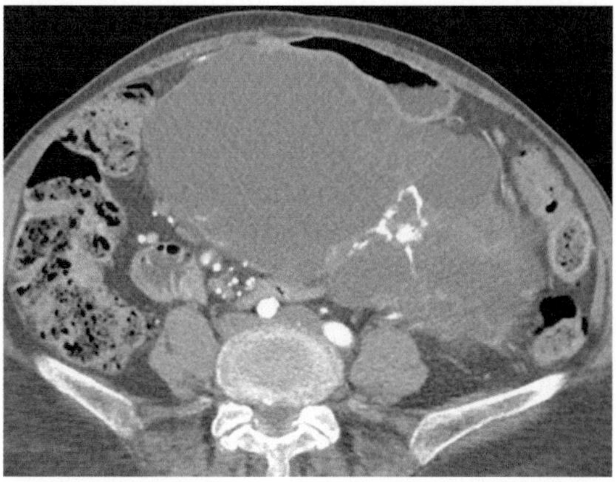

Fig. 4.1 Axial CECT demonstrates a large macrocystic mass with multiple internal septations and large central dystrophic calcifications. This mass was found to be a serous cystadenoma at surgical resection

The macrocystic variant comprises roughly 15–25 % of all cases and presents as a unilocular or oligocystic lesion that may be indistinguishable from other common cystic tumors (such as an IPMN or MCN). This morphologic subtype does not usually demonstrate either a central scar or calcification. While several studies have attempted to delineate imaging features that might demarcate these macrocystic serous cystadenomas from other cystic lesions using such imaging features as cyst location, wall thickness, wall enhancement, and external lobulation, the prospective diagnosis of this type of lesion remains very difficult [10, 11]. Finally, the "solid" variant can be the most confusing and difficult to diagnose prospectively, as these lesions can present as a solid hypervascular mass that avidly enhances on the arterial phase and appears virtually indistinguishable from a pancreatic neuroendocrine tumor. These lesions are thought to result from the avidly vascularized septa of the cystadenoma predominating over the internal cystic component, thus causing the septations to appear as confluent hyperenhancing solid tissue. While these lesions can demonstrate a central scar with calcification, this is quite rare and inadequately specific to allow a confident diagnosis [6, 12].

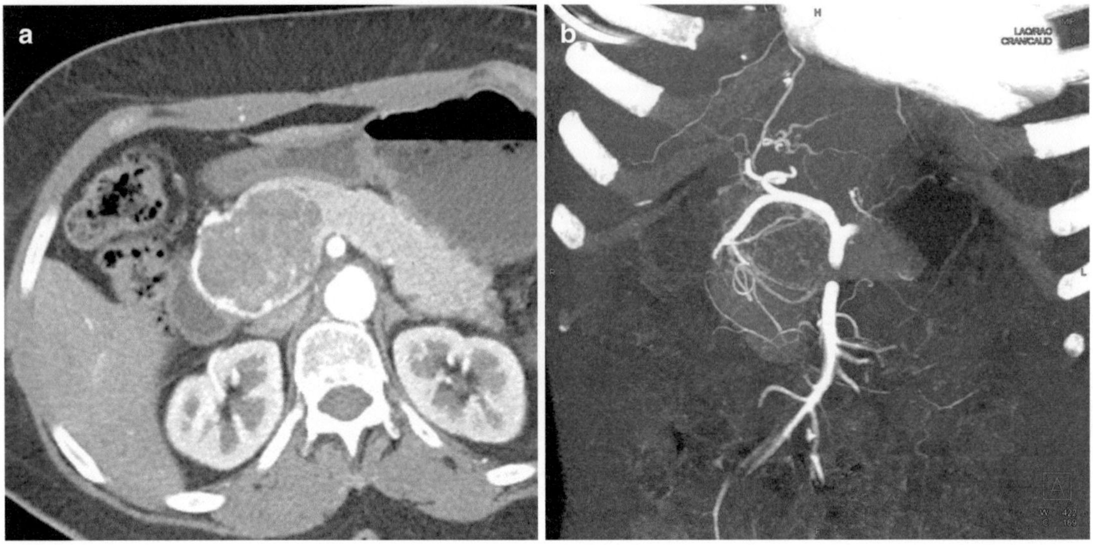

Fig. 4.2 (**a**, **b**) Axial and coronal (with MIP reconstruction) contrast-enhanced CT images demonstrate the classic appearance of a microcystic serous cystadenoma. Notice the prominent peripheral hypervascularity with arteries draped around the margins of the pancreatic head mass

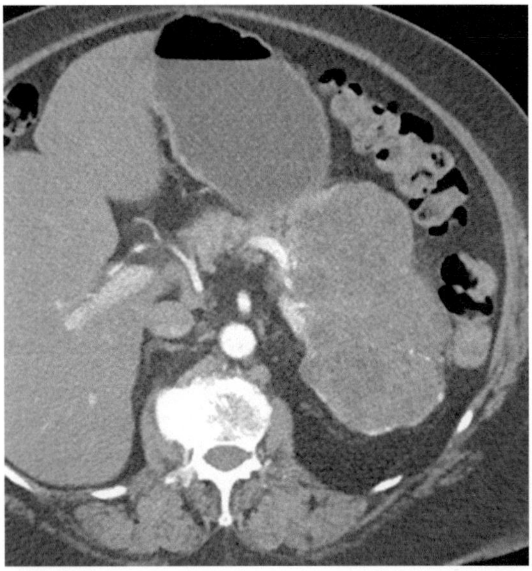

Fig. 4.3 Axial contrast-enhanced CT demonstrates the classic "sponge" appearance of a serous cystadenoma. Notice the lobulated contour of the mass, classic for this entity

Regardless of their morphologic subtype, serous cystadenomas classically demonstrate a "lobulated" contour that can be an important imaging feature in arriving at the correct diagnosis and is not commonly seen with other lesion categories (Fig. 4.3) [5]. These tumors do not communicate with the pancreatic duct and, except in usual cases (or if the mass is very large with significant mass effect), do not obstruct either the pancreatic duct or common bile duct [13]. Arterial phase imaging can be very important, as these are fundamentally hypervascular lesions: Not only can the internal septations of the lesion avidly enhance, but serous cystadenomas characteristically demonstrate prominent peripheral vascularity and rim enhancement, and large feeding vessels (often arising from the gastroduodenal artery or pancreaticoduodenal arcade) may be seen draped around the margins of the cyst on the arterial phase images (often most evident using 3-D reconstructions) (Fig. 4.2) [5]. Calcifications within the lesion are very common and can be peripheral, central, or along septations. Location within the pancreas is generally not a helpful feature: While these lesions are classically thought to be primarily found in the pancreatic head, they can be found in virtually any location within the pancreas, and some recent studies have suggested that serous cystadenomas may be relatively equally distributed throughout the pancreatic head, body, and tail. While serous cystadenomas are one of the few pancreatic cystic neoplasms that can undergo internal hemorrhage, this can be difficult to appreciate on MDCT and is typically easier to perceive on MRI (high signal on pre-contrast T2-weighted images).

In most cases, arriving at a specific diagnosis on imaging may be difficult when lesions are small (particularly when <1 cm). A specific diagnosis is more likely, however, with larger lesions, and lesions with the classic "microcystic" pattern that can be confidently diagnosed do not require any further imaging studies for specific diagnosis. Unfortunately, differentiating the "solid" variant from neuroendocrine tumors can be virtually impossible, and such lesions are almost always diagnosed only after the lesion is surgically resected. Serous cystadenomas are one of the few lesions where MRI does offer a clear advantage over MDCT in providing a specific diagnosis: The internal architecture of these lesions, even when not readily apparent on MDCT, is often very easily delineated on T2-weighted images, which can nicely demonstrate the presence of internal septations and "microcystic" morphology within a T2 hyperintense, cystic mass. When confronted with a lesion on MDCT that is indeterminate, but suspicious for serous cystadenoma, MRI is clearly the test of choice.

In general, imaging has a very important role to play in the management of these lesions, as small serous cystadenomas which can be confidently diagnosed on imaging can generally be conservatively managed with serial imaging follow-up. Lesions that are confidently felt to represent serous cystadenomas are usually only resected when large (>4 cm) or when they cause symptoms [7].

4.4 Mucinous Cystic Neoplasm

Mucinous cystic neoplasms (MCN) are rare (~2.5 % of all exocrine pancreatic tumors) premalignant or frankly malignant pancreatic cystic neoplasms that are virtually always diagnosed in women (with roughly 99.7 % of cases seen in women). These lesions are virtually never found in men, and in those few reports of MCN in males, they tend to present at significantly older ages [14]. Patient age can be helpful in formulating a diagnosis, as MCN occur in a slightly younger age group than serous cystadenomas, with a mean age of roughly 50 years [6]. Given their age and gender predilection, these tumors are frequently referred to as the "mother" tumor. Unfortunately, even though the majority (~72 %) of MCN are benign mucinous cystadenomas, even "benign" MCN harbor the potential for malignancy (with rates of malignancy between 6 and 36 %), and consequently, all MCN should be surgically resected [3, 6]. The key differentiating feature in the pathologic diagnosis of these lesions is the presence of ovarian stroma lining the cyst wall, a feature not seen with any other pancreatic cystic neoplasms [14].

MCN classically present as a unilocular or multilocular encapsulated cystic lesion in the pancreatic body or tail (Figs. 4.4, 4.5, and 4.6) [15]. Lesions tend to be quite large, with an average size of 6–11 cm [14]. Unlike other cystic lesions, where the location of the cyst can be of limited value in formulating a differential diag-

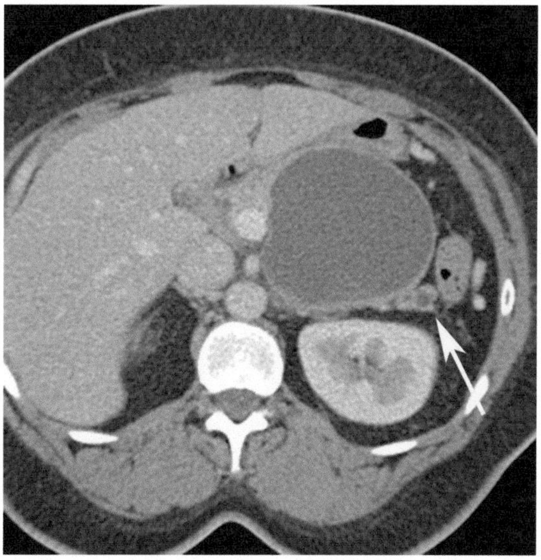

Fig. 4.4 Axial contrast-enhanced CT demonstrates a large cystic mass with a well-defined wall in the pancreatic tail. Note that the pancreatic tail upstream from the mass is atrophic (*arrow*), a sign highly suspicious for malignancy. This was found to be a malignant MCN at surgery

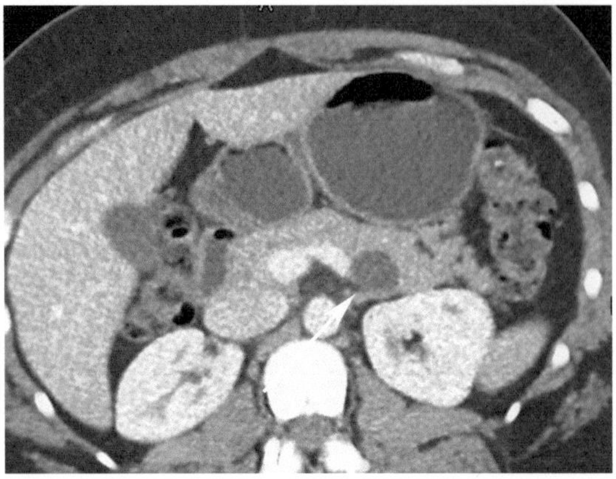

Fig. 4.5 Axial contrast-enhanced CT demonstrates a well-defined cystic lesion (*arrow*) in the pancreatic tail of a middle-aged female. There is no complexity associated with the cyst, and this was found to be a benign MCN at resection

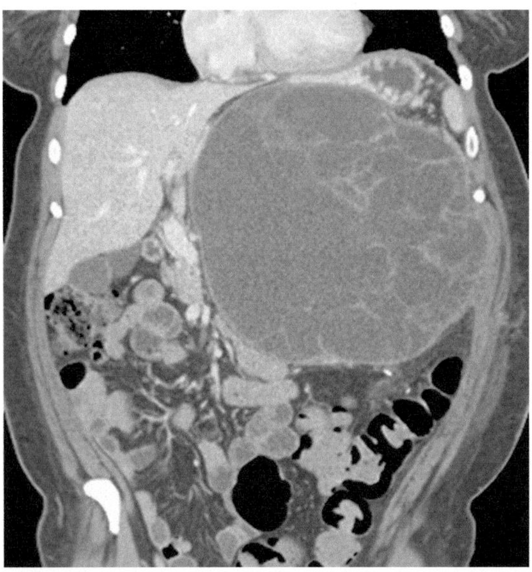

Fig. 4.6 Coronal contrast-enhanced CT demonstrates a classic malignant MCN of the pancreatic tail with extensive internal septations and complexity

nosis, cyst location is vitally important in MCN evaluation, as any cyst in the pancreatic tail should be raised as a concern for a MCN. Unlike serous cystadenomas, which demonstrate a "microcystic" morphology, MCN are macrocystic tumors, appearing as a solitary unilocular cyst or as a cyst with a few (<6) dominant cystic locules (each measuring > 2 cm). The appearance of these lesions can further vary depending on the presence of invasive malignancy or atypia, as malignant MCN do not infrequently demonstrate thick walls, mural nodularity, and irregular septations. Lesions can demonstrate thin or thick calcifications (~15 % of cases) either at the lesion periphery or within septations. Unlike the other major category of pancreatic mucinous neoplasms (i.e., IPMN), MCN do not communicate with the pancreatic duct, and the presence of apparent communication with the pancreatic duct should discourage the diagnosis of a MCN [6].

In addition to diagnosis, MDCT can be a very valuable tool in risk stratifying MCN, and several features can be strongly suggestive of malignancy, including wall thickening, peripheral mural nodularity, thick or irregular septations, calcifications, obstruction of either the pancreatic or common bile ducts, pancreatic parenchymal atrophy upstream from the lesion, or large size (usually > 4 cm) [16]. In some cases, the diagnosis of a malignant MCN is easily made in the presence of a discrete soft tissue mass associated with the cyst that can be locally aggressive and involve the adjacent spleen, stomach, left adrenal gland, or vasculature. Alternatively, "benign" MCN do not infrequently present as a simple unilocular cyst with an imperceptible wall, no internal complexity, and no evidence of pancreatic or biliary ductal obstruction. We have found in our practice that 3-D reconstruction methods can be very valuable in assessing for subtle signs of malignant transformation, as subtle peripheral wall thickening and mural nodularity that might be difficult to perceive on the source axial images are readily visible on the volume-rendered reconstructions.

4.5 Intraductal Papillary Mucinous Neoplasm

Intraductal papillary mucinous neoplasms (IPMN) are mucin-producing neoplasms arising from the ductal epithelium either in the main pancreatic duct or the pancreatic duct side branches. IPMN can range from being benign to frankly malignant, with lesions divided by the World

Health Organization into IPMN with low-grade dysplasia, intermediate-grade dysplasia, high-grade dysplasia, or frank invasive carcinoma. These tumors are classically divided into three major categories: (1) *side-branch IPMN*, which are lesions primarily centered in the pancreatic duct side branch and which carry a variable risk of malignancy depending on the individual features of the cyst (high-grade dysplasia in 25 % and invasive malignancy in 17 %); (2) *main-duct IPMN*, which are lesions centered in the main pancreatic duct and which carry a very high risk of malignancy (close to 60 %); and (3) *mixed-type IPMN*, which share features of both side-branch and main-duct IPMN and which harbor a risk of malignancy comparable to main-duct IPMN [17]. Demographic features are generally less helpful in the diagnosis, given that IPMN are so frequently seen incidentally in all patient groups, although IPMN do tend to be more often seen in elderly patients with a male predominance (70 %) and are accordingly sometimes referred to as "grandfather" tumors. As mentioned in the introduction of this chapter, one of the major dilemmas in abdominal radiology is our increasing incidental identification of pancreatic cysts on CT and MRI examinations performed for completely unrelated indications, and it is undoubtedly true that a very large percentage of these incidental, asymptomatic cysts are side-branch IPMN. The management of IPMN has been a matter of great debate, although it should be noted that the 2012 International Association of Pancreatology international consensus guidelines for the management of mucinous neoplasms places a great deal of emphasis on imaging findings for risk stratification of cysts, including lesion size and morphologic features [18].

Side-branch IPMN (Fig. 4.7) typically present as a well-defined cystic lesion that communicates with the pancreatic duct. While MRI with MRCP has traditionally been thought to be superior for demonstrating duct communication, MDCT images with thin collimation, multiplanar reformations, and 3-D imaging can be reasonably comparable in demonstrating a connection between a cyst and the pancreatic duct. IPMN can have variable morphology, and although many

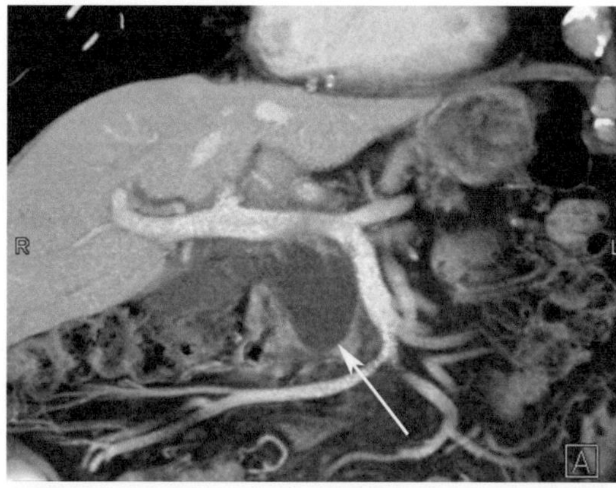

Fig. 4.7 Coronal volume-rendered contrast-enhanced CT demonstrates a large cystic lesion (*arrow*) in the pancreatic head which was shown to communicate with the main pancreatic duct (not shown), compatible with a side-branch IPMN

lesions may appear unilocular, it is not uncommon to see lesions with more complex morphologies, including lesions that appear tubular or as "grapelike" clusters of interconnecting cysts. While side-branch IPMN can appear anywhere in the pancreas, there is a predisposition for the pancreatic head and uncinate process. Unlike the other lesions in this discussion, which inevitably are solitary lesions, IPMN are frequently multiple, and the presence of multiple pancreatic cysts in the same patient should strongly suggest the presence of multiple side-branch IPMN [6]. At least one study has suggested that patients with multiple IPMN may be at higher risk of developing invasive carcinoma [19].

Main-duct IPMN (Figs. 4.8 and 4.9), on the other hand, do not present as a discrete cystic mass, but rather, present as a markedly dilated, tortuous pancreatic duct (usually > 1 cm in size). These lesions can result in either dilatation of the entire duct or just a segment, and it is not uncommon to see "bulging" of the dilated duct into the ampulla, an imaging correlated to the mucin-filled ampulla visible to the endoscopist during an ERCP. Polyploid enhancing nodules may sometimes be visible within the duct itself and are very strong clues to the presence of malignancy, while calcifications (which are often amorphous in morphology) may be seen within

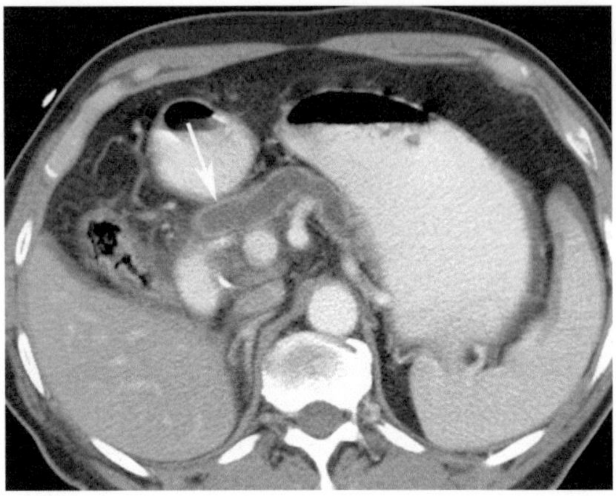

Fig. 4.8 Axial contrast-enhanced CT demonstrates a diffusely dilated main pancreatic duct (*arrow*), compatible with a main-duct IPMN

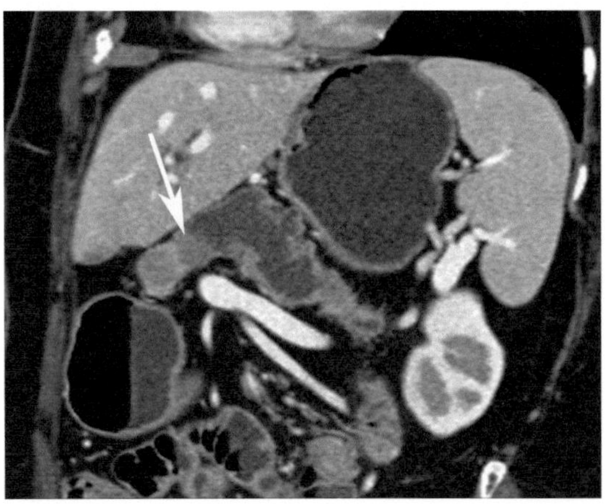

Fig. 4.9 Curved planar reformation from a contrast-enhanced CT demonstrates a markedly dilated main pancreatic duct with intraductal enhancing solid soft tissue (*arrow*), compatible with a malignant main-duct IPMN

the dilated duct as well. In most cases, the pancreas overlying the dilated duct is either frankly atrophic or demonstrates fatty infiltration, but this may not always be present. While a dilated pancreatic duct may represent a main-duct IPMN, it should be recognized that there is significant imaging overlap with findings of both chronic pancreatitis and a small occult mass (such as adenocarcinoma) obstructing the pancreatic duct and ancillary imaging features must be sought out to differentiate these three possibilities. In some cases, endoscopic ultrasound may be necessary to confidently distinguish a main-duct IPMN from chronic pancreatitis or an occult obstructing adenocarcinoma.

As mentioned previously, the 2012 International Association of Pancreatology guidelines for mucinous cyst management place a great deal of stress on imaging features for risk stratification of cysts, and several features are thought to be strongly suspicious for malignancy, including dilatation of the main pancreatic duct (especially ≥ 1 cm), biliary obstruction, enhancing mural nodularity, wall thickening, abrupt change in main pancreatic duct caliber, distal pancreatic atrophy, or large cyst size (typically greater than 3 cm) [18]. It should be noted that IPMN may demonstrate other forms of internal complexity, but there is little data to suggest that such features as thin septations or calcifications provide any degree of increased risk for malignancy.

4.6 Solid Pseudopapillary Neoplasm

Solid pseudopapillary neoplasms (SPEN), also known *Hamoudi* tumors or *Franz* tumors, are rare pancreatic neoplasms which are almost always seen in young women (usually under 35 years of age), with only a small minority of cases diagnosed in men (~12 %). As a result of this age and gender predisposition, these tumors are frequently referred to as "daughter" tumors. Although less certain, some studies have suggested a slightly higher incidence in patients of African or Asian ethnicities [6, 20, 21]. While these lesions are classified as low-grade malignancies, they have an excellent prognosis after surgical resection, with fewer than 10 % of patients demonstrating distant metastases (usually to the liver) or locoregional lymphadenopathy and reported 5-year survival rates as high as 94–97 % [22]. In fact, given the relative indolence of these lesions, it is not surprising that these tumors are increasingly being identified incidentally on imaging, with over 40 % of all cases found in patients undergoing imaging for unrelated reasons. However, despite these incidentally discovered masses, most patients do present with nonspecific symptoms of abdominal pain or discomfort [22].

While the diagnosis of these lesions is largely contingent on patient demographics (especially age and gender), there are several relatively consistent imaging features: SPEN classically present as a well-circumscribed, encapsulated mass that can occur anywhere in the pancreas and which is often relatively large at presentation (average>5 cm) (Figs. 4.10 and 4.11). Lesions can vary in their internal attenuation from appearing mostly cystic to mostly solid, but even apparently "solid" components demonstrate minimal enhancement and may represent intratumoral hemorrhage rather than true enhancing solid tissue. In some cases, the presence of gross intratumoral or peritumoral hemorrhage may be present and is very strongly suggestive of SPEN, although blood within the lesion is often easier to perceive on MRI compared to CT [23, 24]. In rare instances, SPEN can be associated with large retroperitoneal hemorrhage that may result in the patient's presentation. Calcification is very frequent and may be seen either within the center of the lesion or peripherally (Figs. 4.10 and 4.11) [25, 26].

SPEN do not communicate with the pancreatic duct and do not typically cause pancreatic ductal obstruction or pancreatic atrophy, even if the lesion is quite large and bulky. Similarly, even large tumors situated in the pancreatic head do not typically cause biliary obstruction. Lesions are very well defined and often round or oval in shape, with the presence of an enhancing peripheral capsule a consistent feature. SPEN do not demonstrate evidence of vascular encasement, narrowing, occlusion, or invasion [25, 27, 28].

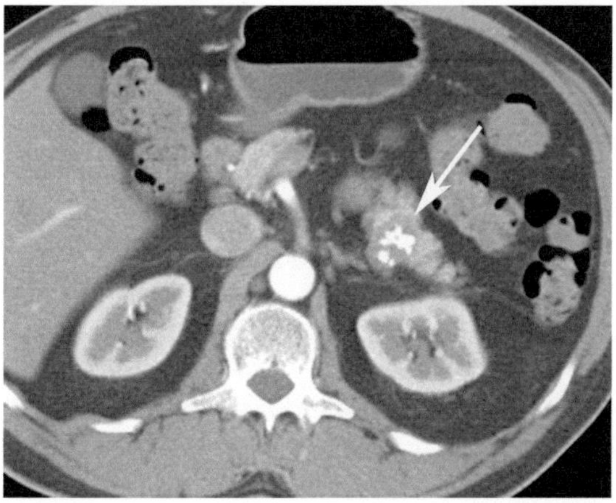

Fig. 4.10 Axial contrast-enhanced CT demonstrates a SPEN tumor (*arrow*) in young women with coarse internal calcifications

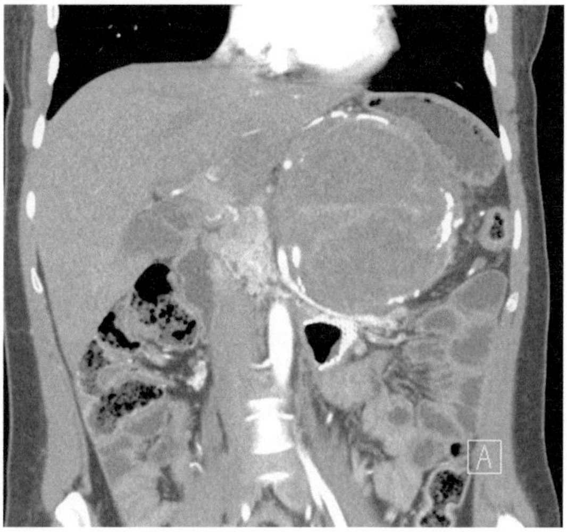

Fig. 4.11 Coronal contrast-enhanced CT in a young woman demonstrates a large cystic pancreatic mass with extensive calcifications and some internal solid components. This mass was found to be a SPEN at resection

4.7 Cystic Neuroendocrine Tumors

Most neuroendocrine tumors present as solid well-marginated hypervascular masses that are most apparent on the arterial phase of imaging. While some lesions, particularly as they grow larger, can demonstrate cystic and necrotic features, it is worth noting that some neuroendocrine tumors can appear as a primarily cystic lesion that can be easily confused with other more common cystic neoplasms (such as an IPMN). Cystic neuroendocrine tumors are most often nonsyndromic (i.e., not associated with a clinical syndrome due to hormone hypersecretion), and in those rare cases that are syndromic, lesions are almost always of the non-insulin-secreting type

[6, 29]. Like other neuroendocrine tumors, cystic neuroendocrine tumors are associated with von Hippel-Lindau syndrome, neurofibromatosis, and multiple endocrine neoplasia (MEN) type I and are more apt to be multiple in the setting of one of these syndromes.

Cystic neuroendocrine tumors almost always demonstrate the presence of either a peripheral "rind" of hypervascular enhancing solid tissue or, alternatively, hyperenhancing mural nodularity along the margins of the cyst (Fig. 4.12) [30]. This diagnosis is one of the primary reasons for the inclusion of arterial phase images in the evaluation of a suspected pancreatic cystic neoplasm, as both the solid rim and mural nodularity associated with these lesions are almost always most conspicuous on the arterial phase and may be more difficult to appreciate on venous phase imaging. Unfortunately, given that the hypervascular components may be less conspicuous on the venous phase, these lesions are not infrequently incorrectly diagnosed as IPMN when only a venous phase is acquired. In addition, the presence of other signs of metastatic dissemination can also be a strong clue to the correct diagnosis, including hyperenhancing liver or lymph node metastases.

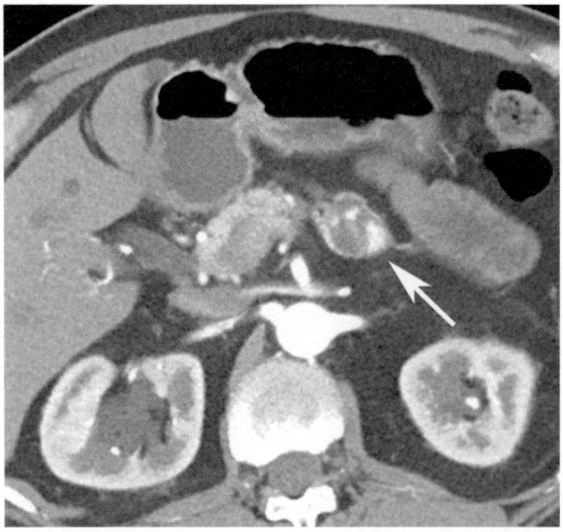

Fig. 4.12 Axial contrast-enhanced CT in the arterial phase demonstrates a small cystic pancreatic lesion (*arrow*) with prominent hyperenhancing soft tissue nodularity along its margin, compatible with a cystic neuroendocrine tumor

4.8 Lymphoepithelial Cysts

Lymphoepithelial cysts are rare (<0.5 % of all pancreatic cystic lesions) benign pancreatic cystic neoplasms that are most commonly seen in elderly men between 50 and 70 years old. These lesions have no malignant potential and are usually an incidental finding seen on imaging studies performed for totally unrelated reasons, although patients can rarely present with nonspecific symptoms of abdominal pain. The exact etiology of these lesions is not well understood, with different theories suggesting they could represent the sequelae of branchial cleft cysts fusing with the pancreatic remnant during embryogenesis or epithelial inclusions within a peripancreatic lymph node with squamous metaplasia [31].

Prospective diagnosis can be extraordinarily difficult, although these lesions do tend to be peripancreatic (abutting and invaginating into the pancreas) rather than being truly of pancreatic origin. If a lesion is suspected to be extrapancreatic, rather than arising from the pancreas itself, lymphoepithelial cyst (along with lymphangioma and pseudocyst) should be considered [31, 32]. While some reports have suggested the presence of microscopic fat within lesions resulting in signal loss on opposed-phase chemical shift gradient-echo MRI images, macroscopic fat is very rarely visible within these lesions on MDCT [31–33].

Conclusion

Multidetector computed tomography now offers a powerful tool for the evaluation, diagnosis, and risk stratification of pancreatic cystic neoplasms. Improvements in image quality and spatial resolution, as well as sophisticated 3-D reconstruction techniques, allow exquisite assessment of the internal architecture of these lesions that not only may allow the radiologist to provide a specific diagnosis but also to assess features that might predict the risk of malignancy.

References

1. Sahani DV, Sainani NI, Blake MA, Crippa S, Mino-Kenudson M, del-Castillo CF. Prospective evaluation of reader performance on MDCT in characterization of cystic pancreatic lesions and prediction of cyst biologic aggressiveness. AJR Am J Roentgenol. 2011;197:W53–61.
2. Visser BC, Yeh BM, Qayyum A, Way LW, McCulloch CE, Coakley FV. Characterization of cystic pancreatic masses: relative accuracy of CT and MRI. AJR Am J Roentgenol. 2007;189:648–56.
3. Sahani DV, Kambadakone A, Macari M, Takahashi N, Chari S, Fernandez-del Castillo C. Diagnosis and management of cystic pancreatic lesions. AJR Am J Roentgenol. 2013;200:343–54.
4. Chaudhari VV, Raman SS, Vuong NL, et al. Pancreatic cystic lesions: discrimination accuracy based on clinical data and high-resolution computed tomographic features. J Comput Assist Tomogr. 2008;32:757–63.
5. Chu LC, Singhi AD, Hruban RH, Fishman EK. Characterization of pancreatic serous cystadenoma on dual-phase multidetector computed tomography. J Comput Assist Tomogr. 2014;38:258–63.
6. Dewhurst CE, Mortele KJ. Cystic tumors of the pancreas: imaging and management. Radiol Clin North Am. 2012;50:467–86.
7. Sakorafas GH, Smyrniotis V, Reid-Lombardo KM, Sarr MG. Primary pancreatic cystic neoplasms revisited. Part I: serous cystic neoplasms. Surg Oncol. 2011;20:e84–92.
8. Lal A, Bourtsos EP, DeFrias DV, Nemcek AA, Nayar R. Microcystic adenoma of the pancreas: clinical, radiologic, and cytologic features. Cancer. 2004;102:288–94.
9. Choi JY, Kim MJ, Lee JY, et al. Typical and atypical manifestations of serous cystadenoma of the pancreas: imaging findings with pathologic correlation. AJR Am J Roentgenol. 2009;193:136–42.
10. Kim SY, Lee JM, Kim SH, et al. Macrocystic neoplasms of the pancreas: CT differentiation of serous oligocystic adenoma from mucinous cystadenoma and intraductal papillary mucinous tumor. AJR Am J Roentgenol. 2006;187:1192–8.
11. Cohen-Scali F, Vilgrain V, Brancatelli G, et al. Discrimination of unilocular macrocystic serous cystadenoma from pancreatic pseudocyst and mucinous cystadenoma with CT: initial observations. Radiology. 2003;228:727–33.
12. Hayashi K, Fujimitsu R, Ida M, et al. CT differentiation of solid serous cystadenoma vs endocrine tumor of the pancreas. Eur J Radiol. 2012;81:e203–8.
13. Khalpey Z, Rajab TK, Ashley SW. Serous cystadenoma causing the double duct sign. J Gastrointest Surg. 2012;16:1282–3.
14. Mortele KJ. Cystic pancreatic neoplasms: imaging features and management strategy. Semin Roentgenol. 2013;48:253–63.
15. Sakorafas GH, Smyrniotis V, Reid-Lombardo KM, Sarr MG. Primary pancreatic cystic neoplasms revisited: part II. Mucinous cystic neoplasms. Surg Oncol. 2011;20:e93–101.
16. Procacci C, Carbognin G, Accordini S, et al. CT features of malignant mucinous cystic tumors of the pancreas. Eur Radiol. 2001;11:1626–30.
17. Raman SP, Fishman EK, Lennon AM. Endoscopic ultrasound and pancreatic applications: what the radiologist needs to know. Abdom Imaging. 2013;38:1360–72.
18. Tanaka M, Fernandez-del Castillo C, Adsay V, et al. International consensus guidelines 2012 for the management of IPMN and MCN of the pancreas. Pancreatology. 2012;12:183–97.
19. Raman SP, Kawamoto S, Blackford A, et al. Histopathologic findings of multifocal pancreatic intraductal papillary mucinous neoplasms on CT. AJR Am J Roentgenol. 2013;200:563–9.
20. Buetow PC, Buck JL, Pantongrag-Brown L, Beck KG, Ros PR, Adair CF. Solid and papillary epithelial neoplasm of the pancreas: imaging-pathologic correlation on 56 cases. Radiology. 1996;199:707–11.
21. Cantisani V, Mortele KJ, Levy A, et al. MR imaging features of solid pseudopapillary tumor of the pancreas in adult and pediatric patients. AJR Am J Roentgenol. 2003;181:395–401.
22. Law JK, Ahmed A, Singh VK, et al. A systematic review of solid-pseudopapillary neoplasms: are these rare lesions? Pancreas. 2014;43:331–7.
23. Ventriglia A, Manfredi R, Mehrabi S, et al. MRI features of solid pseudopapillary neoplasm of the pancreas. Abdom Imaging. 2014;39:1213–20.
24. Guerrache Y, Soyer P, Dohan A, et al. Solid-pseudopapillary tumor of the pancreas: MR imaging findings in 21 patients. Clin Imaging. 2014;38:475–82.
25. Raman SP, Kawamoto S, Law JK, et al. Institutional experience with solid pseudopapillary neoplasms: focus on computed tomography, magnetic resonance imaging, conventional ultrasound, endoscopic ultrasound, and predictors of aggressive histology. J Comput Assist Tomogr. 2013;37:824–33.
26. Sunkara S, Williams TR, Myers DT, Kryvenko ON. Solid pseudopapillary tumours of the pancreas: spectrum of imaging findings with histopathological correlation. Br J Radiol. 2012;85:e1140–4.
27. Liu QY, Lai DM, Zeng YP, Lin XF, Li HG. Computed tomography and magnetic resonance imaging findings of malignant solid pseudopapillary tumors of the pancreas with macroscopic venous tumor thrombosis: a report of 4 cases. J Comput Assist Tomogr. 2014;38:383–90.
28. Palmucci S, Uccello A, Leone G, Failla G, Ettorre GC. Rare pancreatic neoplasm: MDCT and MRI features of a typical solid pseudopapillary tumor. J Radiol Case Rep. 2012;6:17–24.

29. Horton KM, Hruban RH, Yeo C, Fishman EK. Multidetector row CT of pancreatic islet cell tumors. Radiographics. 2006;26:453–64.
30. Paik KY, Choi SH, Heo JS, Choi DW. Solid tumors of the pancreas can put on a mask through cystic change. World J Surg Oncol. 2011;9:79.
31. Sakorafas GH, Smyrniotis V, Reid-Lombardo KM, Sarr MG. Primary pancreatic cystic neoplasms of the pancreas revisited. Part IV: rare cystic neoplasms. Surg Oncol. 2012;21:153–63.
32. Mege D, Gregoire E, Barbier L, Del Grande J, Le Treut YP. Lymphoepithelial cyst of the pancreas: an analysis of 117 patients. Pancreas. 2014;43:987–95.
33. Kavuturu S, Sarwani NE, Ruggeiro FM, et al. Lymphoepithelial cysts of the pancreas. Can preoperative imaging distinguish this benign lesion from malignant or pre-malignant cystic pancreatic lesions? JOP. 2013;14:250–5.

MR in Cystic Tumors of the Pancreas

5

Riccardo Manfredi, Sara Mehrabi, Enrico Boninsegna, and Roberto Pozzi Mucelli

5.1 Introduction

Cystic neoplasms of the pancreas are rare tumors that arise from elements of the epithelial component of the pancreas. They represent 1% of all pancreatic cancers and 10% of all cystic lesions of the gland [1]. Nowadays cystic neoplasms of the pancreas are diagnosed more frequently due to the spread of increasingly accurate imaging techniques. The diagnosis is often incidental because they tend to be asymptomatic or they present nonspecific symptoms.

Although they are considered benign lesions in the early stages, progressive malignant degeneration is possible for the occurrence of dysplastic foci [2].

The WHO classification is based to the histological features of the wall with special reference to the epithelium lining, the main element in the differential diagnosis with nonneoplastic cystic lesions of the pancreas [3]. This classification distinguishes serous cystic neoplasms (SCNs), mucinous cystic neoplasms (MCNs), intraductal papillary mucinous neoplasms (IPMNs), and solid pseudopapillary neoplasms (SPNs).

R. Manfredi, MD, MBA (✉) • S. Mehrabi, MD
E. Boninsegna, MD • R. Pozzi Mucelli, MD
Department of Radiology, Policlinico G. B. Rossi, University of Verona, Verona, Italy
e-mail: riccardo.manfredi@univr.it; saraprinaz@yahoo.it; boninsegnae@gmail.com; roberto.pozzimucelli@univr.it

A correct classification is particularly important because it affects the subsequent choice of therapy that it is not necessarily surgery. Those with a greater potential for malignant transformation are MCNs, IPMNs of the main pancreatic duct, and SPNs, which require a surgical resection, while SCNs and branch-duct IPMNs have a very low malignant potential and can be managed with a radiological follow-up [4].

Pancreatic neuroendocrine tumors (NETs) present as cystic lesions in approximately 5% of cases, with radiological features similar to other cystic lesions of the pancreas. Their appearance can be identical to SCNs, MCN, or SPNs, and often a definitive diagnosis can be obtained only after histological examination.

Magnetic resonance imaging (MRI) is the most important technique in the evaluation of cystic neoplasms of the pancreas, because it allows to analyze the morphology of the lesions, their content, and the relationship with the pancreatic ductal system [5].

With regard to other imaging methods, ultrasonography can in many cases identify a cystic lesion of the pancreas, but it does not have the same spatial and contrast resolution of MRI, it is affected by patient's constitutional factors, and not least it depends from the operator experience [5].

Although the endoscopic ultrasonography may help to overcome some of these limitations, it remains an invasive technique. CT can better depict the presence of calcification, but it does not allow to identify the typical features which

M. Del Chiaro et al. (eds.), *Cystic Tumors of the Pancreas*, DOI 10.1007/978-3-319-31882-0_5

are often essential for the differential diagnosis of these neoplasms [5].

In the following part of the text, the various pancreatic cystic neoplasms will be described, with particular attention to the MRI aspects useful for the differential diagnosis.

5.2 Serous Cystic Neoplasms

5.2.1 Background

Serous cystic neoplasms (SCNs) are divided according to the WHO classification in serous cystadenoma and serous cystadenocarcinoma, although the second was reported in the literature in a very limited number of cases.

SCNs are more frequent in female patients (male/female, 1:3), with an average age of 62 years (range 35–84 years). They can be found in any pancreatic region, but they are more frequent in the head (>50 %). The size can be extremely variable, from 1–2 cm to 20–25 cm (average 6–10 cm) [6].

To date the only established association between SCNs and others neoplasm is von Hippel-Lindau disease, an autosomal dominant condition caused by mutations of suppressor gene VHL.

More than 50 % of serous cystadenomas are asymptomatic and discovered incidentally during diagnostic evaluations conducted for other symptoms (often unrelated). Symptoms are nonspecific: abdominal pain (25 %), anorexia and dyspepsia (10 %), rarely jaundice (7 %), weight loss, and a palpable abdominal mass. Clinical symptoms are commonly seen in serous cystic neoplasms larger than 4 cm [7]. Symptoms are related to a mass-compressing effect and are nonspecific. Even when present, symptoms often do not raise immediate alarm, so it is not uncommon that the onset of symptoms may precede the diagnosis of a few years (average a year and a half). The most common symptom is abdominal pain, but only 35 % of patients who present with symptomatic serous cystadenoma present a typical pancreatic pain ("bar" irradiation).

With regard to laboratory tests, there are no tumor markers or tests indicative of the biological behavior of the lesions [8].

5.2.2 Pathology

Serous cystadenoma frequently appears as a rounded, full of liquid fluid, and transparent cystic mass, with lobulated and well-defined margins. Dimensions may vary in diameter from 1 to 25 cm (average 6–11 cm). They are usually single lesions, but, especially in the von Hippel-Lindau patients, multiple lesions or multifocal and confluent neoplasms can be present. There is no communication between the lesion and the main pancreatic duct. Macroscopically they are divided according to the number and size of cysts into three subtypes: microcystic, macrocystic, and mixed type [1, 6].

In the classical form, microcystic lesions present well-circumscribed lobulated margins. When spongy texture is present, it is formed by multiple (>6) small cysts that vary from 1 to 5 mm in diameter. The cysts are filled with serous transparent fluid. In 30 % of cases, there is a typical central "star-shaped" scar composed of white nodules and fibrosis. The scar often has calcium deposits, which may appear to radiological investigations as starry or punctuated calcifications.

In the macrocystic form, the lesion is characterized by the presence of a small number (<6) of larger cysts. The intracystic fluid can be clear and transparent or a brownish fluid with blood. The cutting surface shows the presence of a quantifiable number of cysts or, sometimes, a single cyst (unilocular variant), with a diameter between 2 and 15 cm. This form typically does not present the central scar [3, 6].

In mixed form, the lesion is characterized by the presence of larger cysts, situated on the periphery of the lesion, and microcysts in the center. There may be a central scar.

Microscopically the different forms of cystadenoma are indistinguishable and show the typical serous epithelium that can vary from cubical to squamous, in which the cells present clear cytoplasm and round nuclei. Cytological atypia and mitotic activity are rare. Typically in these tumors glycogen is intracellular (positive for periodic acid-Schiff) and intracellular mucin is absent. The neoplastic stroma is highly vascularized. The walls that separate the cysts are larger and contain hemosiderin-laden macrophages and sometimes islets of Langerhans and trapped exocrine acini. The fibrous scar characteristic of microcystic variant is also formed by hyalinized tissue, frequently associated with calcification. All variants of serous cystadenoma lack a fibrous pseudocapsule.

Malignant serous cystic neoplasms are rare. Cystic adenocarcinomas are associated with lymphovascular and perineural invasion, extension to adjacent organs, and detection of metastatic disease in the regional lymph nodes and liver. A minimal nuclear atypia and a more prominent papillary architecture have been described in some serous cystadenomas presenting also a positivity for the proliferation marker Ki-67 and an overexpression of the p53 protein. These features are considered premalignant and are associated with a risk of malignant transformation of 3 % [2, 6].

5.2.3 MRI

Magnetic resonance imaging (MRI) plays an important role in the characterization of cystic tumors: the multiplicity of sequences on the various planes of the space and the use of the contrast medium allow to obtain information on the morphology and composition of the lesion. In addition, the use of magnetic resonance cholangiopancreatography (MRCP) allows a better assessment of the relationship between the cystic mass and the main pancreatic duct, helpful in the differential diagnosis between serous cystadenoma and branch-duct intraductal papillary mucinous neoplasm [5].

Microcystic serous cystadenoma (Figs. 5.1 and 5.2) appears hypointense on T1-weighted images in respect to the adjacent parenchyma, with homogeneous signal intensity in the lesion; septa and calcifications are not well visible. Rarely hemorrhagic foci within the mass can be identified. On T2-weighted images, it appears as a group of small cysts, with hyperintense fluid content, without any communication with the main pancreatic duct, separated each other by thin fibrous septa. It can present a pathognomonic central fibrous scar. On T1-weighted images after contrast administration, the information obtained are essentially comparable to those obtainable by computed tomography (CT): contrast enhancement of walls and septa in the arterial phase, allowing optimal visualization of the "honeycomb" structure, which is even better recognizable in the portal venous phase.

T2-weighted images are important to evaluate the content of the cystic lesion (fluid, presence of septa) and pancreatic ductal system. The use of images with fat saturation allows to suppress the high intensity of the signal from the adipose tissue and consequently to increase the representation of the internal structure of the lesion. MRCP sequences give an optimal representation of the pancreatic ductal system. T1-weighted fat saturated images can identify foci of internal bleeding or protein deposits, features more often seen in pseudocysts or degenerated solid tumors of the pancreas. In addition, T1-weighted images are useful for evaluating the adjacent pancreatic parenchyma to identify, for example, signal changes suggestive of chronic pancreatitis, especially in those cases where a pseudocyst is part of the differential diagnosis [3, 5].

Diffusion-weighted imaging (DWI) is nowadays very important in the diagnosis of pancreatic masses. In serous cystadenomas, the values of apparent diffusion coefficient (ADC) are substantially similar to those of simple cysts: in b1000 sequences, the lesion appears hypointense, not presenting signal restriction in ADC. For this reason, information obtained from diffusion images do not allow an adequate differential diagnosis of serous cystadenoma from mucinous cystic neoplasms [9].

The presence of a mass with a spongy appearance and central calcifications in the pancreatic head in a woman is diagnostic for serous cystic neoplasm, especially when the remaining pancreatic parenchyma is normal, without dilation of the Wirsung duct. In this case, you need no other

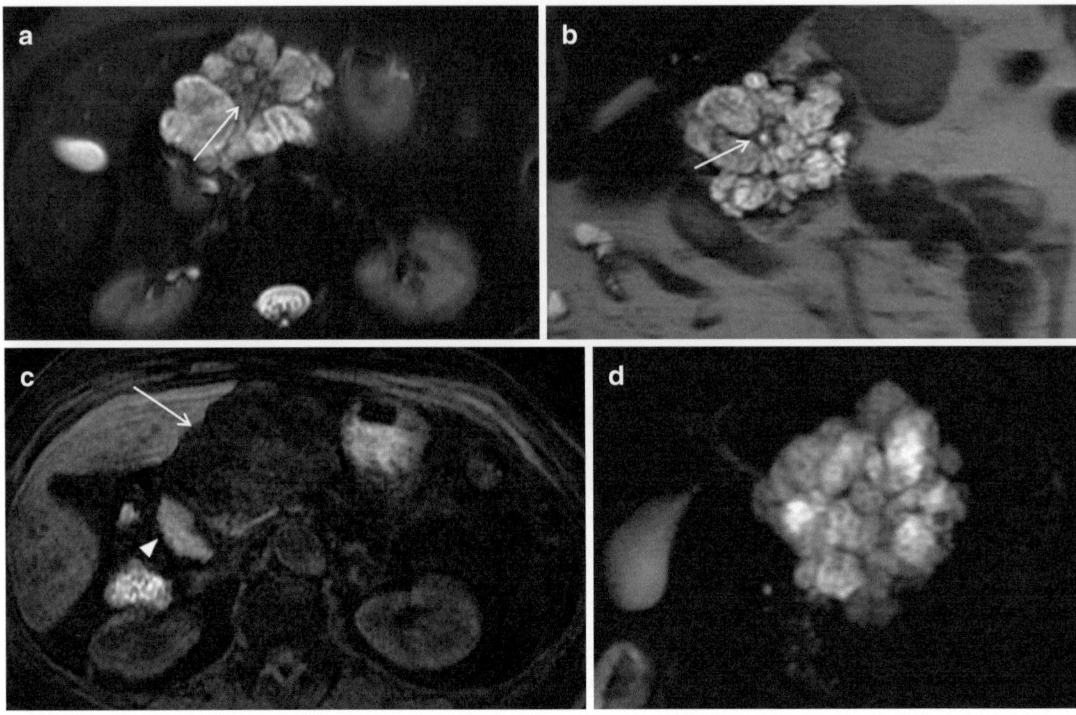

Fig. 5.1 A 69-year-old female patient with serous cystadenoma in the pancreatic head. (**a**, **b**) Axial (**a**) and coronal (**b**) T2-weighted images: the lesion presents multiple hyperintense microcysts, with septa that radiate from the central scar (*arrow*). (**c**) Axial T1-weighted GRE image with fat saturation: the content of the lesion (*arrow*) is homogeneously hypointense compared to the adjacent pancreatic parenchyma (*arrow head*). (**d**) MRCP image: the cystic lesion is well visible; main pancreatic duct cannot be depicted

diagnostic investigations, because the choice of treatment is made on the basis of clinical presentation and the patient's general condition.

Serous cystadenoma is in the differential diagnosis of intraductal papillary mucinous neoplasms (IPMNs), and it is essential to detect a possible communication with the main pancreatic duct, never present in serous cystadenoma.

The diagnosis can also be considered definitive when the lesion shows a mixed micro-macrocystic aspect, with cysts >2 cm at the periphery of the lesion and the microcysts in center.

The most difficult diagnosis is a lesion with oligocystic-macrocystic pattern (number of cysts <6, cyst diameter >2 cm): this variant is very similar to mucinous cystic neoplasms. The presence of papillary projections or mural nodules in the cysts is suspicious for borderline mucinous cystadenoma or mucinous cystadenocarcinoma. These nodules appear as areas of low signal intensity in T2-weighted images and present contrast enhancement.

In the presence of unilocular cystic lesions, the differential diagnosis is with pseudocyst; other possibilities are intraductal papillary mucinous neoplasms and lymphoepithelial cysts. These lesions can be differentiated from pseudocysts because of the lack of clinical, laboratory, and imaging findings (pancreatic inflammation, atrophy or parenchymal calcifications, duct dilation, or intraductal stones) suggestive of pancreatitis [10]. Pseudocysts are also more common in the body-tail of the pancreas and appear hypointense on T1-weighted images and hyperintense (if filled with fluid) or mixed intensity (if filled with fluid and debris) on T2-weighted images. At MRCP pseudocysts appear hyperintense and contiguous to the main pancreatic duct.

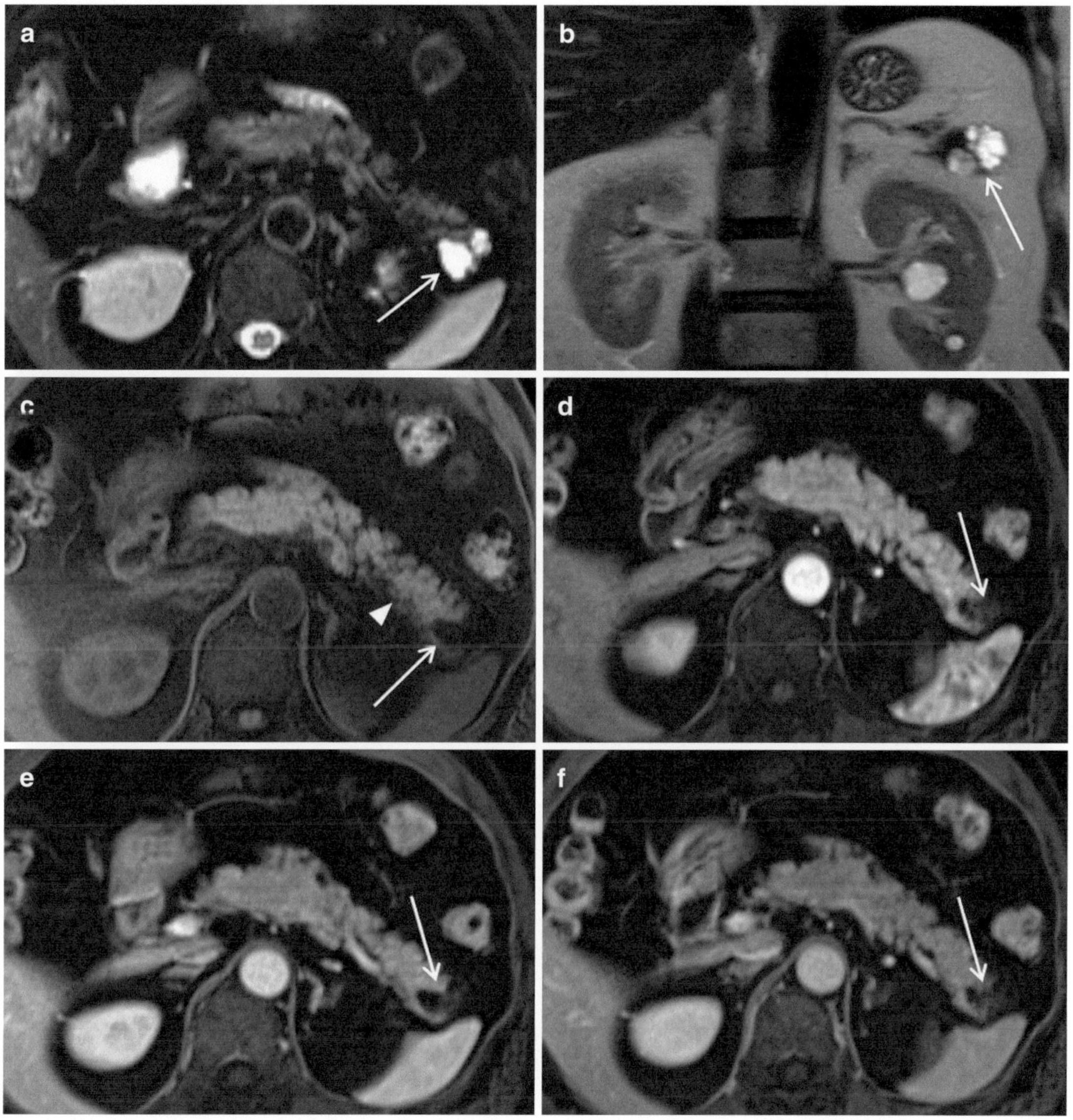

Fig. 5.2 A 56-year-old male patient with serous cystadenoma in the pancreatic tail. (**a**, **b**) Axial (**a**) and coronal (**b**) T2-weighted images: the lesion presents multiple hyperintense microcysts with septa (*arrow*). (**c**) Axial T1-weighted GRE image with fat saturation: the content of the lesion (*arrow*) is homogeneously hypointense compared to the adjacent pancreatic parenchyma (*arrow head*). (**d–f**) Axial T1-weighted GRE images with fat saturation after contrast administration, in pancreatic (**d**), portal (**e**), and late (**f**) phases: a progressive contrast enhancement of septa (*arrow*) is visible

When the differentiation is not possible with diagnostic imaging, symptomatic patients should undergo surgery. Asymptomatic patients with unilocular cyst with thin walls, especially if small, can be monitored over time with CT or MRI [7].

Note, in most cases, serous cystadenoma is presented as a single lesion, except in von Hippel-Lindau patients. In this syndrome, the pancreas is involved in 15–30 % of cases with the presence of multiple serous cystadenomas, without a preferential localization. The average age at diagnosis is 30 in these cases. The diagnosis of von Hippel-Lindau must therefore always be considered when multiple pancreatic cysts are found in an asymptomatic patient without clinical evidence of pancreatitis. In these cases, a complete clinical and radiological evaluation should also include the central nervous system (most common manifestation: cerebellar hemangiomas), eye (retinal hemangiomas), kidneys (cysts, clear cell carcinoma), and adrenal glands (pheochromocytoma).

5.3 Mucinous Cystic Neoplasms

5.3.1 Background

Mucinous cystic neoplasms (MCNs) are rare cystic lesion of the pancreas [2, 5], representing approximately 2–5 % of all exocrine pancreatic tumors and 17 % of cystic neoplasms of the pancreas [11]. They occur almost exclusively in women between the third and eighth decade, with peak incidence in the fifth decade (average age 49). The majority of lesions occur in the body-tail of the pancreas, while the head is only rarely involved.

In recent years, some evidences have suggested the possible origin of MCNs by ectopic primordial ovarian tissue that undergoes malignant degeneration [12].

The possible derivation of the stromal component of MCNs from ovarian primordial gonad is supported by their morphology and the positive immunohistochemical analysis for inhibin, estrogen, and progesterone receptors, indicating precisely stromal luteinization.

In addition, the embryological origin of the pancreas reinforces this hypothesis. The dorsal pancreatic bud, which gives rise to the body and tail of the pancreas and a small part of the pancreatic head, and the left primordial gonad are very close in an early stage of development (fourth to fifth week), unlike the ventral pancreatic bud, which gives rise to most of the pancreatic head, which is separated from the primordial right gonad from the hepatobiliary gem. This makes it plausible that the primordial egg cells could easily be incorporated in the pancreas and would also explain the predilection of MCNs for the body-tail of the pancreas [12].

The clinical presentation depends on the size of the tumor: small tumors are asymptomatic and discovered incidentally; larger tumors produce symptoms by compression of adjacent structures and palpable abdominal mass.

MCNs constitute a category of potentially malignant cystic neoplasms of the pancreas: benign forms such as mucinous cystadenomas (MCAs) are known precursors of invasive forms such as mucinous cystoadenocarcinomas (MCACs) [2, 3].

Consequently, it is crucial to plan a proper diagnostic and therapeutic strategy to differentiate MCNs from other pancreatic cystic tumors with a benign biological behavior addressed to follow-up, such as serous cystadenomas (SCAs) and other cystic lesions of the pancreas, such as pseudocysts and nonneoplastic mucinous cysts.

In addition, MCNs enter into the differential diagnosis with another category of cystic tumors which also have malignant potential such as intraductal papillary mucinous neoplasm (IPMNs) [13].

5.3.2 Pathology

Mucinous cystic neoplasms (MCNs) are characterized by the presence of mucin-secreting epithelial cells, supported by ovarian-type stroma, which delimits a cystic cavity without communication with the pancreatic ductal system [2].

The presence of mucin-secreting columnar epithelium distinguishes MCNs from serous cystadenoma, solid pseudopapillary neoplasm, and cystic neuroendocrine tumor.

The absence of communication with the pancreatic ductal system is fundamental in the distinction between MCNs and IPMNs. In fact, even IPMNs are characterized by the presence of mucin-secreting epithelial cells, and this has led in the past some pathologists to interpret MCNs and IPMNs as a single entity.

According to the degree of epithelial dysplasia, they can be classified into adenoma, borderline tumor, and carcinoma, invasive or noninvasive, although all MCNs of the pancreas should be considered potentially malignant [2].

The progression from cystadenoma to cystadenocarcinoma is also suggested by the average age of onset of two forms: the average age of onset of cystoadenocarcinomas is 54.2 years, while the average age of onset of borderline forms or adenomas is 44.7 years.

MCNs appear as round masses with smooth surface and fibrous pseudocapsule of variable thickness, with frequent calcifications. Tumor size can vary widely in a range between 2 and 35 cm, average between 6 and 10 cm.

MCNs usually are macrocystic and multilocular, rarely unilocular, with cystic spaces ranging from a few to several centimeters in diameter, containing mucin or mucin dense mixed hemorrhagic-necrotic material. The inner surface of unilocular tumors usually appears smooth and shiny, while tumors often show multilocular papillary projections and nodules.

The malignancy of MCNs correlates significantly with the presence of papillary projections and/or nodules.

There is no communication between the tumor and the main pancreatic duct.

MCNs show two distinct components: an inner layer and an outer layer with epithelial cells very similar to ovarian stroma. The epithelium often shows areas with pseudopyloric, gastric, small bowel, and colon differentiation, while ovarian stroma is composed of densely packed cells with round nuclei. About half of the tumors also contain endocrine cells at the base of the columnar cells. The spectrum of cell differentiation varies from columnar benign epithelium to severely atypical epithelium [2].

Mucinous cystadenomas (MCAs) show only mild epithelial dysplasia characterized by a slight increase in the size of nuclei located in lower layers and the absence of mitosis.

Borderline mucinous cystadenomas show moderate dysplasia, characterized by papillary projections or crypts and invaginations with crowding of atypical nuclei and rare mitoses.

Mucinous cystoadenocarcinomas (MCACs) present severe dysplasia/carcinoma in situ which usually occur focally and can only be identified after careful research of multiple sections from different areas of the tumor. The epithelial cells that often form papillae with irregular junctions or arborescence show nuclear stratification, severe nuclear atypia, and frequent mitoses.

MCACs can be further classified into invasive or noninvasive, depending on the presence of stromal invasion. The invasive component usually is similar to the common ductal adenocarcinoma.

5.3.3 MRI

The role of MR Imaging in MCNs includes both the identification and characterization [3, 11].

MCNs appear as oligolocular microcystic or macrocystic lesions, more rarely multilocular, localized in the body-tail (Fig. 5.3). They are rounded in shape and well circumscribed and present a wall with thin internal septa that delimit cystic spaces [5].

On T1-weighted images (performed with fat saturation), the content is homogeneous and hypointense, although the presence of mucin or foci of hemorrhage can increase the intensity of signal.

Because of the fluid content, MCNs are hyperintense on T2-weighted images; the characteristics and the distribution of internal nodularity are well visible in these sequences. The presence of mucin and hemorrhagic foci can make the cyst content inhomogeneous and determines the formation of fluid levels.

Contrast administration makes it easier to recognize the walls, vegetations, or solid components.

Maximum enhancement of wall, mural nodules, and solid components is observed in the venous phase or delayed phase. However, recognition of calcification does not improve after administration of contrast medium.

DWI sequences can facilitate the identification of areas of ADC restriction in correspondence with the solid components of the lesion as the parietal nodules.

The acquisition of images on the coronal plane helps to recognize the characteristics described above.

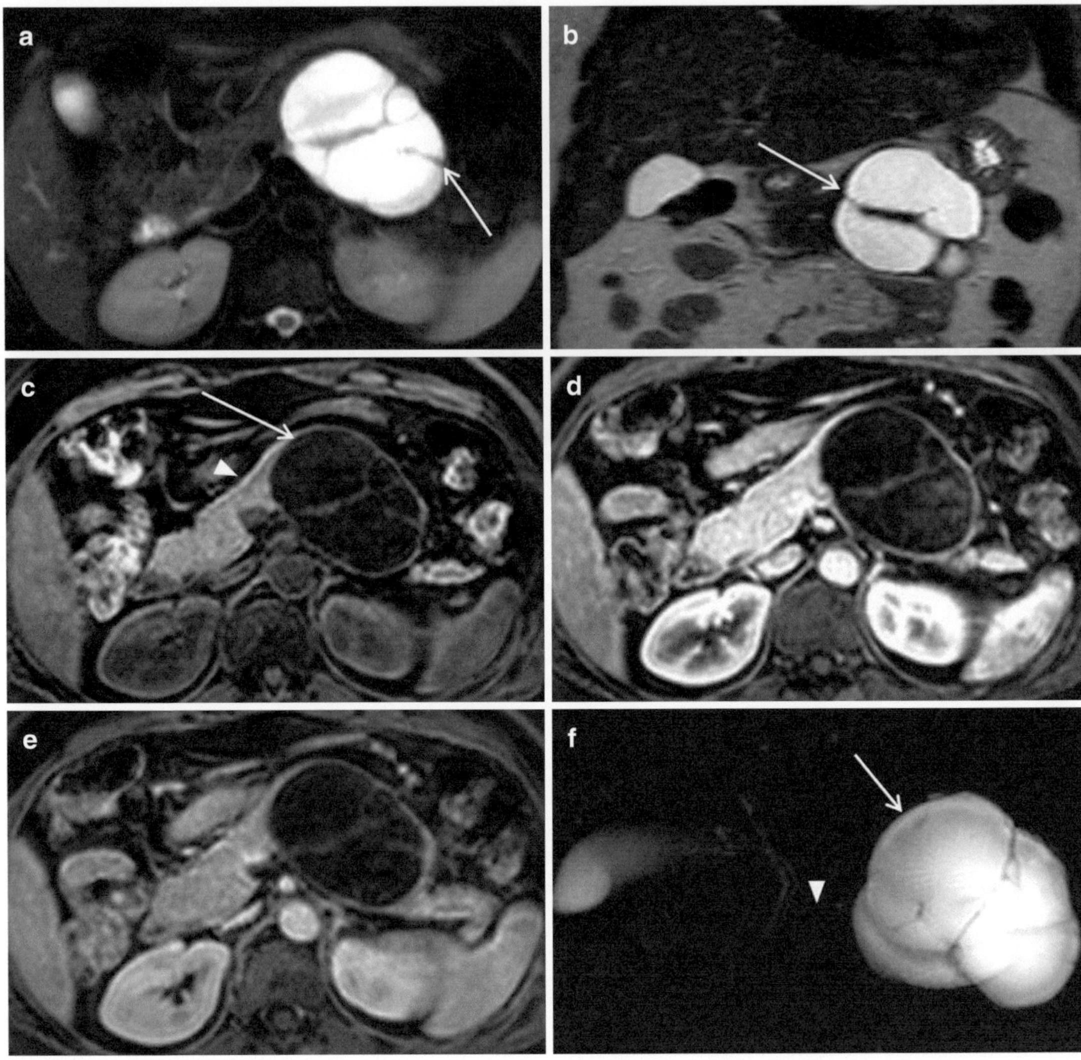

Fig. 5.3 A 76-year-old female patient with mucinous cystadenoma in the body-tail of the pancreas. (**a**, **b**) Axial (**a**) and coronal (**b**) T2-weighted images: a hyperintense cystic mass with septa (*arrow*) is visible. (**c**) Axial T1-weighted GRE image with fat saturation: the content of the lesion (*arrow*) is homogeneously hypointense compared to the adjacent pancreatic parenchyma (*arrow head*). (**d**, **e**) Axial T1-weighted GRE images with fat saturation after contrast administration, in pancreatic (**d**) and portal (**e**) phases: contrast enhancement of walls and septa is visible. (**f**) MRCP image: the cystic lesion is well visible (*arrow*); there is no communication with the main pancreatic duct (*arrowhead*)

The first diagnostic distinction has to be made between mucinous adenomas and adenocarcinomas: adenomas usually present as an oligolocular lesion with septa, while adenocarcinomas tend to have larger size (>4 cm) and a more complex structure.

Cyst walls and septa are typically thicker in adenocarcinomas, which present solid nodules with contrast enhancement.

The content of the cysts in adenomas tends to be more homogeneous, hypointense on T1 images, and hyperintense on T2 images, while fluid inside adenocarcinomas tends to be more heterogeneous and presents a greater hyperintensity on T1 images for the presence of bleeding or solid components. These features are highly suggestive of malignancy of the lesion suggesting surgical resection [14].

In particular, the element which correlates more strongly with the malignancy of MCNs is represented by the presence of parietal nodules.

It can be difficult to differentiate a pseudocyst from a MCN when septa within the lesion are not visible. Otherwise, a positive history of acute or chronic pancreatitis is in favor of pseudocysts [15].

Only a fine-needle aspiration can differentiate with certainty the two cystic lesions: high levels of amylase for pseudocysts and high levels of CEA and CA 19-9 for MCNs.

The classic microcystic form of SCA generally is not a problem for the differential diagnosis, whereas there are rare solid and oligocystic variants of SCA with an appearance that can simulate the MCN. One element that can help in the differential diagnosis between SCAs and MCNs is represented by age, as SCAs tend to occur at a later age than the MCNs.

Branch-duct IPMNs may have a cystic appearance and mimic MCNs. However, the demonstration of communication with the pancreatic ductal system allows to make the differential diagnosis [13, 14]. T2-weighted images (highly sensitive to fluids) are optimal to see the Wirsung duct; the examination can also be completed with MRCP images.

In addition, IPMNs occurred more commonly in men.

5.4 Intraductal Papillary Mucinous Neoplasms

5.4.1 Background

Intraductal papillary mucinous neoplasms (IPMNs) are cystic lesions of the pancreas developing from the mucinous epithelium of the pancreatic ductal system. The cellular atypia is responsible for excessive production of mucin, resulting in dilation of the main pancreatic duct or formation of cystic enlargement of branch ducts.

IPMNs, once considered rare injury, presented in recent years a considerable increase in the incidence, because of technological advancement in diagnostic imaging, currently constituting about 27 % of all cystic neoplasms of the pancreas [11, 16].

Elderly males are mainly affected, with a peak of incidence between 60 and 70 years.

Clinically, nearly half of patients are asymptomatic, and the neoplasm is an incidental finding during an ultrasound examination, CT, or MRI carried out for reasons not correlated to the presence of a cystic pancreatic neoplasm or abdominal pain. Symptoms of IPMNs are nonspecific: in most cases, abdominal pain is present, more rarely jaundice, weight loss, and diabetes.

The role of MR Imaging, currently considered the gold standard in the study of these neoplasms, is to identify the typical signs of IPMNs, to differentiate from other cystic lesions, and to distinguish the various forms of IPMNs, because main-duct IPMNs have a high potential risk of malignancy, significantly greater than branch-duct IPMNs. Therefore, MRI is the first choice technique to monitor these tumors over time, in order to detect any signs of malignant progression [17].

Main-duct IPMN is characterized by exclusive dilation of the main pancreatic duct, which may be involved in focal or diffuse sense. In most patients with segmental forms, the tumor is located at the body-tail of the pancreas.

Branch-duct IPMNs are characterized by papillary proliferation and mucin hypersecretion within the lumen of the branch ducts. They can present as a single lesion or as multiple cystic lesions (multifocal branch-duct IPMN).

Mixed IPMNs, as the central, predominantly affect male patients (56 % men, 44 % women) and are characterized by the involvement of the main pancreatic duct and one or multiple secondary ducts [11].

5.4.2 Pathology

IPMNs have very wide a spectrum of aggressiveness that depends on the degree of cellular atypia: according to the current WHO classification, they are classified as intraductal papillary mucinous adenoma, borderline IPMN (with moderate dysplasia), and intraductal papillary mucinous carcinoma, noninvasive (in situ) or invasive.

The adenoma is characterized by the presence of columnar epithelium composed of mucin-secreting cells with low-grade atypia. The borderline IPMN is characterized by low degree of dysplasia with epithelial cells that have lost the normal polarity, characterized by the presence of nuclear pyknosis. The intraductal papillary mucinous carcinoma is instead characterized by a high degree of epithelial cell atypia without or with invasion of adjacent tissues (carcinoma in situ and invasive carcinoma, respectively). Within the same tumor, different degrees of dysplasia can be found, suggesting a progressive degeneration from malignant adenoma to borderline tumor, up to carcinoma in situ and finally to invasive carcinoma [2].

The pathologic features suspicious then for dysplastic changes are loss of cell polarity, altered tissue differentiation, high mucin concentration in the cytoplasm, nuclear enlargement, and high rate of mitosis [2].

With regard to immunohistochemical analysis, IPMNs are divided into gastric, intestinal, and biliary neoplasms. The gastric type is primarily associated with branch-duct IPMNs (98 % of cases) and correlates with high-grade dysplasia or invasive carcinoma in only 8 % of cases. The intestinal type, on the contrary, is associated mainly to main-duct IPMNs (73 % of cases) and is correlated to a significantly higher frequency of malignancy (80 %) [57]. Finally, main-duct IPMNs and mixed IPMNs are characterized by a high potential for degeneration with a risk of malignancy of 70 % (57–92 %), while branch-duct IPMNs present a significantly lower risk of degeneration (25 %; average 6–46 %) with a percentage of 15 % developing to invasive carcinoma. In the latter case, the prognosis is comparable to pancreatic adenocarcinoma [18, 19].

5.4.3 MRI

Although computed tomography has a higher spatial resolution, magnetic resonance imaging, in addition to an anatomical representation of the pancreatic parenchyma comparable to CT, presents higher contrast resolution and with MRCP images allows the representation of the ductal system [20].

On T1-weighted images, IPMNs appear as single or multiple ductal dilations, homogeneously hypointense compared with the surrounding pancreatic parenchyma (Fig. 5.4). Hypointensity is more evident in the sequences performed with fat saturation due to the higher signal from the adjacent pancreatic parenchyma. On T2-weighted images, the content of the cyst fluid is markedly hyperintense compared to the surrounding parenchyma. A more accurate evaluation is possible with MRCP images which allow to obtain an anatomical representation of pancreatic-biliary ductal system. MRCP images can evaluate the localization and extension of the cystic lesion, the presence of dilated side branches, or intraluminal filling defects.

Finally, the dynamic phase after administration of contrast medium is essential for the assessment of signs of degeneration. Mural nodules closely adherent to the cystic part of the tumor are associated with malignant degeneration. The greatest difficulty is to identify these nodules when they are still small in size, in order to make an early diagnosis of IPMN with aggressive potential. Another radiological sign predictive of malignancy is the contrast enhancement of the IPMN walls [10, 17, 21].

Main-duct IPMNs appear as focal or diffuse dilation of the main pancreatic duct (Fig. 5.5). They generally have a fusiform appearance and walls consisting of ductal epithelium. In focal forms, the involvement of the body-tail is characterized by the presence of localized dilation in the distal part of the pancreas, leaving the parenchyma of the head unscathed; on the contrary, the involvement of the pancreatic head is often accompanied by dilation of the entire upstream duct. The localization of the dilation of the main pancreatic duct is not related to the biological behavior of the tumor [17].

Main-duct IPMNs enter into the differential diagnosis mainly with different causes of ductal dilation. In particular, in the presence of diffuse forms of main-duct IPMN, the pancreas may be very similar to a picture of chronic obstructive pancreatitis. The presence of mucin deposits

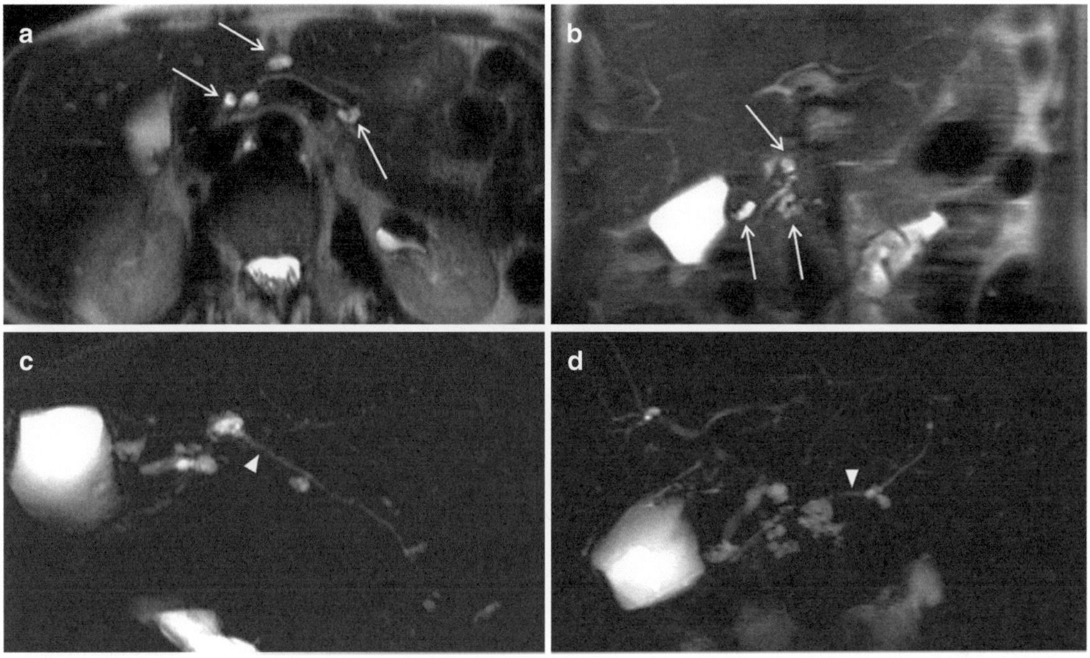

Fig. 5.4 A 57-year-old female patient with multifocal branch-duct IPMNs. (**a**, **b**) Axial (**a**) and coronal (**b**) T2-weighted images: multiple cystic dilations of pancreatic branch ducts (*arrows*) are visible along the whole gland, hyperintense compared to the surrounding parenchyma. (**c**, **d**) Axial (**c**) and coronal (**d**) MRCP images: IPMNs are depicted in pancreatic head, body, and tail; the connection with the main pancreatic duct (*arrowhead*) is well visible for all the cysts

within the cyst is characteristic of IPMNs. These deposits appear as filling defects mildly hyperintense on T1-weighted images and markedly hypointense on T2 images compared to the fluid content of the lesion; on the contrary, the presence of diffuse calcifications is associated mainly with the presence of chronic pancreatitis.

Mixed IPMNs are characterized by the presence of diffuse dilation of the main pancreatic duct and one or multiple dilated side ducts (Fig. 5.5).

Side-branch IPMNs appear as single or multiple cystic lesions, round or oval, communicating with the lumen of the main pancreatic duct, which presents normal caliber.

Imaging appearance of branch-duct IPMNs may be similar to other cystic neoplasms, such as mucinous cystic neoplasms (MCNs). While MCNs preferentially affect women (95 % of cases) with an age range between 40 and 50 and are located in most of the cases in the body-tail, IPMNs primarily affect elder male patients; Furthermore, the presence of multiple cystic dilations throughout the pancreatic parenchyma is more indicative of IPMN [21].

The definitive diagnosis of branch-duct IPMN occurs, however, with the demonstration of communication between the cystic lesion and the main pancreatic duct. MRCP images are the best for the evaluation of such communication.

In the past, several studies have been conducted on the use of pharmacological stimulation with secretin for a better view of the ductal system, but in almost all cases, the communication with the main pancreatic duct can be depicted on MCRP images in basal conditions, without the need of secretin stimulation [14, 22].

Another important role of diagnostic imaging is to monitor over time these tumors in order to identify early signs suggestive of malignant degeneration.

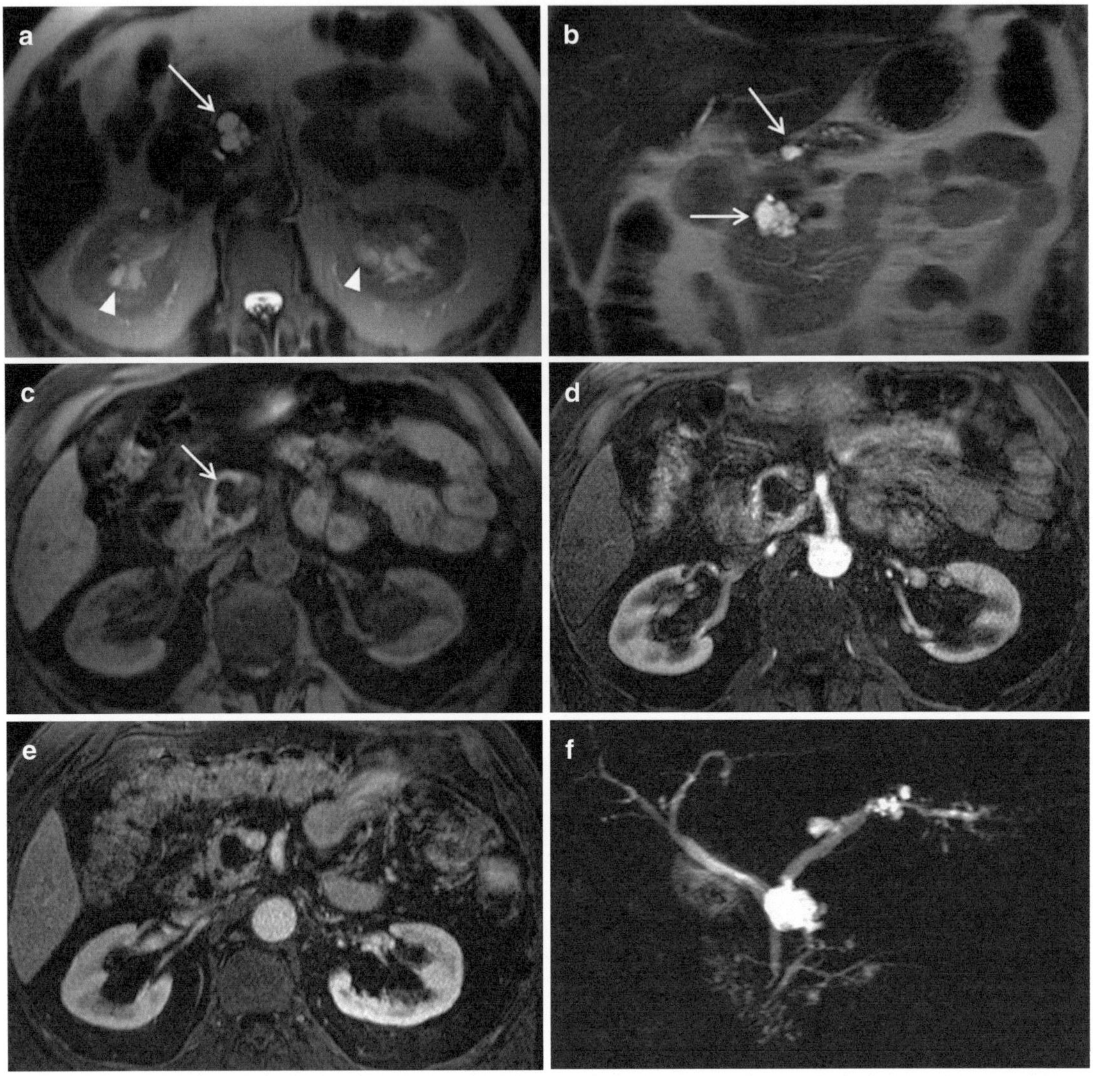

Fig. 5.5 A 57-year-old female patient with multifocal branch-duct IPMNs and main-duct IPMN (mixed IPMN). (**a**, **b**) Axial (**a**) and coronal (**b**) T2-weighted images: multiple cystic dilations of pancreatic branch ducts (*arrows*) are visible along the whole gland, hyperintense compared to the surrounding parenchyma; main pancreatic duct is dilated, too; note the presence of multiple cysts in the kidneys (*arrowheads*). (**c**) Axial T1-weighted GRE image with fat saturation: IPMNs (*arrow*) appear hypointense compared to the surrounding pancreatic parenchyma. (**d**, **e**) Axial T1-weighted GRE images with fat saturation after contrast administration, in pancreatic (**d**) and portal (**e**) phases: there are no mural nodules within cystic lesions. (**f**) MRCP image: IPMNs are depicted in pancreatic head, body, and tail; the connection with the main pancreatic duct, greatly dilated, is well visible for all the cysts

The signs that better correlate with the degeneration are (1) the presence of cystic lesions >3 cm in diameter, (2) the presence of vegetations or mural nodules >3 mm in diameter, (3) contrast enhancement of the walls of the pancreatic duct involved, and (4) dilation of the main pancreatic duct >18 mm.

5.5 Solid Pseudopapillary Neoplasms

5.5.1 Background

Solid pseudopapillary neoplasms (SPNs) of the pancreas are rare lesions with a frequency between 0.9 and 2.7 % of all pancreatic tumors and 4 % of cystic neoplasms [23, 24].

SPN was described for the first time in 1959 by Franz and characterized by Haimoudi in 1970. Only in 1996, the World Health Organization has reclassified according to its pathologic features this solid-cystic neoplasm giving it the name of "solid pseudopapillary tumor" of the pancreas and renamed in 2010 "solid pseudopapillary neoplasm," name accepted and internationally recognized [23].

SPN preferentially affects young women (incidence peak between 20 and 30 years), with a male to female ratio of 1:9 [24].

The pathogenesis of this tumor remains unknown; some authors have suggested the association with pregnancy or polycystic ovaries. The prevalence in females during puberty has in the past suggested the existence of a relationship between tumor growth and female sex hormones [25, 26].

The lesions can be localized in any region of the gland, and the diagnosis usually occurs in discrete sizes: 8–10 cm in average with a range between 0.5 and 25 cm [26]. The tumor size at diagnosis does not correlate directly with increased malignancy or with a worse prognosis. There is no clinical evidence of a correlation between the tumor occurrence and some extrinsic factors such as alcohol, coffee, and cigarette smoke [24].

Although it can usually remain asymptomatic, due to its considerable size, SPN can determine clinical symptoms of stomach compression such as nausea, fullness, or dull epigastric pain [27]. Rarely weight loss, dyspepsia, and jaundice can also be observed, and occasionally lesions are identified directly on physical examination as palpable masses. In some cases, the disease is diagnosed incidentally during the execution of clinical and instrumental examinations performed for other reasons. Laboratory data are not diagnostic; these tumors do not seem to be associated with any marker in use [23].

At diagnosis most SPNs are localized only in the pancreatic gland without infiltration of the surrounding structures, characterizing it as a benign neoplasm. In 5–15 % of patients, however, liver metastases are present at diagnosis; but even in these cases, the low degree of aggressiveness of SPN determines a good prognosis [25]. The 5-year survival rate is currently over 90 % in all those patients who have undergone a radical tumor resection [25].

5.5.2 Pathology

SPN usually manifests as a solitary intrapancreatic mass. Rare is the infiltration of adjacent structures; at diagnosis usually SPNs present with considerable size. Macroscopically, the neoplasm appears as a round or oval well-circumscribed lesion with sharp margins, separated from the surrounding healthy pancreas by a fibrous capsule [28]. Sometimes calcification and septa can be found within the lesion although these are not diagnostic [23]. The tissue inside the neoplasm is usually more or less parenchymatous with presence of cystic areas due to necrotic-bleeding phenomena.

SPN in fact origins a solid mass, and only after months/years its increase in volume, poorly supported by an adequate blood supply, causes a gradual loss of neoplastic tissue with consequent formation of pseudopapillae, necrosis, and bleeding [29, 30]. The alternation of solid and cystic areas results in the pathognomonic aspect of the lesion, even if the relationship between the two components is very variable. Histologically two main types of cells are found: in the solid areas, a layer of neoplastic cells, and in the pseudopapillary component, a fibrovascular axis, surrounded by one or two layers of columnar epithelium [31].

5.5.3 MRI

SPN of the pancreas is a rare expansive lesion that can occur at any site of the pancreatic parenchyma, with sizes ranging from small to very big. The lesion is generally round or oval, with sharp edges and a thin wall; in smaller lesions, the wall may be difficult to appreciate [23, 29, 31] (Fig. 5.6).

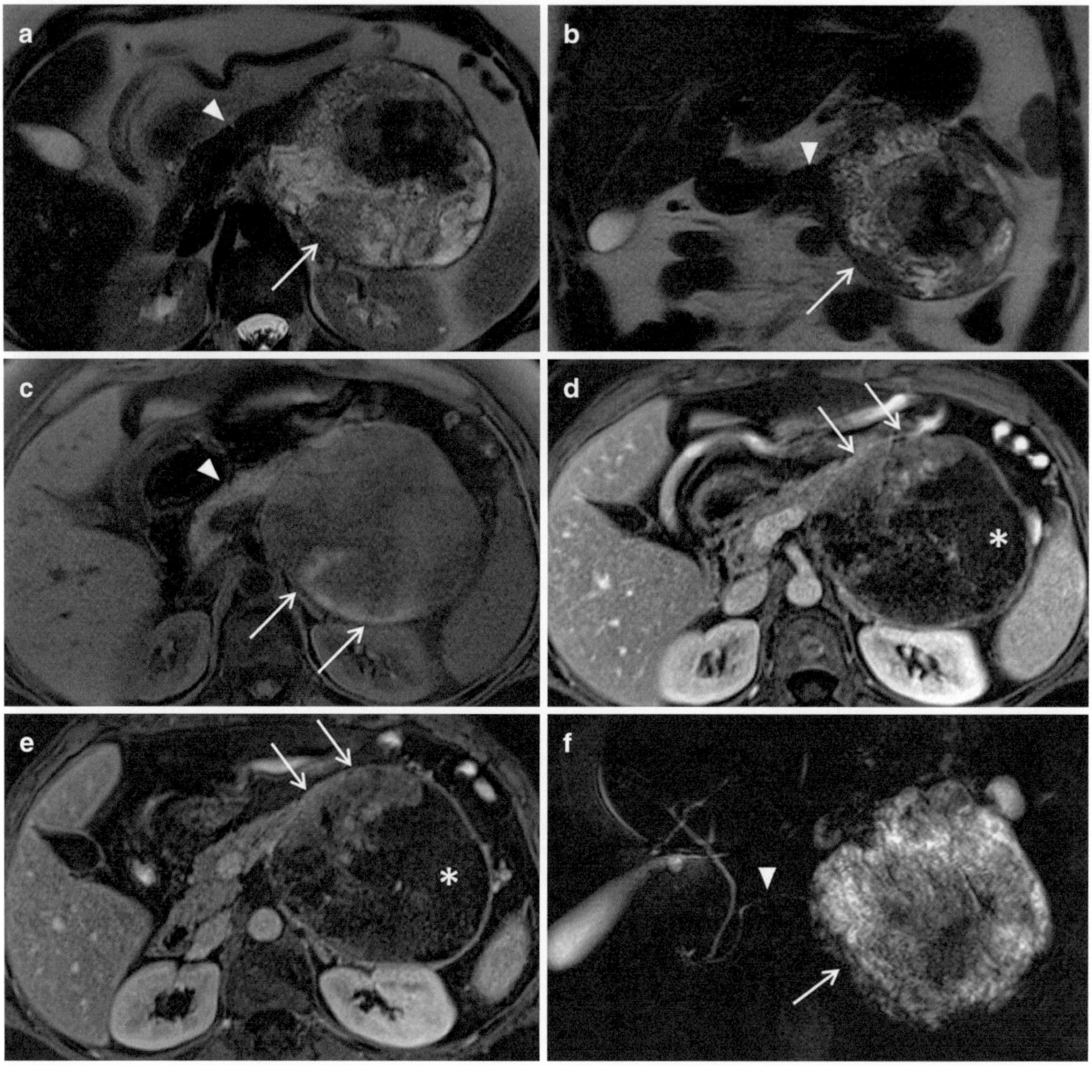

Fig. 5.6 A 43-year-old female patient with solid pseudopapillary neoplasm (SPN). (**a**, **b**) Axial (**a**) and coronal (**b**) T2-weighted images: a cystic lesion (*arrow*) is present in the tail of the pancreas; it is heterogeneously hyperintense compared to the surrounding pancreatic parenchyma (*arrowhead*). (**c**) Axial T1-weighted GRE image with fat saturation: the neoplasm is hypointense compared to the surrounding pancreatic parenchyma (*arrowhead*); hyperintense areas correspond to intralesional hemorrhage (*arrows*). (**d**, **e**) Axial T1-weighted GRE images with fat saturation after contrast administration, in pancreatic (**d**) and portal (**e**) phases: the capsule and the solid portion of the lesion (*arrow*) show contrast enhancement; cystic and hemorrhagic regions appear hypointense (*asterisk*). (**f**) MRCP image: the large cystic component of the mass (*arrow*) presents an intermediate signal in relation to the hemorrhagic intralesional component; main pancreatic duct is not dilated (*arrowhead*)

The mass is hypointense on T1-weighted images and heterogeneously hyperintense on T2-weighted images compared to the surrounding healthy pancreatic parenchyma; its signal is homogeneous or heterogeneous in relation to the different percentage of solid and cystic/hemorrhagic components [23, 24]. MRI is therefore the most effective technique to identify the presence of intralesional blood; the hemorrhagic areas present a signal variability related to the hemoglobin degradation [28]. The presence of an intralesional hyperintense zone on T1-weighted fat-suppressed images with low signal on T2 images indicates the presence of various metabolites of hemoglobin, such as methemoglobin and hemosiderin [32]. Note the appearance of these necrotic-hemorrhagic portions is usually uneven and sometimes fluid levels can also be observed [24, 28]. In addition to these aspects, it is necessary to remember that in large tumors there is a significant presence of cystic component, which appears hypointense on T1 images and markedly hyperintense on T2 images. In these images, it is easy to recognize the thick wall and the solid portion of the neoplasm represented by pseudopapillae [23, 29].

The fibrous capsule on T1-weighted images is hardly distinguishable from the lesion because of the small size and the hypointense signal; it presents low signal intensity on T2-weighted images, separating the lesion from the healthy adjacent pancreatic parenchyma [23, 29]. After contrast injection, the wall and the solid components present contrast enhancement. Solid areas, better identified after contrast administration, are noticed mainly at the periphery, while the cystic components are located most frequently in the center of the lesion [5, 23, 29].

The internal solid and cystic architecture is clearly visible both on MRI and CT images, but bleeding is more clearly delineated on MRI [29]. The presence of calcification instead represents a rare occurrence; in this case, CT is the first-line investigation.

Only rare cases of liver metastases from SPN of the pancreas have been described; even more rarely involvement and dilation of the main pancreatic duct upstream the lesion with pancreatic parenchyma atrophy have been observed. These features together with the presence of a fibrous capsule and hemorrhagic areas are key elements to differentiate SPNs from other cystic lesions of the pancreas [23, 29, 31].

When this neoplasm has an important cystic component, it can be confused with a mucinous cystic neoplasm. The latter, however, is localized preferentially in the body-tail, and it may be responsible for compressive phenomena, with dilation of the main pancreatic duct.

Serous cystadenoma compared to SPN is more frequently polycystic and microcystic; its margins are lobulated and contrast enhancement of the septa within the lesion can be observed. The presence of a central fibrous scar, not typical of SPN, with or without calcifications, indicates the presence of serous cystadenoma [5].

At diagnosis nonfunctioning neuroendocrine tumors can grow to considerable size, with consequent increase in the incidence of calcification, cystic degeneration, or central areas of necrosis and hemorrhage. However, their marked hypervascularity during the arterial phase of the dynamic study is useful for the differential diagnosis [23, 29].

Mucinous cystic neoplasms, serous cystadenoma, and neuroendocrine tumors are lesions that must always be considered in the differential diagnosis with solid pseudopapillary neoplasm in the presence of a cystic/solid pancreatic mass [3, 15].

5.6 Neuroendocrine Tumors

5.6.1 Background

Pancreatic neuroendocrine tumors (NETs) are rare tumors, 2–10 % of all primary tumors of the pancreas. They originate from multipotent stem cells of the ductal epithelium and show endocrine differentiation.

The mortality rate is significantly lower compared to pancreatic adenocarcinoma with a median survival of 7.1 years after complete resection; survival is reduced to 5.2 in cases of locally advanced disease without metastases and 2.1 years in presence of metastases.

Pancreatic NETs have no predilection for age or sex and are located in any portion of the pancreas; preferential locations depend on the histological type [33].

In 10–30 % of cases, NETs are found in patients with hereditary syndromes: MEN (multiple endocrine neoplasia) or von Hippel-Lindau syndrome (VHL).

Clinically NETs are classified as “functioning” and “nonfunctioning” tumors, in relation to the presence or absence of a specific clinical syndrome induced by hormone secretion.

Nonfunctioning NETs are the most common (60–80 % of all NETs); insulinomas and gastrinomas are the most common functioning NETs.

Clinically, these two types of cancer occur in very different ways: functioning NETs show the effects of increase hormone secretion; nonfunctioning NETs present symptoms related to compression or to the presence of metastases. In MEN-1 patients (characterized by pituitary adenomas, endocrine tumors, and hyperparathyroidism), pancreatic NETs are found in 40–80 % of patients, mainly nonfunctioning NETs. Multiple pancreatic NETs are found in 10–15 % of patients with von Hippel-Lindau syndrome [34].

Although NETs tend to be less aggressive than adenocarcinoma, they often metastasize to the liver. At diagnosis, except for insulinomas, 50–60 % of NETs present liver metastases.

5.6.2 Pathology

According the World Health Organization (WHO) classification, pancreatic NETs are divided in well-differentiated and poorly differentiated tumors.

Well-differentiated NETs have the characteristic "organoid" aspect of tumor cells, with trabecular features. Cells are generally uniform and produce abundant neurosecretory granules, reflecting the marked and diffuse immunoexpression of neuroendocrine markers such as A chromogranin A and synaptophysin.

Poorly differentiated NETs have a chaotic architecture, with irregular nuclei and poor cytoplasmic granularity. The immunoexpression of neuroendocrine markers is typically limited.

In 2006 the European Neuroendocrine Tumor Society (ENETS) proposed a classification based on the expression of mitotic index Ki67. The classification was adopted and extended by WHO in 2010:

- G1: $\leq$ 2 mitoses per 2 mm^2 and Ki-67 index $\leq$ 2%
- G2: = 2–20 mitoses per 2 mm^2 or Ki-67 index between 3 and 20 %
- G3: $\geq$ 21 mitoses per 2 mm^2 or Ki-67 index > 20%

G1 and G2 (low and intermediate grades) correspond to well-differentiated NETs and show the expression of chromogranin A and synaptophysin; G3 (high grade) indicates a poorly differentiated tumor (endocrine carcinoma) [34].

The 5-year survival rate for nonfunctioning well-differentiated NET is between 60 and 100 %; for poorly differentiated carcinomas it is 29 %.

Generally pancreatic NETs occur as solid rounded single lesions, with or without a capsule. Their dimensions are 0.5–1 cm for insulinomas and up to 10 cm for nonfunctioning NETs.

In rare cases, these masses appear considerably hemorrhagic, with bluish-purple color and soft texture. Sometimes fibrosis is massive and gives hard consistency and a whitish color.

Necrotic foci can be found within the lesions, especially in malignant masses; necrosis, if abundant, gives a cystic aspect to the neoplasm. In these cases, the differential diagnosis with cystic tumor or pseudopapillary neoplasm can be difficult.

NETs can sometimes show aspects of malignant tumors: irregular margins; infiltration of perivisceral adipose tissue, mainly through satellite nodules; and infiltration of the duodenal wall, common bile duct, spleen, or vessels. The involvement of splenic vessels with vascular thrombosis can cause splenic infarcts.

The cytological examination of material obtained by FNAB (fine-needle biopsy) is the most widely used technique for the diagnosis of pancreatic masses.

In most cases, the histological appearance of the tumors is sufficient to suggest the endocrine origin.

The presence of amyloid extracellular deposits is frequently observed in insulinomas. Because these tumors usually grow slowly, the normal structures such as ducts and pancreatic islets can be trapped inside the tumor.

5.6.3 MRI

Magnetic resonance imaging (MRI) is frequently used for the identification of pancreatic NETs and it is complementary to CT; MRI can be used to confirm a CT finding or to locate a suspicious lesion not depicted at CT. MRI advantages are the high contrast resolution, the high sensitivity of dynamic study, and the optimal visualization of pancreatic ductal system.

Nowadays MRI devices allow rapid breath-hold acquisitions, even after contrast administration, with significant reduction of motion artifacts. Diffusion-weighted imaging (DWI) is helpful for the identification of small pancreatic NETs. During the same examination, the liver can also be examined, and MRI presents higher accuracy to depict liver metastases compared to CT [35, 36].

NETs generally have hypointense signal on T1-weighted images with fat suppression and hyperintense signal on T2-weighted images compared to surrounding pancreatic tissue [37].

After contrast administration, there is a typical marked and homogeneous contrast enhancement of the lesion in both pancreatic and portal phases, which reflects the high vascularization of the tumor; in cystic NETs, there is contrast enhancement of the peripheral rim (Fig. 5.7).

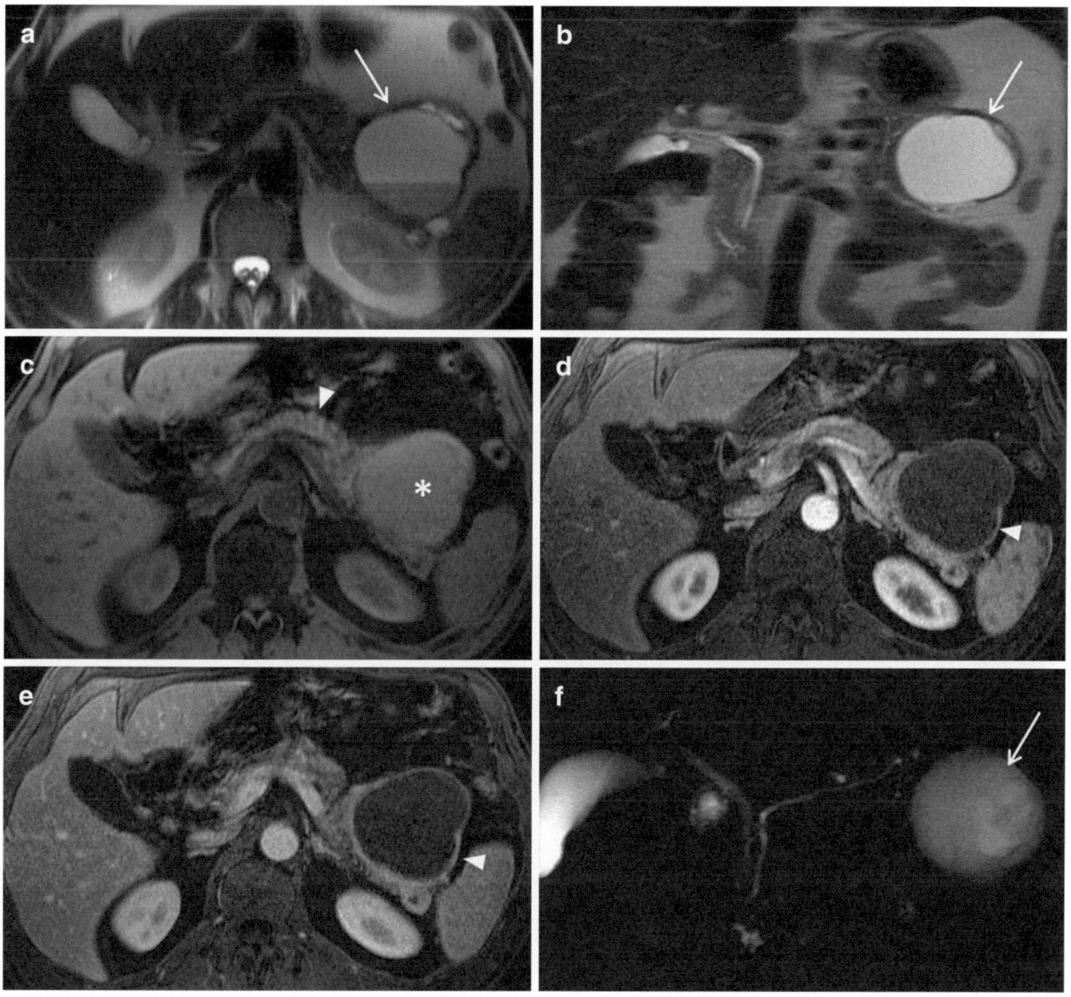

Fig. 5.7 A 58-year-old patient with cystic pancreatic neuroendocrine tumor. (**a, b**) Axial (**a**) and coronal (**b**) T2-weighted images: a hyperintense cystic mass (*arrow*) is visible in the pancreatic tail; intracystic fluid contains blood and presents two different signal intensities, because of the presence of different hemoglobin metabolites. (**c**) Axial T1-weighted GRE image with fat saturation: intracystic fluid (*asterisk*) is isointense to pancreatic parenchyma (*arrowhead*) because of the presence of blood inside the cyst. (**d, e**) Axial T1-weighted GRE images with fat saturation after contrast administration, in pancreatic (**d**) and portal (**e**) phases: cystic walls are hypervascularized (*arrowhead*). (**f**) MRCP image: cystic lesion is hyperintense (*arrow*) and it does not communicate with the main pancreatic duct

Larger tumors show a more heterogeneous contrast enhancement.

At DWI sequences, NETs usually present hyperintense signal at high-b-value images and hypointensity on ADC maps, with ADC values significantly lower than healthy pancreas [8, 9]. ADC value may vary according to specific histopathological features, such as the differentiation degree, the coexistence of intralesional hemorrhage, necrosis, and the cellularity degree. Some studies show that apparent diffusion coefficient (ADC) correlates with Ki-67 value, showing a decrease in ADC value in tumors with high expression of Ki-67 [38].

NET metastatic lesions reflect the characteristics of the primary tumor. Their most common site is the liver. Liver metastases generally are hypointense on T1-weighted images and hyperintense on T2-weighted images. In the dynamic study after contrast administration, metastatic lesions are hyperintense in the arterial phase and relatively hypointense in the portal venous phase.

In approximately 5 % of cases, pancreatic NETs present as cystic lesions (Fig. 5.7), and this aspect is found more frequently in MEN-1 patients. Cystic degeneration can also occur, mainly in functioning NET [39].

There are two forms of cystic NETs:

- Macrocystic form, characterized by the presence of a limited number (<3) of cysts with islands of neuroendocrine cells within the wall: these forms are very similar to mucinous cystic neoplasms.
- Microcystic form, characterized by the presence of numerous small cavitations localized within the tumor mass and surrounded by tumor cells; these forms are very similar to serous cystadenomas.

The preoperative diagnosis can be difficult because, although often these tumors secrete glucagon, sometimes they are nonfunctioning.

The fluid inside the cysts is hypointense on T1-weighted images and hyperintense on T2-weighted images; the wall thickness is variable. The appearance is identical to other cystic lesions of the pancreas, and often a definitive diagnosis can be obtained only after histological examination. The wall sometimes is calcified and presents early contrast enhancement in the arterial phase.

The prognosis of cystic forms is better than solid pancreatic NETs [40]. The presence of calcifications and the lack of ductal stenosis and vascular invasion can be useful aspects to differentiate NETs from adenocarcinomas.

References

1. Adet A, Miquel R, Bombi JA, Gines A, Fernandez-Esparrach G, De Juan C, et al. Incidence and characteristics of pancreatic cystic neoplasms. Gastroenterol Hepatol. 2010;33(8):563–8.
2. Zamboni G, Scarpa A, Bogina G, Iacono C, Bassi C, Talamini G, et al. Mucinous cystic tumors of the pancreas: clinicopathological features, prognosis, and relationship to other mucinous cystic tumors. Am J Surg Pathol. 1999;23(4):410–22.
3. Morana G, Guarise A. Cystic tumors of the pancreas. Cancer Imaging Off Publ Int Cancer Imaging Soc. 2006;6:60–71.
4. Salvia R, Crippa S, Falconi M, Bassi C, Guarise A, Scarpa A, et al. Branch-duct intraductal papillary mucinous neoplasms of the pancreas: to operate or not to operate? Gut. 2007;56(8):1086–90.
5. Kalb B, Sarmiento JM, Kooby DA, Adsay NV, Martin DR. MR imaging of cystic lesions of the pancreas. Radiographics Rev Publ Radiol Soc North Am Inc. 2009;29(6):1749–65.
6. Sakorafas GH, Smyrniotis V, Reid-Lombardo KM, Sarr MG. Primary pancreatic cystic neoplasms revisited. Part I: serous cystic neoplasms. Surg Oncol. 2011;20(2):e84–92.
7. Tseng JF. Management of serous cystadenoma of the pancreas. J Gastrointest Sur Off J Soc Surg Aliment Tract. 2008;12(3):408–10.
8. Bassi C, Salvia R, Gumbs AA, Butturini G, Falconi M, Pederzoli P. The value of standard serum tumor markers in differentiating mucinous from serous cystic tumors of the pancreas: CEA, Ca 19-9, Ca 125, Ca 15-3. Langenbeck's Arch Surg/Deutsche Gesellschaft fur Chirurgie. 2002;387(7-8):281–5.
9. Boraschi P, Donati F, Gigoni R, Salemi S, Bartolozzi C, Falaschi F. Diffusion-weighted MRI in the characterization of cystic pancreatic lesions: usefulness of ADC values. Magn Reson Imaging. 2010;28(10):1447–55.
10. Guarise A, Faccioli N, Ferrari M, Salvia R, Mucelli RP, Morana G, et al. Evaluation of serial changes of pancreatic branch duct intraductal papillary mucinous neoplasms by follow-up with magnetic resonance imaging. Cancer Imaging. 2008;8:220–8.

11. Kosmahl M, Pauser U, Peters K, Sipos B, Luttges J, Kremer B, et al. Cystic neoplasms of the pancreas and tumor-like lesions with cystic features: a review of 418 cases and a classification proposal. Virchows Archiv Int J Pathol. 2004;445(2):168–78.
12. Zamboni G, Bonetti F, Scarpa A, Pelosi G, Doglioni C, Iannucci A, et al. Expression of progesterone receptors in solid-cystic tumour of the pancreas: a clinicopathological and immunohistochemical study of ten cases. Virchows Arch A Pathol Anat Histopathol. 1993;423(6):425–31.
13. Procacci C, Graziani R, Bicego E, Zicari M, Bergamo Andreis IA, Zamboni G, et al. Papillary cystic neoplasm of the pancreas: radiological findings. Abdom Imaging. 1996;21(3):554–8.
14. Manfredi R, Bonatti M, D'Onofrio M, Mehrabi S, Salvia R, Mantovani W, et al. Incidentally discovered benign pancreatic cystic neoplasms not communicating with the ductal system: MR/MRCP imaging appearance and evolution. Radiol Med. 2013;118(2):163–80.
15. Kim YH, Saini S, Sahani D, Hahn PF, Mueller PR, Auh YH. Imaging diagnosis of cystic pancreatic lesions: pseudocyst versus nonpseudocyst. Radiographics Rev Publ Radiol Soc North Am Inc. 2005;25(3):671–85.
16. Tanaka M, Chari S, Adsay V, Fernandez-del Castillo C, Falconi M, Shimizu M, et al. International consensus guidelines for management of intraductal papillary mucinous neoplasms and mucinous cystic neoplasms of the pancreas. Pancreatology Off J Int Assoc Pancreatol. 2006;6(1-2):17–32.
17. Manfredi R, Graziani R, Motton M, Mantovani W, Baltieri S, Tognolini A, et al. Main pancreatic duct intraductal papillary mucinous neoplasms: accuracy of MR imaging in differentiation between benign and malignant tumors compared with histopathologic analysis. Radiology. 2009;253(1):106–15.
18. Salvia R, Crippa S, Partelli S, Armatura G, Malleo G, Paini M, et al. Differences between main-duct and branch-duct intraductal papillary mucinous neoplasms of the pancreas. World J Gastrointest Surg. 2010;2(10):342–6.
19. Vullierme MP, d'Assignies G, Ruszniewski P, Vilgrain V. Imaging IPMN: take home messages and news. Clin Res Hepatol Gastroenterol. 2011;35(6-7):426–9.
20. Irie H, Honda H, Aibe H, Kuroiwa T, Yoshimitsu K, Shinozaki K, et al. MR cholangiopancreatographic differentiation of benign and malignant intraductal mucin-producing tumors of the pancreas. AJR Am J Roentgenol. 2000;174(5):1403–8.
21. Manfredi R, Mehrabi S, Motton M, Graziani R, Ferrari M, Salvia R, et al. MR imaging and MR cholangiopancreatography of multifocal intraductal papillary mucinous neoplasms of the side branches: MR pattern and its evolution. Radiol Med. 2008;113(3):414–28.
22. Carbognin G, Pinali L, Girardi V, Casarin A, Mansueto G, Mucelli RP. Collateral branches IPMTs: secretin-enhanced MRCP. Abdom Imaging. 2007;32(3):374–80.
23. Ventriglia A, Manfredi R, Mehrabi S, Boninsegna E, Negrelli R, Pedrinolla B, et al. MRI features of solid pseudopapillary neoplasm of the pancreas. Abdom Imaging. 2014.
24. Sun CD, Lee WJ, Choi JS, Oh JT, Choi SH. Solid-pseudopapillary tumours of the pancreas: 14 years experience. ANZ J Surg. 2005;75(8):684–9.
25. Coleman KM, Doherty MC, Bigler SA. Solid-pseudopapillary tumor of the pancreas. Radiographics Rev Publ Radiol Soc North Am Inc. 2003;23(6):1644–8.
26. Cooper JA. Solid pseudopapillary tumor of the pancreas. Radiographics Rev Publ Radiol Soc North Am Inc. 2006;26(4):1210.
27. Hav M, Lem D, Chhut SV, Kong R, Pauwels P, Cuvelier C, et al. Clear-cell variant of solid-pseudopapillary neoplasm of the pancreas: a case report and review of the literature. Malays J Pathol. 2009;31(2):137–41.
28. Papavramidis T, Papavramidis S. Solid pseudopapillary tumors of the pancreas: review of 718 patients reported in English literature. J Am Coll Surg. 2005;200(6):965–72.
29. Yu MH, Lee JY, Kim MA, Kim SH, Lee JM, Han JK, et al. MR imaging features of small solid pseudopapillary tumors: retrospective differentiation from other small solid pancreatic tumors. AJR Am J Roentgenol. 2010;195(6):1324–32.
30. Zhang H, Liang TB, Wang WL, Shen Y, Ren GP, Zheng SS. Diagnosis and treatment of solid-pseudopapillary tumor of the pancreas. Hepatobiliary Pancreat Dis Int HBPD INT. 2006;5(3):454–8.
31. Yao X, Ji Y, Zeng M, Rao S, Yang B. Solid pseudopapillary tumor of the pancreas: cross-sectional imaging and pathologic correlation. Pancreas. 2010;39(4):486–91.
32. Choi JY, Kim MJ, Kim JH, Kim SH, Lim JS, Oh YT, et al. Solid pseudopapillary tumor of the pancreas: typical and atypical manifestations. AJR Am J Roentgenol. 2006;187(2):W178–86.
33. Ehehalt F, Saeger HD, Schmidt CM, Grutzmann R. Neuroendocrine tumors of the pancreas. Oncologist. 2009;14(5):456–67.
34. Klimstra DS, Modlin IR, Coppola D, Lloyd RV, Suster S. The pathologic classification of neuroendocrine tumors: a review of nomenclature, grading, and staging systems. Pancreas. 2010;39(6):707–12.
35. Rockall AG, Reznek RH. Imaging of neuroendocrine tumours (CT/MR/US). Best Pract Res Clin Endocrinol Metab. 2007;21(1):43–68.
36. Hayashi D, Tkacz JN, Hammond S, Devenney-Cakir BC, Zaim S, Bouzegaou N, et al. Gastroenteropancreatic neuroendocrine tumors: multimodality imaging features with pathological correlation. Jpn J Radiol. 2011;29(2):85–91.
37. Chang S, Choi D, Lee SJ, Lee WJ, Park MH, Kim SW, et al. Neuroendocrine neoplasms of the gastrointestinal tract: classification, pathologic basis, and imaging features. Radiographics Rev Publ Radiol Soc North Am Inc. 2007;27(6):1667–79.

38. Schmid-Tannwald C, Schmid-Tannwald CM, Morelli JN, Neumann R, Haug AR, Jansen N, et al. Comparison of abdominal MRI with diffusion-weighted imaging to 68Ga-DOTATATE PET/CT in detection of neuroendocrine tumors of the pancreas. Eur J Nucl Med Mol Imaging. 2013;40(6):897–907.
39. Kadota Y, Shinoda M, Tanabe M, Tsujikawa H, Ueno A, Masugi Y, et al. Concomitant pancreatic endocrine neoplasm and intraductal papillary mucinous neoplasm: a case report and literature review. World J Surg Oncol. 2013;11:75.
40. Scoazec JY, Vullierme MP, Barthet M, Gonzalez JM, Sauvanet A. Cystic and ductal tumors of the pancreas: diagnosis and management. J Visc Surg. 2013;150(2):69–84.

Endoscopic Ultrasound (EUS) of Cystic Tumors of the Pancreas

6

Stephan L. Haas, Urban Arnelo, J. Matthias Löhr, and Julio Iglesias-Garcia

6.1 Introduction

The rising number of cystic lesions diagnosed in the pancreas is mimicking a parallel development that was observed when computed tomography was increasingly used two decades ago. In a rising number of subjects, adrenal tumors were detected. Eventually, we learned that many of these lesions are completely benign. Consequently, these adrenal lesions were coined incidentalomas [1]. It is still a challenging task to identify those pancreatic cysts which are benign and completely harmless and those which are preneoplastic or already harboring malignant cell transformations.

EUS is a minimally invasive procedure allowing high-resolution diagnostic imaging of the pancreas, both parenchyma and duct system. Radial echoendoscopes display a 360° cross-sectional image that is perpendicular to the long axis of the scope, whereas the image of linear echoendoscopes is parallel to the long axis of the scope.

S.L. Haas, MD, PhD (✉) • U. Arnelo, MD, PhD
J.M. Löhr, MD, PhD
Center for Digestive Diseases, Karolinska University Hospital, Stockholm 14186, Sweden
e-mail: stephan.haas@karolinska.se; st.haas@ki.se; urban.arnelo@ki.se; matthias.lohr@ki.se

J. Iglesias-Garcia, MD, PhD
Department of Gastroenterology, Foundation for Research in Digestive Diseases, University Hospital Santiago de Compostela,
Santiago de Compostela, Spain
e-mail: julioiglesiasgarcia@gmail.com

Compared to radial echoendoscopes, linear echoendoscopes allow fine needle aspiration of pancreatic cysts and sampling of suspicious solid lesions and are therefore the preferred device for patients of most EUS centers when examining patients with pancreatic cysts.

In general, sedoanalgesia is used during the examination, whereas intubation and introduction of anesthesia are performed in some centers when a longer examination time is anticipated or when patients previously did not tolerate endoscopic examinations despite proper i.v. sedation.

EUS is a safe procedure with a very low complication rate. Known complications encompass perforations (e.g., hypopharynx, esophagus, duodenal bulb), complications associated with sedation, and complications due to the fine-needle aspirations.

EUS has the highest sensitivity to detect minimal changes in the pancreas but has a limited accuracy to characterize pancreatic cysts correctly.

The diagnostic accuracy of EUS to differentiate mucinous versus nonmucinous cysts was rather low in a multicenter study by Brugge and coworkers (the sensitivity, specificity, and accuracy were 56 %, 45 %, 51 %, respectively) [2].

M. Del Chiaro et al. (eds.), *Cystic Tumors of the Pancreas*, DOI 10.1007/978-3-319-31882-0_6

Operator dependency and low interobserver agreement are reasons for the limited diagnostic accuracy of EUS: Interobserver agreement was only fair ($\kappa=0.24$) for differentiation of neoplastic versus nonneoplastic cysts [3]. Agreement was moderately good ($\kappa=0.46$) for the diagnosis of SCA, but only fair for the remaining cystic lesions.

Overlapping morphological features between different PCN together with limited interobserver agreement are the main reasons that EUS alone has limited accuracy for correct cyst characterization.

6.2 EUS Morphology

A thorough examination of cystic lesions of the pancreas by EUS encompasses the evaluation of the following features: cyst type (unilocular/oligolocular/multilocular; micro-/macrocystic), cyst shape (lobulated, regular), cyst size, exact location of the cyst in the pancreas, cyst wall thickness and regularity, the presence of thin/thick septations, mural nodules, and cyst content (anechogenic, echogenic).

Moreover, the communication of the cyst with the pancreatic duct system should be assessed, and dilatation of the main pancreatic duct has to be ruled out. In any patient with a pancreatic cyst, suspicious local lymph nodes should be ruled out that could represent a pancreatic malignancy with lymph node metastasis.

The key questions for the endosonographer are: Is the pancreatic cyst a nonneoplastic (e.g., pseudocyst) or a neoplastic cyst? What is the specific entity of a neoplastic pancreatic cyst (e.g., IPMN, MCN, SCN). Is this a mucinous or a nonmucinous pancreatic cyst? Is the cyst malignant or nonmalignant?

Unfortunately, the endoscopic ultrasound has a rather low accuracy to answer these questions.

One reason for this low accuracy to differentiate different pancreatic cystic neoplasms is that the morphologic appearance is not confined to one neoplasm with some important morphological overlaps which have to be kept in mind.

Another reason is the relatively low interobserver agreement and a strong operator dependency.

In the following, the characteristic endoscopic findings of pancreatic cysts are discussed.

6.2.1 Pseudocysts

The main differential diagnosis to neoplastic cysts are pseudocysts and walled-off necroses which are found in patients with acute or chronic pancreatitis. Middle-aged men with alcohol overconsumption are often affected. Pseudocysts represent approximately 80 % of all pancreatic cysts (Fig. 6.1). The wall of pseudocysts is in the early stage thin and can become thicker during "maturation." Infrequently, septations can be found in pseudocysts. Pseudocyst with a communication with the pancreatic duct contains anechogenic pancreatic juice. Pseudocysts and especially walled-off necroses (WON) can also contain debris comprising fibrin and necrotic tissue which has an irregular echogenicity, and this necrotic material has to be differentiated from mural nodules which are adherent to the cyst wall and exhibit vascular perfusion. Debris can float within the cyst which can be detected by changing the position of the patient. Vascular perfusion of mural nodules or of irregular thickened cyst walls can be visualized by applying the color Doppler imaging. Of note, the power

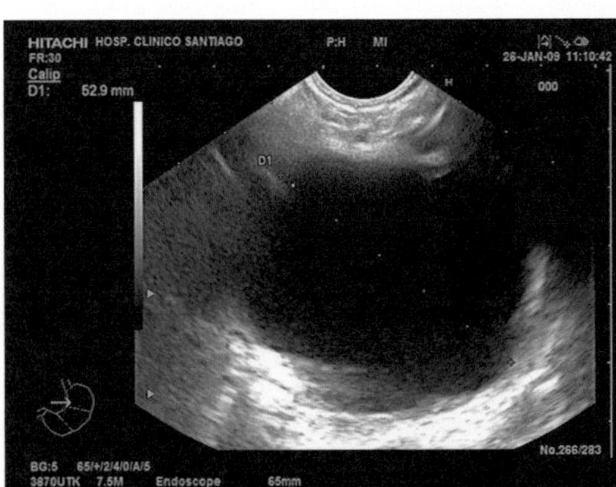

Fig. 6.1 EUS of a pseudocyst (an anechogenic unilocular cyst showing no septations)

Doppler mode has a higher sensitivity to detect small vessels with low velocity blood flow compared to the standard Doppler mode.

When the diagnosis of a pseudocyst is inconclusive, FNA can be performed to rule out MCN as the main differential diagnosis (pseudocyst: amylase >5000 U/mL, CEA <5 mg/L).

6.2.2 Congenital Simple Pancreatic Cysts

Typically this monolocular round or slightly oval cyst has thin regular cyst wall with a complete anechogenic cyst content and is found in a pancreas with no other abnormalities such as signs of chronic pancreatitis. These simple cysts can be a manifestation of a von Hippel-Lindau syndrome or are associated with polycystic kidney disease.

An EUS-FNA is usually not performed when these cysts are >1 cm large. Low amylase and CEA levels can be expected in the cyst fluid.

6.2.3 Serous Cystic Neoplasm (SCN)

Serous cystic neoplasms are most often (>80 %) found in the body and tail of female subjects (Fig. 6.2). This benign cystic neoplasm is composed of numerous microscopic (<2 mm) cysts (multilocular, microcystic) and can be misdiagnosed as a lobular-shaped solid tumor when a CECT is performed. A central calcification represented by a strong echogenic signal is considered as pathognomonic but is found only in less than 20 % of cases. In contrast to IPMN, no communication to the pancreatic duct system is present, and neither the main pancreatic duct (MPD) nor the side branches are dilated.

The oligocystic SCN subtype is composed of larger cysts and can have a similar appearance to mucinous cystic neoplasms (MCN). The diagnosis of SCN can frequently be made with high accuracy so that FNA is only in a small number of patients indicated. In contrast, to establish the correct diagnosis of a atypical oligocystic SCN, FNA is frequently required for further cyst characterization. In small cysts, fine-needle aspiration of cyst fluid can pose a problem. If FNA is successful, cyst fluid analysis demonstrates low CEA and low amylase levels, cellularity is often sparse and can demonstrate glycogen positive cuboidal cells.

6.2.4 Mucinous Cystic Neoplasm (MCN)

Mucinous cystic neoplasms (MCN) are characteristically found in middle-aged woman (90 %) representing an unilocular or oligolocular cyst (single cyst or few macrocysts) in the body and tail of the pancreas (Fig. 6.3). In around 15 % of cases, calcifications of the cyst wall or calcified

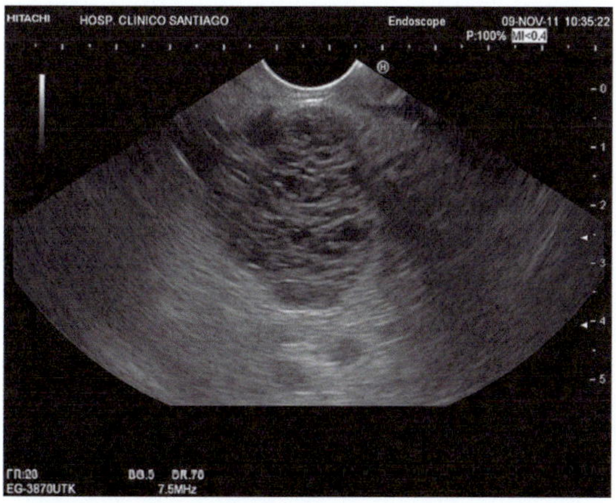

Fig. 6.2 EUS of a serous cystic neoplasm (SCN) demonstrating numerous microcysts

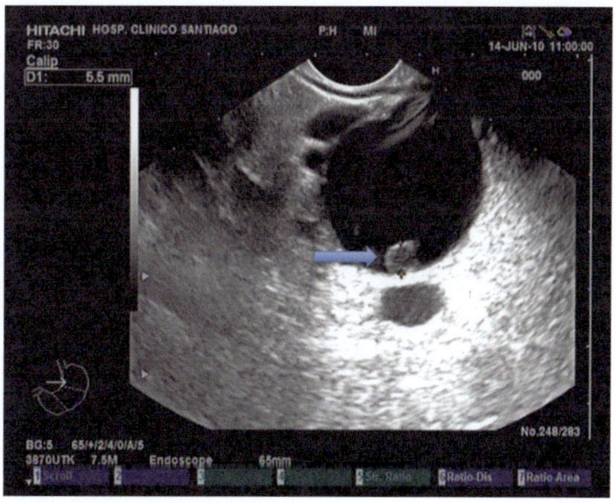

Fig. 6.3 EUS of a mucinous cystic neoplasm (MCN) with a mural nodule (*arrow*)

septations are visible. These cystic tumors are preneoplastic lesions or have already progressed to malignancy.

Warning signs indicating malignancy are large diameter (>3 cm), mural nodules, a thick and irregular cyst wall, thick septations, and an obstructed pancreatic duct. Irregular hypoechogenic lesions adjacent to a MCN indicate malignant infiltration.

EUS-FNA can confirm the suspicion of a mucinous cystic neoplasm by the evidence of an intracystic elevation of CEA (192 ng/mL) and the detection of mucin. Very high CEA levels indicate malignancy, but in some malignant MCN, CEA is low. High viscosity is a key feature of both MCN and IPMN and hampers aspiration of cyst fluid. Viscous mucin-rich cyst fluid can easily be appreciated by the so-called string sign [4]. Cystic subtypes of pancreatic neuroendocrine tumors (NET) are rare but can resemble a MCN. of note, they can show a very thick wall (Fig. 6.4).

6.2.5 Intraductal Papillary Mucinous Neoplasia (IPMN)

Mucinous cystic neoplasm and intraductal papillary mucinous neoplasia (IPMN) are the two mucinous cystic tumors with a clear risk for malignancy. The goal is to diagnose these two tumors with high accuracy. IPMN is most often localized in the pancreatic head and represents a multilocular, multicystic tumor which can have grapelike appearance (Figs. 6.5 and 6.6). Most often patients with IPMN are seen by the endoscopists when the cysts were incidentally detected by cross-sectional imaging or during the workup of recurrent pancreatitis.

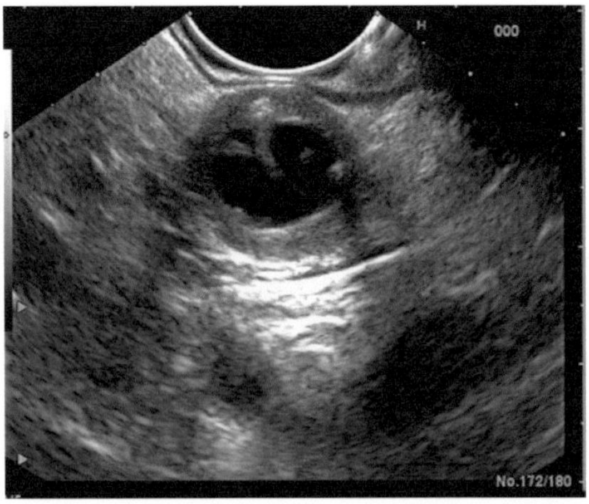

Fig. 6.4 EUS of cystic pancreatic neuroendocrine tumor (NET) with a prominent wall

Endoscopy can reveal in 25–50 % of patients a gaping fishmouth papilla with protruding viscous mucus [5]. Visualization of the papilla is easier with a radial echoendoscope than a linear echoendoscope.

The delineation of a communication between the cystic lesion and the main/side duct branches is sometimes difficult but is an important feature to differentiate IPMN from MCN. Dilatation of the main duct can be moderate or marked and segmental or diffuse. A dilatation of the MPD >5 mm without other causes of obstruction should raise the suspicion for main-duct (MD)-IPMN [6].

Due to obstruction, parenchymal changes can be observed in patients with IPMN that can resemble sonographic signs of chronic pancreatitis. A thorough inspection of the whole pancreas is mandatory to rule out multifocal IPMN. IPMN features of a potential malignancy are localization of the cyst in the main pancreatic duct (MD-IPMN), a prominent dilatation of the main pancreatic duct (MPD > 10 mm), a diameter of >3 cm of a side-branch IPMN, mural nodules (>10 mm) within the cysts, and solid lesions adjacent to the cyst [7]. Of note, EUS is the most sensitive method to detect mural nodules [8–11].

EUS-guided fine-needle aspiration of cyst fluid can be challenging due to the viscous nature of the cyst fluid and when IPMN is located in the pancreatic head. CEA levels in the cyst fluid are generally elevated. No definite cutoff is established, but a cutoff of ≥192–200 ng/mL enables the diagnosis of a mucinous cyst with an accuracy of approximately 80 % [2, 6, 12]. Importantly, a low CEA level does not exclude IPMN. Due to the communication of IPMN with pancreatic duct system, amylase levels in IPMN (like in pseudocysts) are high (>250 U/L). This is an important feature when differentiating IPMN from MCN. The accuracy of EUS-FNA to diagnose IPMN was in one study very high (sensitivity of 82 %, a specificity

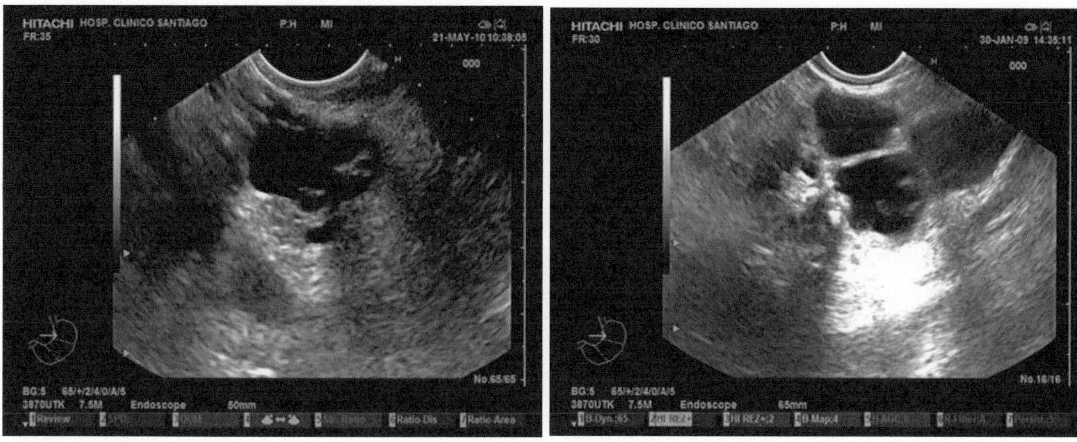

Figs. 6.5 and 6.6 EUS of a branch-duct IPMN with a grapelike cystic structure

of 100 %, positive predictive value of 100 %, negative predictive value of 92 %, and accuracy of 94 %) [13].

Other studies could not replicate these very positive results [2, 14, 15].

Apart from morphological features, CEA cyst levels and cytology can contribute to identify malignancy in IPMN. Suspicious mural nodules and solid areas should also be sampled. In a study from Indianapolis/the USA, the sensitivity, specificity, and accuracy of EUS-FNA for the diagnosis of malignancy in IPMNs were 75 %, 91 %, and 86 %, respectively, while the level of CEA has of limited prognostic value [16]. In a similar study which used a cyst fluid CEA > 200 ng/mL as cutoff, CEA had a low accuracy to detect malignant IPMN (sensitivity, specificity, positive predictive value, negative predictive value, and accuracy of a cyst fluid were 52.4 %, 42.3 %, 42.3 %, 52.4 %, and 46.8 %, respectively) [17].

6.3 EUS-Fine-Needle Aspiration (EUS-FNA)

A meta-analysis of 51 articles with a total of 10,941 patients confirmed that EUS-FNA is a relatively safe procedure with a low complication risk profile [18]. The overall complication rate of EUS in combination with FNA is higher than EUS without FNA, and the complication rate of EUS-FNA of pancreatic cysts is higher than EUS-FNA of solid pancreatic lesions (2.75 % versus 0.82 %). After EUS-FNA, pancreatitis was seen in 1.1 %, bleeding in 0.3 %, infection in 0.2 %, abdominal pain in 0.8 %, and fever in 0.3 %.

EUS-FNA for pancreatic cysts may have a higher risk of infection compared with EUS-FNA of solid masses, and a retrospective study demonstrated an infection rate of 1.1 % in patients with antibiotic prophylaxis versus 0.6 % in patients without antibiotic use [19]. Prospective studies are lacking but are warranted. Despite the lack of strong evidence, the prophylactic of a single shot of antibiotic prior to EUS-FNA followed by 3–5 days of oral antibiotics is a daily practice and recommended for EUS-FNA for pancreatic cysts (fluoroquinolones or beta-lactam antibiotics).

Rarely, fine-needle aspirations of the pancreatic cyst can lead to an intracystic or retroperitoneal bleeding or acute pancreatitis but is usually self-limited. In most cases, pancreatitis after EUS was mild, but one developed a fatal severe pancreatitis [18].

Due to the close proximity of the echoendoscope to the pancreas, tumor seeding occurs very rarely, and few cases are reported in the literature including one patient with peritoneal tumor seeding after EUS-FNA of IPMN [20].

Even if only cytology can be obtained, besides the diagnostic evaluation of the cells, analysis of the mucous is very valuable. To safely place the needle within the cyst, a minimum size of 1 cm is suggested. Cyst fluid is usually aspirated with a single pass using a G22 or G25 aspiration needle. In larger cysts and if mucus is likely, the use of a G19 needle might be advantageous.

With a rather simple test directly after EUS-FNA, cyst fluid can be tested for viscous mucin, suggesting the presence of mucinous cystic neoplasms (IPMN and MCN): a drop is taken between two fingers and is pulled apart. A string forms in a drop of cyst fluid spread between two gloved fingers. A distraction of 3.5 mm has been suggested to be consistent with a mucinous cyst. Mucinous cyst fluid had a median string length of 3.5 mm in an analysis of 50 mucinous and 29 nonmucinous cysts [21]. Importantly, there is an overlap of the string sign: the string length ranged from 0 to 9 mm in nonmucinous cyst fluid and from 2 to 20 mm in mucinous cyst fluid.

In a study of 98 histologically proven pancreatic cysts, the string sign was highly specific (95 %) for the diagnosis of mucinous pancreatic cysts (length of the string, 10 mm) [4]. Without any further testing, a positive string sign was found to be 11 times more likely in a patient with a mucinous pancreatic cyst than in a patient with a nonmucinous cyst. It has to be kept in mind that a negative string sign does not exclude a mucinous cyst due to relatively low sensitivity with a low negative predictive value (sensitivity, 58 %; specificity, 95 %; positive predictive value, 94 %; negative predictive value, 60 %) [4].

6.4 Contrast-Enhanced Endoscopic Ultrasound

Contrast-enhanced transabdominal ultrasound (CEUS) and contrast-enhanced endoscopic ultrasound (CE-EUS) can be applied to further characterize the microperfusion of pancreatic lesions. In Europe hexafluoride microbubbles (SonoVue, Bracco UK Ltd., UK) are most widely used in an off-label setting. The perfusion of pancreatic lesions can be increased or decreased in comparison to the rest of the pancreas [22]. After the intravenous application of a contrast agent, a pancreatic cyst is non-perfused but the microvascularization of the cyst wall, thicker septations, or mural nodes can be visualized by an enhancement. Solid hypoechogenic areas of malignancy can be demonstrated by a reduced perfusion (reduced enhancement after i.v. administration of the contrast agent).

Particularly the detection of mural nodules in mucinous cystic neoplasms (IPMN, MCN) is of critical importance as these nodules represent a warning sign for potential malignancy. These mural nodules can be mimicked by debris and necrotic material in a pancreatic cyst. In a large study from Japan, 581 patients with pancreatic cysts received standard EUS followed by CEUS. In this study, CEUS was superior in discriminating mural nodules from mucus clots and distinguished more accurately malignant from benign pancreatic cysts [23]. The detection of mural nodules by CEUS had an excellent reproducibility, and interobserver agreement was higher in CEUS than standard EUS (kappa coefficient 0.83 versus 0.69).

6.5 Probe-Based Confocal Laser Endomicroscopy (pCLE)

Probe-based confocal laser endomicroscopy enables the in vivo and real-time microscopic evaluation of the epithelium throughout the gastrointestinal tract and can even be used in combination with ERCP and EUS [24]. During EUS, a mini probe (0.632 mm of diameter) is introduced through a G19 needle into a cyst (needle-based CLE or nCLE) [25, 26].

First feasibility results proved the safety of this method (21924718). In the INSPECT study, the villous structures of IPMN were characterized by nCLE with a 3 % risk for acute pancreatitis and an overall complication risk of 9 % [27]. Diagnosing IPMN by the identification of epithelial villous structures by nCLE had a limited sensitivity of 59 %, a rather low negative predictive value of 50 % but a very high specificity of 100 % and a high positive predictive value of 100 %.

Moreover, this method has a high accuracy for the diagnosis of serous cystic neoplasms (SCA) with good interobserver agreement: by the detection of the characteristic dense subepithelial capillary vascularization of the cyst wall, nCLE had a sensitivity, specificity, and accuracy of 69, 100, and 87 % in a recent study with 31 patients [28]. This has the potential to reduce unnecessary surgical resections or follow-up imaging in SCA patients.

Recently, nCLE criteria for other pancreatic cyst entities such as pseudocysts, MCN, and cystic neuroendocrine tumors (NET) were presented which correlated with pathological specimens: MCN, gray epithelial band with a thin dark line; pseudocysts, field of bright, gray and black particles; and cystic NEN, dark spots surrounded by gray areas [28].

Conclusion

Surgeons and gastroenterologists are confronted with an increasing number of patients with pancreatic cysts. In most centers, MRT/MRCP is regarded as the primary imaging method of choice. When diagnosis is inconclusive, EUS especially in combination with EUS-FNA is a valuable tool to further characterize cystic pancreatic neoplasms. Combination of additional EUS tools such as contrast enhancement and elastography has the potential to further increase the accuracy of EUS in the detection of cystic and solid lesion of the pancreas.

References

1. Anagnostis P, Karagiannis A, Tziomalos K, Kakafika AI, Athyros VG, Mikhailidis DP. Adrenal incidentaloma: a diagnostic challenge. Hormones (Athens). 2009;8(3):163–84.
2. Brugge WR, Lewandrowski K, Lee-Lewandrowski E, Centeno BA, Szydlo T, Regan S, et al. Diagnosis of pancreatic cystic neoplasms: a report of the cooperative pancreatic cyst study. Gastroenterology. 2004;126(5):1330–6.
3. Ahmad NA, Kochman ML, Brensinger C, Brugge WR, Faigel DO, Gress FG, et al. Interobserver agreement among endosonographers for the diagnosis of neoplastic versus non-neoplastic pancreatic cystic lesions. Gastrointest Endosc. 2003;58(1):59–64.
4. Bick BL, Enders FT, Levy MJ, Zhang L, Henry MR, Abu Dayyeh BK, et al. The string sign for diagnosis of mucinous pancreatic cysts. Endoscopy. 2015;47(7):626–31.
5. Inui K, Nakazawa S, Yoshino J, Yamachika H, Kanemaki N, Wakabayashi T, et al. Mucin-producing tumor of the pancreas – intraluminal ultrasonography. Hepatogastroenterology. 1998;45(24):1996–2000.
6. Tanaka M, Fernandez-del Castillo C, Adsay V, Chari S, Falconi M, Jang JY, et al. International consensus guidelines 2012 for the management of IPMN and MCN of the pancreas. Pancreatology. 2012;12(3):183–97.
7. Kubo H, Chijiiwa Y, Akahoshi K, Hamada S, Harada N, Sumii T, et al. Intraductal papillary-mucinous tumors of the pancreas: differential diagnosis between benign and malignant tumors by endoscopic ultrasonography. Am J Gastroenterol. 2001;96(5):1429–34.
8. Lim LG, Itoi T, Lim WC, Mesenas SJ, Seo DW, Tan J, et al. Current status on the diagnosis and management of pancreatic cysts in the Asia-Pacific region: role of endoscopic ultrasound. J Gastroenterol Hepatol. 2011;26(12):1702–8.
9. Kobayashi G, Fujita N, Noda Y, Ito K, Horaguchi J, Takasawa O, et al. Mode of progression of intraductal papillary-mucinous tumor of the pancreas: analysis of patients with follow-up by EUS. J Gastroenterol. 2005;40(7):744–51.
10. Baba T, Yamaguchi T, Ishihara T, Kobayashi A, Oshima T, Sakaue N, et al. Distinguishing benign from malignant intraductal papillary mucinous tumors of the pancreas by imaging techniques. Pancreas. 2004;29(3):212–7.
11. Ohno E, Hirooka Y, Itoh A, Ishigami M, Katano Y, Ohmiya N, et al. Intraductal papillary mucinous neoplasms of the pancreas: differentiation of malignant and benign tumors by endoscopic ultrasound findings of mural nodules. Ann Surg. 2009;249(4):628–34.
12. Park WG, Mascarenhas R, Palaez-Luna M, Smyrk TC, O'Kane D, Clain JE, et al. Diagnostic performance of cyst fluid carcinoembryonic antigen and amylase in histologically confirmed pancreatic cysts. Pancreas. 2011;40(1):42–5.
13. Fernandez-Esparrach G, Pellise M, Sole M, Soria MT, Miquel R, Mata A, et al. EUS FNA in intraductal papillary mucinous tumors of the pancreas. Hepatogastroenterology. 2007;54(73):260–4.
14. Centeno BA, Warshaw AL, Mayo-Smith W, Southern JF, Lewandrowski K. Cytologic diagnosis of pancreatic cystic lesions. A prospective study of 28 percutaneous aspirates. Acta Cytol. 1997;41(4):972–80.
15. de Jong K, Bruno MJ, Fockens P. Epidemiology, diagnosis, and management of cystic lesions of the pancreas. Gastroenterol Res Pract. 2012;2012: 147465.
16. Pais SA, Attasaranya S, Leblanc JK, Sherman S, Schmidt CM, DeWitt J. Role of endoscopic ultrasound in the diagnosis of intraductal papillary mucinous neoplasms: correlation with surgical histopathology. Clin Gastroenterol Hepatol. 2007;5(4):489–95.
17. Kucera S, Centeno BA, Springett G, Malafa MP, Chen YA, Weber J, et al. Cyst fluid carcinoembryonic antigen level is not predictive of invasive cancer in patients with intraductal papillary mucinous neoplasm of the pancreas. JOP. 2012;13(4):409–13.
18. Wang KX, Ben QW, Jin ZD, Du YQ, Zou DW, Liao Z, et al. Assessment of morbidity and mortality associ-

ated with EUS-guided FNA: a systematic review. Gastrointest Endosc. 2011;73(2):283–90.
19. Guarner-Argente C, Shah P, Buchner A, Ahmad NA, Kochman ML, Ginsberg GG. Use of antimicrobials for EUS-guided FNA of pancreatic cysts: a retrospective, comparative analysis. Gastrointest Endosc. 2011;74(1):81–6.
20. Hirooka Y, Goto H, Itoh A, Hashimoto S, Niwa K, Ishikawa H, et al. Case of intraductal papillary mucinous tumor in which endosonography-guided fine-needle aspiration biopsy caused dissemination. J Gastroenterol Hepatol. 2003;18:1323–4. Australia.
21. Leung KK, Ross WA, Evans D, Fleming J, Lin E, Tamm EP, et al. Pancreatic cystic neoplasm: the role of cyst morphology, cyst fluid analysis, and expectant management. Ann Surg Oncol. 2009;16(10):2818–24.
22. D'Onofrio M, Biagioli E, Gerardi C, Canestrini S, Rulli E, Crosara S, et al. Diagnostic performance of contrast-enhanced ultrasound (CEUS) and contrast-enhanced endoscopic ultrasound (ECEUS) for the differentiation of pancreatic lesions: a systematic review and meta-analysis. Ultraschall Med. 2014;35(6):515–21.
23. Kamata K, Kitano M, Omoto S, Kadosaka K, Miyata T, Yamao K, et al. Contrast-enhanced harmonic endoscopic ultrasonography for differential diagnosis of pancreatic cysts. Endoscopy. 2016;48(1):35–41.
24. Löhr JM, Lonnebro R, Stigliano S, Haas SL, Swahn F, Enochsson L, et al. Outcome of probe-based confocal laser endomicroscopy (pCLE) during endoscopic retrograde cholangiopancreatography: A single-center prospective study in 45 patients. United Eur Gastroenterol J. 2015;3(6):551–60.
25. Tsujino T, Yan-Lin Huang J, Nakai Y, Samarasena JB, Lee JG, Chang KJ. In vivo identification of pancreatic cystic neoplasms with needle-based confocal laser endomicroscopy. Best Pract Res Clin Gastroenterol. 2015;29(4):601–10.
26. Giovannini M. Needle-based confocal laser endomicroscopy. Endosc Ultrasound. 2015;4(4):284–8.
27. Konda VJ, Meining A, Jamil LH, Giovannini M, Hwang JH, Wallace MB, et al. A pilot study of in vivo identification of pancreatic cystic neoplasms with needle-based confocal laser endomicroscopy under endosonographic guidance. Endoscopy. 2013;45(12): 1006–13.
28. Napoleon B, Lemaistre AI, Pujol B, Caillol F, Lucidarme D, Bourdariat R, et al. In vivo characterization of pancreatic cystic lesions by needle-based confocal laser endomicroscopy (nCLE): proposition of a comprehensive nCLE classification confirmed by an external retrospective evaluation. Surg Endosc. 2015 [Epub ahead of print].

7 Endoscopy in Cystic Tumors of the Pancreas

Andrea Tringali and Guido Costamagna

7.1 Introduction

The main endoscopic approach to cystic tumors of the pancreas is today represented by EUS.

Endoscopic evaluation of the papilla of Vater and visualization of the pancreatic ductal system by ERCP and/or peroral pancreatoscopy (POPS) can have a role in pancreatic cystic tumors (mainly IPMN) communicating with the main pancreatic duct (MPD).

The diagnostic role of ERCP in IPMN for pancreatic juice sampling or MPD brushings is not routinely recommended and should be reserved in the context of research [1].

A therapeutic role of endoscopic pancreatic sphincterotomy (EPS) can be considered to reduce the episodes of pancreatitis recurrence due to mucus-related MPD obstruction.

Another role of endoscopy in cystic tumors of the pancreas is the identification of synchronous and metachronous gastrointestinal malignancies; despite there are no screening recommendations at present [1], screening of colorectal polyps and cancer in patients with IPMN was proposed [2, 3].

A. Tringali, MD, PhD (✉)
G. Costamagna, MD, FACG
Digestive Endoscopy Unit, Fondazione Policlinico Gemelli – Catholic University, Rome, Italy
e-mail: andrea.tringali@rm.unicatt.it; gcostamagna@rm.unicatt.it

7.2 Duodenoscopy

Visualization of the papilla of Vater with the side-viewing endoscope permits to diagnose IPMN when a swollen papilla with mucous secretion ("fish-eye appearance") (Fig. 7.1) is identified. This finding can also have clinical and therapeutic implications.

Episodes of acute pancreatitis seem to be significantly more common in cases of IPMN with a dilated papilla with mucin extrusion [4]. The "fish-eye appearance" of the papilla could be also a factor to predict intestinal-type IPMN [4, 5], in

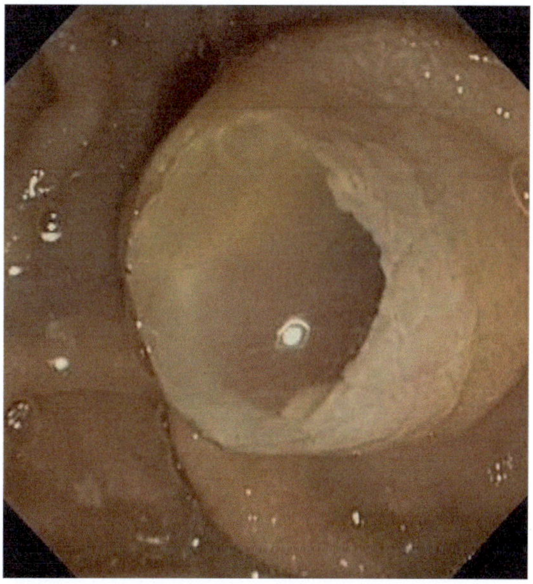

Fig. 7.1 Fish-eye appearance of the papilla of Vater

M. Del Chiaro et al. (eds.), *Cystic Tumors of the Pancreas*, DOI 10.1007/978-3-319-31882-0_7

both main-duct (MD) and branch-duct (BD) IPMN [5]. Intestinal-subtype IPMN seems to have higher grades of dysplasia but a better prognosis after resection, compared with nonintestinal types [6]; a preoperative diagnosis of intestinal-subtype IPMN can be considered to shorten the surveillance interval and to recommend surgical resection [5]. Nevertheless, these interesting observations are obtained from retrospective studies.

The possible correlation between the papilla of Vater aspect and IPMN prognosis needs to be carefully evaluated in prospective studies.

7.3 ERCP

The diagnostic role of ERCP in IPMN is limited to the possibility for pancreatic juice sampling by MPD aspiration, brush, and lavage. A recent meta-analysis [7] showed a 97 % specificity and 35 % sensitivity for ERCP-based pancreatic juice cytology to distinguish benign from malignant IPMN; this poor sensitivity does not justify the ERCP-related risks of complications for diagnostic purposes.

To overcome the low sensitivity of cytology, a cutoff value of 30 ng/mL for carcinoembryonic antigen in pancreatic juice was proposed obtaining an 84 % sensitivity [8]. Another small series [9] showed an 89 % sensitivity to distinguish benign from malignant IPMN using the dosage of MUC1 mRNA on pancreatic juice.

Pancreatic juice collection in IPMN is therefore limited to the research [1] of novel biomarkers of neoplastic degeneration.

EPS can have a therapeutic role in IPMN. Recurrent pancreatitis in IPMN can be related to MPD hypertension secondary to viscous mucus. EPS can reduce MPD obstruction especially in the absence of a patulous papilla (Fig. 7.2). EPS is a "symptomatic" maneuver that can have an indication in patients with IPMN not candidate to surgery or under follow-up when the surgical decision is not undertaken. Few data were published regarding the role of EPS in IPMN; according to a small series [10], EPS resulted effective in reducing the rate of pancreatitis recurrence due to IPMN after a 4-year follow-up. Future prospective evaluation can better define the role of EPS in symptomatic IPMN not candidate to surgery.

7.4 Pancreatoscopy

Peroral pancreatoscopy (POPS) was described 40 years ago, but it still is a complex and expensive technique. Technological refinements lead to the availability of ultrathin pancreatoscopes with enhanced image capabilities (i.e., narrow band imaging) and the possibility for direct tissue acquisition with biopsy forceps. POPS during the last years gained more widespread use after the introduction of a disposable, single-operator miniscope (SpyGlass) which recently significantly improved the quality of the pictures with digital technology (SpyGlass DS).

In a series of 31 patients undergoing surgery for IPMN, pancreatoscopy resulted feasible in 60 % of cases (93 % for main-duct IPMN) [11]. The reported success rate of POPS in IPMN with the SpyGlass system was >90 % [12, 13].

Many studies have evaluated pancreatoscopy to characterize IPMN as a preoperative staging tool [14, 15] or even during duodenopancreatectomy [16].

In a large cohort, the correlation between pancreatoscopic appearance of IPMN and histological samples after surgery was described [17]. Lesions were classified in five types: I (granular type) and II (fish-egg-like type without vascular images) were never associated to malignancy; III (fish-egg-like images with vascular images), IV (villous type), and V (vegetative type) were associated in 90 % of the cases with malignancy. In this study, the accuracy of POPS to differentiate malignant from benign IPMN was 88 % for MD-IPMN and 67 % for BD-IPMN.

Initially, pancreatoscopy-assisted pancreatic fluid aspiration was reported to be more accurate than nasopancreatic tube insertion by ERCP and fluid aspiration in the detection of carcinoma in situ of the pancreas by cytology [18]. Later, a comparative study disclosed similar results for the

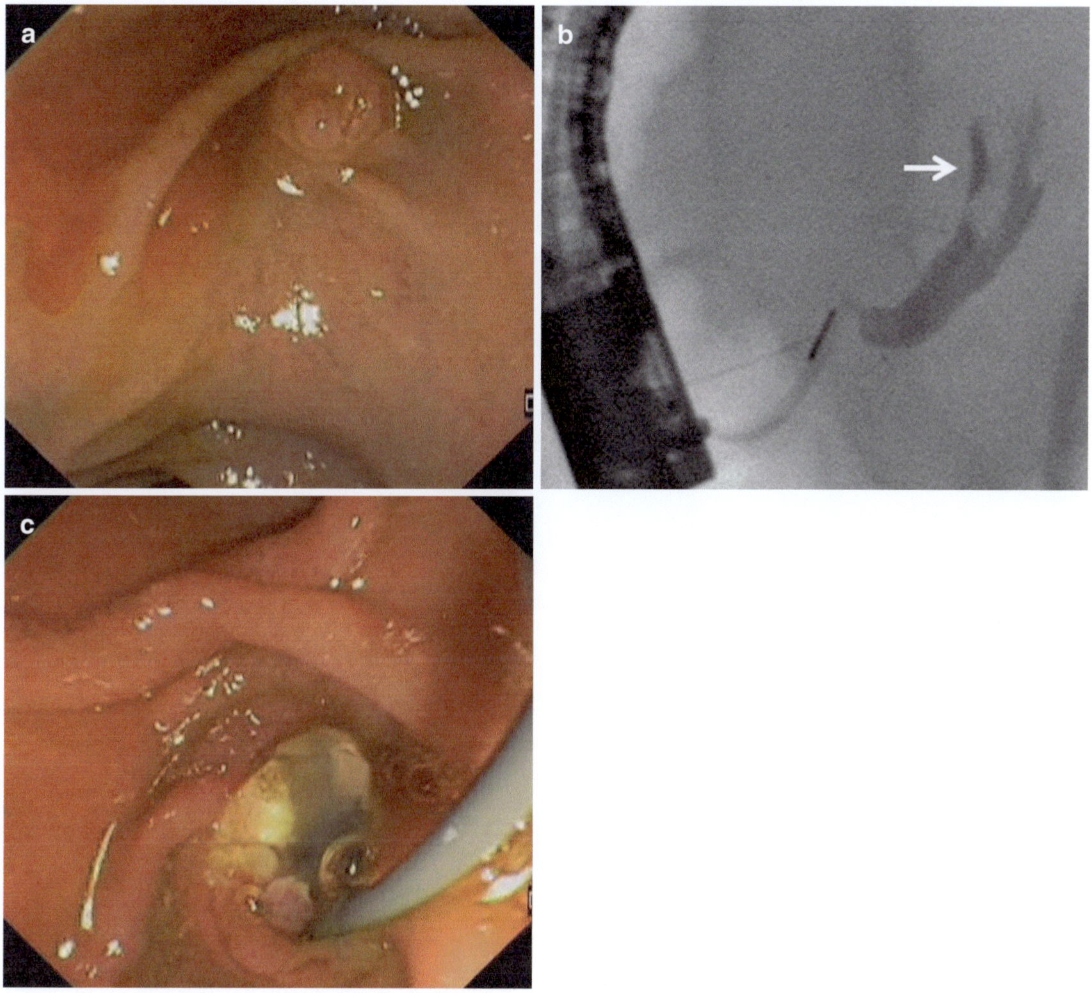

Fig. 7.2 Normal-appearing papilla in a case of branch-duct IPMN (**a**). Pancreatography shows a mucus-related filling defect in the main pancreatic (*arrow*) (**b**). After endoscopic pancreatic sphincterotomy, mucus passage is visible (**c**)

detection of malignancy among IPMN by POPS compared to nasopancreatic tube collection [19]. More recently, few series with new pancreatoscopes and ultrathin forceps have reported the realization of pancreatic ductal biopsies under direct visualization by POPS, but their accuracy in histological sample is unknown [20, 21].

Video pancreatoscopes with NBI seem to provide a better identification of malignant IPMN [11], but further evaluations are needed.

POPS-aided assessment of the excision margin during pancreatectomy for IPMN was described in small series [13, 14] but was never compared to preoperative frozen section.

Preoperative identification of main-duct IPMN (Fig. 7.3) and the possibility for "tattooing" the resection margin [22] can be a topic for future studies.

Intraoperative pancreatoscopy was described [16] but is not recommended due to the risk of mucin leakage [1].

The main complication of POPS is pancreatitis which was reported in 10–12% of the cases and mainly consisted of mild pancreatitis [23].

Despite being a promising technique, today no evidence exists regarding the usefulness of pancreatoscopy in the management of cystic tumors of the pancreas [24].

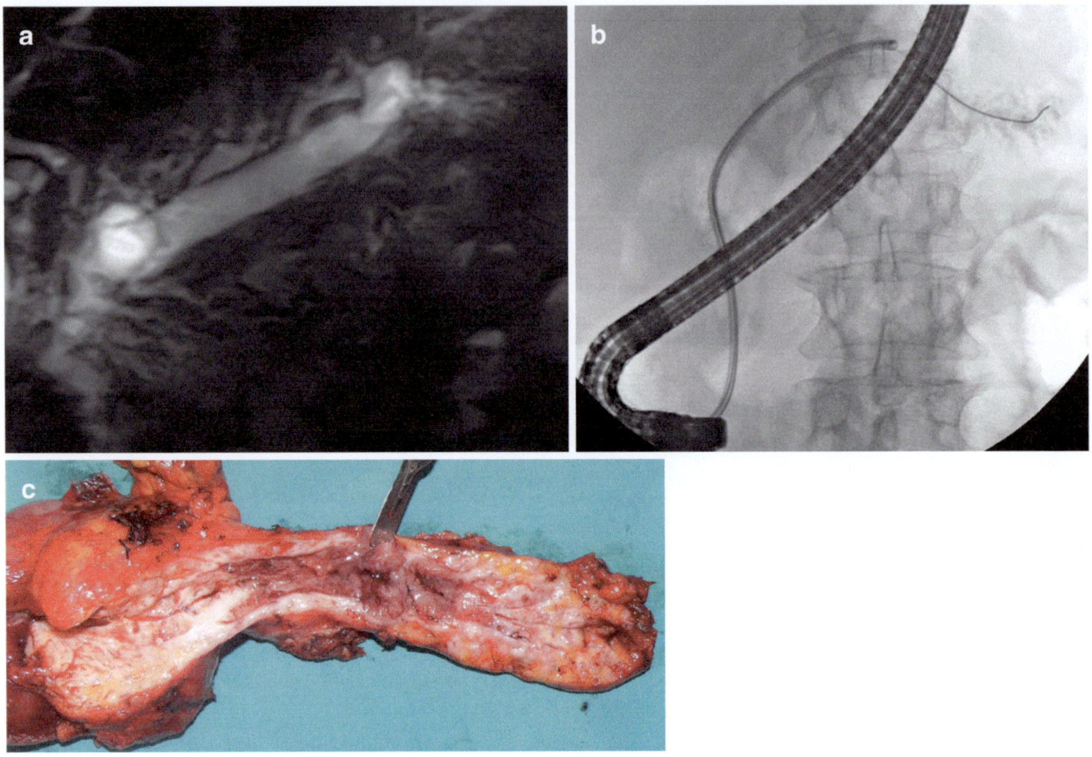

Fig. 7.3 Magnetic resonance cholangiopancreatography shows a main-duct IPMN (**a**). Peroral pancreatoscopy identified the site of the lesion at the body/tail of the pancreas (**b**). Indication for total pancreatectomy is confirmed on the surgical specimen (**c**)

References

1. Tanaka M, Fernández-del Castillo C, Adsay V, Chari S, Falconi M, Jang JY, Kimura W, Levy P, Pitman MB, Schmidt CM, Shimizu M, Wolfgang CL, Yamaguchi K, Yamao K, International Association of Pancreatology. International consensus guidelines 2012 for the management of IPMN and MCN of the pancreas. Pancreatology. 2012;12(3):183–97.
2. Reid-Lombardo KM, Mathis KL, Wood CM, Harmsen WS, Sarr MG. Frequency of extrapancreatic neoplasms in intraductal papillary mucinous neoplasm of the pancreas: implications for management. Ann Surg. 2010;251(1):64–9.
3. Khan S, Sclabas G, Reid-Lombardo KM. Population-based epidemiology, risk factors and screening of intraductal papillary mucinous neoplasm patients. World J Gastrointest Surg. 2010;2(10):314–8.
4. Hata T, Sakata N, Okada T, Aoki T, Motoi F, Katayose Y, Egawa S, Unno M. Dilated papilla with mucin extrusion is a potential predictor of acute pancreatitis associated with intraductal papillary mucinous neoplasms of pancreas. Pancreatology. 2013;13(6):615–20.
5. Aso T, Ohtsuka T, Ideno N, Kono H, Nagayoshi Y, Mori Y, Ohuchida K, Ueda J, Takahata S, Morimatsu K, Aishima S, Igarashi H, Ito T, Ishigami K, Mizumoto K, Tanaka M. Diagnostic significance of a dilated orifice of the duodenal papilla in intraductal papillary mucinous neoplasm of the pancreas. Gastrointest Endosc. 2012;76(2):313–20.
6. Sadakari Y, Ohuchida K, Nakata K, Ohtsuka T, Aishima S, Takahata S, Nakamura M, Mizumoto K, Tanaka M. Invasive carcinoma derived from the non-intestinal type intraductal papillary mucinous neoplasm of the pancreas has a poorer prognosis than that derived from the intestinal type. Surgery. 2010;147(6):812–7.
7. Suzuki R, Thosani N, Annangi S, Komarraju A, Irisawa A, Ohira H, Obara K, Fleming JB, Guha S, Bhutani MS. Diagnostic yield of endoscopic retrograde cholangiopancreatography-based cytology for distinguishing malignant and benign intraductal papillary mucinous neoplasm: systematic review and meta-analysis. Dig Endosc. 2014;26(4):586–93.
8. Hirono S, Tani M, Kawai M, Okada K, Miyazawa M, Shimizu A, Kitahata Y, Yamaue H. The carcinoembryonic antigen level in pancreatic juice and mural nodule size are predictors of malignancy for branch duct type intraductal papillary mucinous neoplasms of the pancreas. Ann Surg. 2012;255(3):517–22.

9. Shimamoto T, Tani M, Kawai M, Hirono S, Ina S, Miyazawa M, Shimizu A, Uchiyama K, Yokoyama S, Tsutsumi M, Yamaue H. MUC1 is a useful molecular marker for malignant intraductal papillary mucinous neoplasms in pancreatic juice obtained from endoscopic retrograde pancreatography. Pancreas. 2010;39(6):879–83.
10. Tringali A, Spera G, Mutignani M, Familiari P, Spada C, Perri V, Riccioni ME, Costamagna G. Intraductal papillary mucinous tumor (IPMT) of the pancreas: review of 30 cases. Gut. 2003;52(Suppl VI):A49.
11. Mukai H, Yasuda K, Nakajima M. Differential diagnosis of mucin-producing tumors of the pancreas by intraductal ultrasonography and peroral pancreatoscopy. Endoscopy. 1998;30 Suppl 1:A99–102.
12. Arnelo U, Siiki A, Swahn F, Segersvärd R, Enochsson L, del Chiaro M, Lundell L, Verbeke CS, Löhr JM. Single-operator pancreatoscopy is helpful in the evaluation of suspected intraductal papillary mucinous neoplasms (IPMN). Pancreatology. 2014;14(6):510–4.
13. Nagayoshi Y, Aso T, Ohtsuka T, Kono H, Ideno N, Igarashi H, Takahata S, Oda Y, Ito T, Tanaka M. Peroral pancreatoscopy using the SpyGlass system for the assessment of intraductal papillary mucinous neoplasm of the pancreas. J Hepatobiliary Pancreat Sci. 2014;21:410–7.
14. Miura T, Igarashi Y, Okano N, Miki K, Okubo Y. Endoscopic diagnosis of intraductal papillary-mucinous neoplasm of the pancreas by means of peroral pancreatoscopy using a small-diameter videoscope and narrow-band imaging. Dig Endosc. 2010;22(2):119–23.
15. Atia GN, Brown RD, Alrashid A, Halline AG, Helton WS, Venu RP. The role of pancreatoscopy in the preoperative evaluation of intraductal papillary mucinous tumor of the pancreas. J Clin Gastroenterol. 2002;35(2):175–9.
16. Yelamani A, Mansard MJ, Dama R, Rebela P, Rao GV, Reddy DN. Intraoperative pancreatoscopy with narrow band imaging: a novel method for assessment of resection margins in case of intraductal papillary mucinous neoplasm. Surg Endosc. 2012;26(12):3682–5.
17. Hara T, Yamaguchi T, Ishihara T, Tsuyuguchi T, Kondo F, Kato K, Asano T, Saisho H. Diagnosis and patient management of intraductal papillary-mucinous tumor of the pancreas by using peroral pancreatoscopy and intraductal ultrasonography. Gastroenterology. 2002;122(1):34–43.
18. Uehara H, Nakaizumi A, Tatsuta M, Lishi H, Kitamura T, Ohigashi H, Ishikawa O, Takenaka A. Diagnosis of carcinoma in situ of the pancreas by peroral pancreatoscopy and pancreatoscopic cytology. Cancer. 1997;79(3):454–61.
19. Yamaguchi T, Shirai Y, Ishihara T, Sudo K, Nakagawa A, Ito H, Miyazaki M, Nomura F, Saisho H. Pancreatic juice cytology in the diagnosis of intraductal papillary mucinous neoplasm of the pancreas. Cancer. 2005;104(12):2830–6.
20. Itoi T, Sofuni A, Itokawa F, Kurihara T, Tsuchiya T, Ishii K, Tsuji S, Ikeuchi N, Arisaka Y, Moriyasu F. Initial experience of peroral pancreatoscopy combined with narrow-band imaging in the diagnosis of intraductal papillary mucinous neoplasms of the pancreas (with video). Gastrointest Endosc. 2007;66(4):793–7.
21. Brauer BC, Chen YK, Ringold DA, Shah RJ. Peroral pancreatoscopy via the minor papilla for diagnosis and therapy of pancreatic diseases. Gastrointest Endosc. 2013;78(3):545–9.
22. Tringali A, Lemmers A, Meves V, Terheggen G, Pohl J, Manfredi G, Häfner M, Costamagna G, Devière J, Neuhaus H, Caillol F, Giovannini M, Hassan C, Dumonceau JM. Intraductal biliopancreatic imaging: European Society of Gastrointestinal Endoscopy (ESGE) technology review. Endoscopy. 2015;47(8):739–53.
23. Yamao K, Ohashi K, Nakamura T, Suzuki T, Sawaki A, Hara K, Fukutoni A, Baba T, Okubo K, Tanaka K, Moriyama I, Fukuda K, Matsumoto K, Shimizu Y. Efficacy of peroral pancreatoscopy in the diagnosis of pancreatic diseases. Gastrointest Endosc. 2003;57(2):205–9.
24. Del Chiaro M, Verbeke C, Salvia R, Klöppel G, Werner J, McKay C, Friess H, Manfredi R, Van Cutsem E, Löhr M, Segersvärd R, European Study Group on Cystic Tumours of the Pancreas. European experts consensus statement on cystic tumours of the pancreas. Dig Liver Dis. 2013;45(9):703–11.

8 PET Scan in Cystic Tumors of the Pancreas

Claudio Pasquali and Anna Caterina Milanetto

8.1 Introduction

Cystic tumors of the pancreas (CTPs) have been increasingly detected over the two past decades, due to the widespread use of high-resolution noninvasive abdominal imaging. CTPs are mostly detected incidentally when abdominal imaging is performed for unrelated indications and the prevalence of incidental pancreatic cystic lesion in adults ranges from 2.8 to 13.5 % [1, 2]. Autopsy series report a CTP prevalence of 23.5 %, ranging from 8 % below 70 years of age to 35 % in >90-year-old people, increasing also in the number and size of the cystic lesions according to age [3]. CTPs include a variety of neoplasms with different prognoses from benign to premalignant or malignant behavior [4]. The WHO 2010 classification of CTP is reported in Table 8.1 [5].

Four types of neoplasms included in Table 8.1 account for approximately 90 % of all cystic tumors of the pancreas: intraductal papillary mucinous neoplasms (IPMNs) either main duct, branch duct, or mixed, mucinous cystic neoplasms (MCNs), serous cystic neoplasms (SCNs) either microcystic or oligocystic variant, and pseudopapillary neoplasms.

The cystic feature, at imaging studies, of pseudopapillary neoplasms, neuroendocrine neoplasms, secondary tumors, or, occasionally, ductal adenocarcinomas is due to degenerative changes. Pseudocysts and other rare nonneoplastic cysts may enter in the differential diagnosis with CTP. Characterization of the cystic lesion with reliable, noninvasive methods is crucial to distinguish benign from malignant CTP and to decide the treatment option or follow-up planning. Preoperative evaluation of pancreatic cystic lesion includes abdominal ultrasound (US), computed tomography (CT), magnetic resonance imaging (MRI), endoscopic ultrasonography (EUS) with fine-needle aspiration cytology (FNAC), and finally US-guided percutaneous FNAC. Despite these diagnostic tools and many evidence-based practice guidelines [6–8] being published, controversial issues still exist in the evaluation and management of CTP, particularly concerning lesion size, the presence of high-risk lesion features, the role of different diagnostic techniques, and the accuracy of markers and cytology for CTP definition. Conflicting results are reported in clinical practice when matching preoperative diagnosis and pathologic results, and even in high-volume centers for pancreatic surgery, the correct diagnosis rate in CTP does not exceed 68 % of operated patients [9].

C. Pasquali, MD (✉) • A. C. Milanetto, MD
Department of Surgery, Oncology, Gastroenterology, Policlinico – University of Padova, Padova, Italy

Unit of Pancreatic and Digestive Endocrine Surgery, Clinica Chirurgica 1, Via Giustiniani 2, Padova 35128, Italy
e-mail: claudio.pasquali@unipd.it; ac.milanetto@email.it

M. Del Chiaro et al. (eds.), *Cystic Tumors of the Pancreas*, DOI 10.1007/978-3-319-31882-0_8

Table 8.1 WHO 2010 classification of cystic pancreatic tumors

Epithelial tumors
Benign
Acinar cell cystadenoma
Serous cystadenoma
Premalignant lesions
Intraductal papillary mucinous neoplasm (IPMN)
Mucinous cystic neoplasm (MCN)
Malignant lesions
Acinar cell cystadenocarcinoma
Intraductal papillary mucinous neoplasm (IPMN) with an associated invasive carcinoma
Mucinous cystic neoplasm (MCN) with an associated invasive carcinoma
Serous cystadenocarcinoma
Solid pseudopapillary neoplasm
Neuroendocrine neoplasms with cystic degeneration
Mesenchymal tumors
Lymphangioma, NOS
Secondary tumors with cystic degeneration

Epithelial tumors are divided according to tumor behavior [5]

8.2 Positron Emission Tomography

2-[18F]-Fluoro-2-deoxy-D-glucose positron emission tomography (18-FDG-PET) is a scintigraphy technique based on the detection of hypermetabolic lesions due to excess glucose consumption from the tumor cells.

Glycolysis in neoplastic cells is increased due to their ability in glucose transportation through the membrane and increased activity of the glycolytic enzymes. The glucose analog (deoxyglucose) radiolabeled with 18 F (a positron emitter), injected 1 h before examination (350–450 Mbq) intravenously, in the patient who fasted for 6 h, is transported into the cell after binding with cell-membrane transporter proteins and then is metabolized by hexokinase into FDG-6-phosphate. FDG-6-phosphate is not further metabolized in the glycolysis pathway and then it remains trapped into the tumor cell. So the FDG-6-phosphate molecule labeled with the radiotracer (18 F) may be detected using a gamma camera. Details of the methods and equipment currently used in our center have been previously published [10]. The radioactivity detected by the gamma camera is coupled with the imaging of a CT scan (hybrid system PET/CT), in order to give a more accurate anatomical information on the site of hypermetabolism. To perform a quantitative analysis, the standardized uptake value (SUV) is calculated in the suspected cancer focus. For the SUV analysis, a circular region of interest is placed over the area of maximal focal uptake and the mean radioactivity values are obtained. The upper normal limit of the SUV may vary in different centers. As described in our previous papers, in our center the focal uptake with an SUV >2.5 is considered positive [10, 11]. In order to avoid false-negative results, patients with diabetes were tested just before FDG injection, having a glycemia of 120–130 mg% (eventually adjusted with insulin). Use of 18-FDG-PET/CT for oncologic imaging is well established and widely accepted for many malignancies [12] including pancreatic cancer [13, 14].

8.3 FDG-PET in Cystic Tumor of the Pancreas

There is little information on the use of FDG-PET in evaluating the malignant potential of the pancreatic cystic lesions despite the first report being published in 2001 from our center. Reviewing the literature only 10 papers have been published so far, if we include only studies with at least 30 patients investigated, in order to compare a significant number of cases of malignant versus benign pancreatic cyst. In Table 8.2 we reported the results in terms of sensitivity and specificity of either FDG-PET or PET/CT. The studies are heterogeneous in terms of case mixing of CTP, design of the study, being most of them retrospective, inclusion of nonneoplastic cysts in the benign group, and finally inclusion of only histologically proven cases or considering follow-up without morphological changes as benign behavior.

About 550 patients having a CTP were investigated in the series published in 13 years from the first study on FDG-PET scan; less than 400

Table 8.2 Sensitivity and specificity of FDG-PET or FDG-PET/CT in differential diagnosis between malignant and benign cystic lesions

Center	Ref.	Type of study	Year	Number of pts	Benign/malignant	All CTP/IPMN	Sensitivity %	Specificity %
Padova, Italy	[11]	R, PET	2001	56	39/17	CTP	94	97
Padova, Italy	[15]	P, PET	2005	50	33/17	CTP	94	94
New York (NY)	[16]	R, PET	2006	68	14/7[a]	CTP	57	85
Indianapolis (IN)	[17]	R, PET	2007	30	23/7	CTP	57	65
Padova (Italy)	[18]	R, PET	2007	64	21/26[a]	IPMN	92	95
Seoul (South Korea)	[19]	R, PET/CT	2010	31	15/16	IPMN	100	87
Osaka (Japan)	[20]	R, PET, PET/CT	2010	72	14/14[a]	IPMN	93	100
Padova (Italy)	[10]	R, PET, PET/CT	2011	145	33/36[a]	IPMN	83	100
Brescia (Italy)	[21]	P, PET/CT	2012	44	32/12	IPMN	83	100
Chiba (Japan)	[22]	R, PET/CT	2013	48	16/32	IPMN	88	88

P prospective, *R* retrospective, *CTP* cystic tumor of the pancreas, *IPMN* intraductal papillary mucinous neoplasm

[a]Results expressed for patients (pts) with proven histology

cases had a confirmed histology with about 160 malignant CTPs included in these studies. As shown in Table 8.2, four of these studies came from our group of investigators accounting of 40 % of cases studied. The papers published by our group in 2007 and 2011 [10, 18] focusing on IPMN, include in part patients reported in the previous 2 studies [11, 15]. Most of the studies were retrospective and only patients investigated more recently had a PET/CT scan (hybrid equipment). Four papers were dealing with all varieties of CPT (overall 157 patients evaluated of which 48 with proven malignancy), and they were investigated with FDG-PET or fusion imaging [17]. Sperti reported a sensitivity of 94 % and a specificity of 94–97 % in distinguishing benign from malignant CTP with an accuracy of 94 %.

When FDG-PET was compared with results of CT imaging in the Italian studies, contrast-enhanced CT had lower sensitivity and specificity (65 % and 87–88 %, respectively) irrespective of the use of multidetector CT equipment in the latter study. The two studies from the USA found a 57 % sensitivity with a specificity of 65–85 %, respectively [16, 17]; however they enrolled a low number of patients (57 of which 14 malignant) with smaller size of lesions.

Six studies reported in Table 8.2 were dealing with IPMNs of the pancreas and the issue of detecting malignancy in this subset of patients. Most of the patients were studied with PET-CT equipment and compared results obtained by MRI and/or CT scan, and in total 220 patients were investigated (cases in the study by Sperti et al. [18] were all included in the most recent paper by Pedrazzoli et al. [10]) with 110 malignant ones.

Sensitivity of FDG-PET/CT to distinguish malignant IPMN ranged from 83 to 100 % and specificity from 87 to 100 %; so 97/110 (88 %) malignant IPMNs investigated had a positive FDG-PET/CT scan. Moreover when considering noninvasive cancer in IPMNs (cancer in situ, CIS) reported in four of these papers, 21/27 cases (78 %) had a positive FDG-PET/CT scan. It is noteworthy that in IPMNs with this technique, we can found most of the cancers in early stage, not yet invasive, than potentially curable with surgical resection.

8.4 Serous Cystic Neoplasms and FDG-PET

Serous cystadenomas (SCAs) account for about 16 % of resected cystic tumors of the pancreas [23]. SCAs are benign, slow-growing tumors. Very few cases of malignant SCA, on the basis of the presence of concomitant tumors in the liver or other extrapancreatic sites, have been described; they represent <1 % of cases [24]. They affect mainly women (approximately 75 %). Mean age of patients who underwent surgery for SCAs was 62 years in the USA [24] and 52 and 56 years in Italian and French series [25, 26]. The typical SCA is formed by many tiny cysts lined by a cuboidal epithelium that is glycogen rich and has a honeycomb appearance, microcystic tumor, defined as having cysts <2 cm in diameter. The cysts are filled with serous fluid, do not communicate with pancreatic ducts, and are often arranged around a central dense fibrous scar with thin fibrous septa radiating to the periphery occasionally calcified in the center [5]. An SCA variant called macrocystic (or oligocystic) with few cysts of more than 2 cm. in size up to 8 cm., without central scar, has been described and comprises 10 to 24 % of cases [23, 25]. They are difficult to differentiate on imaging with mucinous cystadenomas (MCAs). Fifty-six percent of SCAs are asymptomatic and they are resected if the diagnosis based on imaging is uncertain or because of growth. Patients with von Hippel-Lindau syndrome often develop multiple oligocystic SCAs. In our previously published paper, we had 21 SCAs investigated with FDG-PET up to 2003; all of them had a negative PET scan and 15/21 patients had histology (or biopsy)-proven SCA. From 2004 to 2013 in our unit, we operated on 25 more SCAs who had a preoperative PET scan, 20 % of them had a macrocystic variant. Only 1 microcystic SCA had a positive PET scan.

Therefore in case of difficult differential diagnosis between SCA and mucinous cyst as in the macrocystic variant of SCA, FDG-PET may help to establish the benign nature of the CTP at time of first assessment, since in our experience on 46 SCA patients, only one had a false-positive result (2 %) in this subset of patients.

8.5 Mucinous Cystic Neoplasms and FDG-PET

Mucinous cystic neoplasms (MCNs) account for up to 23 % of CTP resected [27]. The risk of malignancy is 17.5–27 % of cases with carcinoma in situ or invasive cancer (mucinous cystadenocarcinoma). They occur mainly in women and in the distal pancreas, being always a single lesion. Histologically they are composed of mucin-producing columnar epithelium associated with ovarian-type stroma. The cyst (unilocular or with septa) does not communicate with the ductal system and occasionally shows calcifications. Mean age at diagnosis is 45 years [28], and patients with associate invasive carcinoma are 5–10 years older and have larger cysts (more than 4 cm. in size) and eventually mural nodules or eggshell calcifications, thick wall, or thick septa. Patients treated with surgical resection have excellent prognosis unless invasive carcinomas with extracapsular growth are found.

In total, including the four studies published (see Table 8.2) and cases unpublished from our center (operated on from 2004 to 2012), 36 MCNs were collected, and 3 false-negative results on PET scan were found, out of 17 malignant MCNs (82 % sensitivity).

8.6 Intraductal Papillary Mucinous Neoplasms and FDG-PET

Intraductal papillary mucinous neoplasms (IPMNs) are defined as macroscopic (cystic or mass-forming) epithelial neoplasms with ductal differentiation that grow primarily within the ductal system of the pancreas [5]. These neoplasms are usually slow growing and they often have a large size when they are diagnosed and still asymptomatic. Histologically they are characterized by a papillary growth pattern and significant luminal presence of mucin, and they may progress from low-grade dysplasia to intermediate- and high-grade dysplasia and then invasive carcinoma. The incidence of IPMNs in the general population is estimated to account for 20 % of CTP but the rate is currently increasing due to widespread use of imaging, and small IPMNs are incidentally detected during the evaluation of patients for other conditions. IPMNs are fairly more common in the elderly [2] with mean age at diagnosis of about 66 years; patients with invasive carcinoma are 3–5 years older, suggesting progression from dysplasia to carcinoma. Basically the tumor may arise in the main pancreatic duct or in the side branches of the ductal system or either in the side branches or the main duct (mixed type). The risk of malignancy in the main-duct type (and mixed type) is high, with invasive carcinoma found in 45 % and cancer in situ in additional 20 % of patients. Predominant in males, the most common presentation of main-duct IPMN is abdominal pain (55 %), with weight loss (45 %), jaundice (17 %), and acute pancreatitis (15 %), due to transient obstruction of the main duct from the mucin secreted by the tumor. Due to the high risk of malignancy, main-duct and mixed-type IPMNs are treated by surgical resection. Branch-duct IPMNs (BD-IPMN), occasionally symptomatic, in some patients present with pancreatitis. Their imaging features range from an isolated pancreatic cyst <1 cm. in size to larger solitary collections of pancreatic cysts. Diffuse multifocal disease occurs in about 40 % of patients having multiple BD-IPMNs of varying sizes, scattered through their pancreas [29].

The risk of malignancy of BD-IPMNs can vary, based on size and associated features, such as nodules, multiplicity, and epithelial subtype. The mean frequency of malignancy (defined as high-grade dysplasia and invasive cancer) for surgically resected BD-IPMNs is 25.5 % [6]. In a cumulative series of patients who underwent surveillance for presumed BD-IPMNs, the surgical intervention rate was <10 %, and the risk of finding an associated malignancy was <2.5 % in 41 months median follow-up, indicating that the overall risks are low, even in a highly selected group of patients [23].

As reported above (see Table 8.2), in the literature a total of 110 malignant IPMNs were investigated with FDG-PET/CT scan with an overall sensitivity of 88 % and still 78 % positivity in 27 patients with noninvasive cancer (CIS). It is not surprising that a "functional" technique like the FDG-PET may detect a focal increase in glucose metabolism even when the disease is limited to microscopic changes, as it occurs in different diseases (i.e., hyperplastic diseases) detected with other types of scintigraphy investigations. This opportunity to detect preinvasive cancers gives us an extraordinary chance as pancreatologists: to identify some high-risk patient with IPMN, with mandatory indication to surgery and to resect cancers with curative intent before the overt spread of disease, having the same dismal prognosis of a pancreatic ductal adenocarcinoma. In our experience [10] PET is more effective than any other procedure in the differential diagnosis of benign and malignant lesions in patients diagnosed with IPMN, and when compared with the international consensus guidelines defined in the Sendai conference [30] that have a high sensitivity (93 %), but low specificity and accuracy (22 and 61 %, respectively), PET scan showed better results (specificity 100 %, accuracy 91 %). Then we concluded that FDG-PET scan may help in the first assessment of IPMNs.

Moreover in 24 % of our patients with IPMN, a preoperative negative PET/CT scan allowed a more conservative pancreatic resection, ruling out the risk of dealing with a cancer when operating on these patients (often with multifocal disease). PET/CT scan is crucial, in our opinion, even in those cases (mainly BD-IPMN) where patients are placed under surveillance to be sure they are cancer-free, avoiding a mandatory evaluation with an endoscopic ultrasound (EUS) with fine-needle cyst fluid aspiration for cytology and tumor marker determination; the role of these investigations has been extensively debated and reviewed in CTP management and particularly in IPMNs [23]. EUS and FNA are also included and recommended in the Fukuoka guidelines for management of BD-IPMNs and MCN [6], but we think that the use of FDG-PET/CT represents a useful, less invasive alternative to EUS-FNA, an operator-dependent technique that may have bias from inconclusive responses from cytology and uncertain results from tumor marker assay in the cyst fluid. In our paper [10] we reported 59 BD-IPMNs (diagnosis based on MRI and without histology) placed under surveillance having a negative FDG-PET/CT. After a mean follow-up of 20 months, 5 cases (8 %) underwent surgery (for symptoms or imaging changes): all were found benign. None of the other 54 patients with BD-IPMN developed malignant disease during a mean 25.5 months of follow-up.

Therefore we suggest the use of FDG-PET/CT in the first assessment of all IPMNs particularly those BD-IPMNs with worrisome features according to the Fukuoka conference [6].

In the literature we could not find any indication about use and timing of FDG-PET/CT in the follow-up of patients placed under surveillance, being mostly BD-IPMNs. In our previous study [10] we usually repeated the investigation every year or in case of changes in the (MR) imaging of the lesion(s), rise in serum CA 19-9, or occurrence of symptoms, but if no worrisome feature is present, the interval may be lengthened every 2 years. Due to low risk for malignancy in BD-IPMN with cysts <1 cm., they can be managed only with conventional imaging unless they show changes in size.

8.7 Solid Pseudopapillary Neoplasms and FDG-PET

Solid pseudopapillary neoplasms (SPNs) of the pancreas are uncommon accounting less than 5 % of resected PCTs. They predominantly affect women (up to 90 %) at median ages of 30–38 years [31], and they account for 30 % of all pancreatic neoplasms in patients <40 years.

SPNs appear as a well-demarcated heterogeneous mass with solid and cystic components. Histologically they are defined as low-grade malignant neoplasms composed of poorly cohesive monomorphic epithelial cells forming solid and pseudopapillary structures; frequently they undergo hemorrhagic cystic degeneration. Usually they form round, solitary, and large (average size 8 cm.) masses [5]. Behavior of these neoplasms is not predictable by the common histologic features and occasionally they may be mistaken for neuroendocrine tumors. Rarely they extend into the stomach or duodenum or spleen. Metastases occur in 5–15 % of cases in the liver or peritoneum. After complete surgical resection 90 % of patients are cured. Recently two papers dealing only with SPN have been published [32, 33]; irrespective of the real behavior, all the SPNs appear to have high metabolism, and the mean (max) SUV was 8.9 with a direct relationship with the proliferative index (Ki-67) and tumor cellularity, according to Dong's experience [32]. Kang et al. [33] who reported a series of 37 cases studied with FDG-PET/CT reviewed all the literature including report of single cases, collecting other 24 SPNs. We added to these series 7 unpublished cases operated on in our center, and in total out of 69 cases, only 2 (3 %) were PET negative. The high rate of FDG-PET positivity even in SPNs with benign behavior makes this test useless in the differential diagnosis between benign and malignant (metastatic) neoplasms in this subset of CTPs; however in those with distant metastases, it may help to stage the cancer.

8.8 Cystic Pancreatic Neuroendocrine Neoplasms (CPNNs) and PET

Cystic pancreatic endocrine neoplasms (CPNNs) represent about 8 % of resected cystic tumors of the pancreas [27] and 10–17 % of resected pancreatic neuroendocrine tumors [34, 35]. Most of them are discovered incidentally and are nonfunctional. CPNNs are more likely to develop in patients with multiple endocrine neoplasia type I [36]. They are generally diagnosed in people aging 60–70 years old. At CT scan, they appear as cystic lesions, frequently with a hypervascular rim and occasionally with septation or containing a solid component. As for all pancreatic neuroendocrine tumors (pNETs), malignancy is difficult to predict based only on biopsy (either cytology or core biopsy). Currently, surgical resection is recommended for all patients; >85 % survive long term.

In our experience FDG-PET was positive in 3 malignant CPNNs and negative in other 3 benign lesions. Despite the high rate of positivity of FDG-PET in neuroendocrine neoplasms with aggressive behavior (78 % sensitivity in malignant pNETs and 83 % specificity, in our experience) [37, 38], this investigation did not enter in the clinical practice to differentiate malignant versus benign pNETs. The 68-gallium – tracers (DOTATOC and DOTANOC) used as somatostatin receptor agonists, are now widely used in PET investigations [39]. Gallium PET is positive in 93–96 % of NETs and represents the "standard" imaging for staging this disease; however both in cystic and non-cystic lesions, the gallium PET is not able to differentiate malignant from benign lesions (unless lymph nodes or distant metastases occur and are detected).

Conclusions

Summarizing, the worldwide experience on the use of PET and its diagnostic role in cystic tumors of the pancreas is somehow limited. Few reports have been published in the last 14 years since our first paper in 2001 dealing with the diagnosis of malignancy in CTP [11]. Since 2001, all over the world, less than 700 patients with different varieties of CTP (including short series and personal unpublished data) have been submitted to PET studies and about 40 % of them in our center. From our first study the results in terms of sensitivity, specificity, and accuracy of FDG-PET were found to be better than conventional CT or MR imaging to detect malignancy in these heterogeneous neoplasms. Despite confirmatory results coming out from our prospective study [15] (in total the 2 studies had more than 100 patients enrolled), two different studies from the USA [16, 17], with a small population enrolled, did not find our encouraging results, reporting only 57 % sensitivity in detecting malignancy in CTP. The subset of CTP patients in which the diagnosis of malignancy is crucial is certainly the IPMNs, because most of them do not need resection but only surveillance, particularly those with branch-duct IPMN, often with multifocal disease. The risk to overlook a cancer or a malignant noninvasive lesion is relatively low, but once the tumor is invasive, its behavior is similar to that of a ductal adenocarcinoma. This explains why it is suggested to submit those patients to EUS and FNA in order to reduce this risk. The FDG-PET showed the ability to detect even "cancer in situ" in IPMNs with high sensitivity (78 % as reported above from our data and literature), and then we strongly recommend FDG-PET/CT as a noninvasive alternative to EUS and FNA to rule out the risk of a malignancy in IPMNs. Currently, even the Italian consensus guidelines for the diagnostic workup and follow-up of cystic pancreatic neoplasms [8] recommend the use of FDG-PET/CT, only when conventional imaging techniques are inconclusive to rule out the cancer diagnosis. We believe, on the basis of the results reported above, that this indication should be extended to all patients with CTP with suspected malignancy undergoing operation and those non-operated, followed up, at first assessment.

From 2007 to 2008 the improvement of the PET equipment with hybrid system PET/CT allowed a better resolution, anatomical localization, and imaging of the focus of hypermetabolism in the abdomen, and since then, the reports showing good results (83–100 % sensitivity) of FDG-PET/CT in CTP are coming from many centers of nuclear medicine all over the world. The limited diffusion of PET/CT equipment, the lack of this facility close to centers dealing with pancreatic surgery, and the cost of this scintigraphy may be in part responsible for the low number of subjects with CTP investigated with this technique.

There are few open questions about the use of FDG-PET/CT in the follow-up of patients with IPMN or in the patients already resected for CTP (particularly IPMNs and those with multifocal disease). We do not have data about the timing to repeat an FDG-PET/CT after the first one, or after surgery, since the risk of malignancy in BD-IPMN is unclear and the risk of recurrence after resection depends on the degree and extent of dysplasia left behind in the residual pancreas. We found it reasonable to submit our patients (at risk) every 2 years to a new FDG-PET/CT, depending on the imaging (worrisome) features and the histology if available and taking into account the age of the patients and the general conditions (most IPMNs are >80 years old). Since a 21–30 % prevalence of extrapancreatic cancers has been reported in patients with IPMN, developed in the course of their lives [40, 41], an FDG-PET/CT may be a good investigation to detect (incidentally) even other cancers as it occurred in 8 % of our patients at first assessment or in the follow-up [42].

Finally, in some variety of CTP, the FDG-PET seems less important to define malignancy. In the SPN, nearly all patients (>95 %) are strongly positive to FDG-PET (with high SUV) independently from the real behavior and prognosis of the tumor. In the rare CPNNs the clinical impact of FDG-PET is limited to those advanced cases in which the FDG uptake with high SUV means poorly differentiated lesion(s) and may help to choose the therapeutic option, giving chemotherapy to the patient.

References

1. Laffan TA, Horton KM, Klein AP, Berlanstein B, Siegelman SS, Kawamoto S, et al. Prevalence of unsuspected pancreatic cysts on MDCT. Am J Roentgenol. 2008;191:802–7.
2. Lee KS, Sekhar A, Rofsky NM, Pedrosa I. Prevalence of incidental pancreatic cysts in the adult population on MR imaging. Am J Gastroenterol. 2010;105:2079–84.
3. Kimura W, Nagai H, Kuroda A, Muto T, Esaki Y. Analysis of small cystic lesions of the pancreas. Int J Pancreatol. 1995;18:197–206.
4. Kloppel G, Solcia E, Longnecker DS, Cappella C, Sobin LH. Histological typing of tumours of the exocrine pancreas. 2nd ed. Berlin: World Health Organization/Springer; 1996.
5. Bosman FT, Carneiro F, Hruban RH, Theise ND. WHO classification of tumours of the digestive system. 4th ed. Lyon: International Agency for Research on Cancer; 2010.

6. Tanaka M, Fernandez-Del Castillo C, Adsay V, Chari S, Falconi M, Jang J-Y, et al. International consensus guidelines 2012 for the management of IPMN and MCN of the pancreas. Pancreatology. 2012;12:183–97.
7. Del Chiaro M, Verbeke C, Salvia R, Klöppel G, Werner J, McKay C, et al. European experts consensus statement on cystic tumours of the pancreas. Dig Liver Dis. 2013;45:703–11.
8. Italian Association of Hospital Gastroenterologists and Endoscopists, Italian Association for the Study of the Pancreas, Buscarini E, Pezzilli R, Cannizzaro R, De Angelis C, et al. Italian consensus guidelines for the diagnostic work-up and follow-up of cystic pancreatic neoplasms. Dig Liver Dis. 2014;46:479–93.
9. Correa-Gallego C, Ferrone CR, Thayer SP, Wargo JA, Warshaw AL, Fernandez-Del Castillo C. Incidental pancreatic cysts: do we really know what we are watching? Pancreatology. 2010;10:144–50.
10. Pedrazzoli S, Sperti C, Pasquali C, Bissoli S, Chierichetti F. Comparison of international consensus guidelines versus 18-FDG PET in detecting malignancy of intraductal papillary mucinous neoplasms of the pancreas. Ann Surg. 2011;254:971–6.
11. Sperti C, Pasquali C, Chierichetti F, Liessi G, Ferlin G, Pedrazzoli S. Value of 18-fluorodeoxyglucose positron emission tomography in the patients with cystic tumors of the pancreas. Ann Surg. 2001;234:675–80.
12. Hustinx R, Benard F, Alavi A. Whole-body FDG-PET imaging in the management of patients with cancer. Semin Nucl Med. 2002;32:35–46.
13. Heinrich S, Goerres GW, Schäfer M, Sagmeister M, Bauerfeind P, Pestalozzi BC, et al. Positron emission tomography/computed tomography influences on the management of resectable pancreatic cancer and its cost-effectiveness. Ann Surg. 2005;242:235–43.
14. Orlando LA, Kulasingam SL, Matchar DB. Meta-analysis: the detection of pancreatic malignancy with positron emission tomography. Aliment Pharmacol Ther. 2004;20:1063–70.
15. Sperti C, Pasquali C, Decet G, Chierichetti F, Liessi G, Pedrazzoli S. 18-FDG PET in differentiating malignant from benign pancreatic cysts: a prospective study. J Gastrointest Surg. 2005;9:22–9.
16. Mansour JC, Schwartz L, Pandit-Taskar N, D'Angelica M, Fong Y, Larson SM, et al. The utility of F-18 fluorodeoxyglucose whole body PET imaging for determining malignancy in cystic lesions of the pancreas. J Gastrointest Surg. 2006;10:1354–60.
17. Tann M, Sandrasegaran K, Jennings SG, Skandarajah A, McHenry L, Schmidt CM. Positron-emission tomography and computed tomography of cystic pancreatic masses. Clin Radiol. 2007;62:745–51.
18. Sperti C, Bissoli S, Pasquali C, Frison L, Liessi G, Chierichetti F, Pedrazzoli S. 18-Fluorodeoxyglucose positron emission tomography enhances computed tomography diagnosis of malignant intraductal papillary mucinous neoplasms of the pancreas. Ann Surg. 2007;246:932–9.
19. Hong HS, Yun M, Cho A, Choi J-Y, Kim M-J, Kim KW, et al. The utility of F-18 FDG PET/CT in the evaluation of pancreatic intraductal papillary mucinous neoplasm. Clin Nucl Med. 2010;35:776–9.
20. Tomimaru Y, Takeda Y, Tatsumi M, Kim T, Kobayashi S, Marubashi S, et al. Utility of 2-[18F] fluoro-2-deoxy-d-glucose positron emission tomography in differential diagnosis of benign and malignant intraductal papillary-mucinous neoplasm of the pancreas. Oncol Rep. 2010;24:613–20.
21. Baiocchi GL, Bertagna F, Gheza F, Grazioli L, Calanducci D, Giubbini R, et al. Searching for indicators of malignancy in pancreatic intraductal papillary mucinous neoplasms: the value of 18FDG-PET confirmed. Ann Surg Oncol. 2012;19:3574–80. doi:10.1245/s10434-012-2234-5.
22. Saito M, Ishihara T, Tada M, Tsuyuguchi T, Mikata R, Sakai Y, et al. Use of F-18 fluorodeoxyglucose positron emission tomography with dual-phase imaging to identify intraductal papillary mucinous neoplasm. Clin Gastroenterol Hepatol. 2013;11:181–6. doi:10.1016/j.cgh.2012.10.037.
23. Farrell JJ, Fernández-del Castillo C. Pancreatic cystic neoplasms: management and unanswered questions. Gastroenterology. 2013;144:1303–15. doi:10.1053/j.gastro.2013.01.073.
24. Galanis C, Zamani A, Cameron JL, Campbell KA, Lillemoe KD, Caparrelli D, et al. Resected serous cystic neoplasms of the pancreas: a review of 158 patients with recommendations for treatment. J Gastrointest Surg. 2007;11:820–6.
25. Bassi C, Salvia R, Molinari E, Biasutti C, Falconi M, Pederzoli P. Management of 100 consecutive cases of pancreatic serous cystadenoma: wait for symptoms and see at imaging or vice versa? World J Surg. 2003;27:319–23.
26. Le Borgne J, de Calan L, Partensky C. Cystadenomas and cystadenocarcinomas of the pancreas: a multiinstitutional retrospective study of 398 cases. Ann Surg. 1999;230:152–61.
27. Valsangkar NP, MoralesOyarvide V, Thayer SP, Ferrone CR, Wargo JA, Warshaw AL, Fernández-del CC. 851 resected cystic tumors of the pancreas: a 33-year experience at the Massachusetts General Hospital. Surgery. 2012;152 Suppl 1:S4–S12. doi:10.1016/j.surg.2012.05.033.
28. Goh BK, Tan YM, Chung YF, Chow PK, Cheow PC, Wong WK, Ooi LL. A review of mucinous cystic neoplasms of the pancreas defined by ovarian-type stroma: clinicopathological features of 344 patients. World J Surg. 2006;30:2236–45.
29. Rodriguez JR, Salvia R, Crippa S, Warshaw AL, Bassi C, Falconi M, et al. Branch-duct intraductal papillary mucinous neoplasms: observations in 145 patients who underwent resection. Gastroenterology. 2007;133:72–9.
30. Tanaka M, Chari S, Adsay V, Fernandez-del Castillo C, Falconi M, Shimizu M, et al. International consensus guidelines for management of intraductal papillary mucinous neoplasms and mucinous cystic neoplasms of the pancreas. Pancreatology. 2006;6:17–32.

31. Reddy S, Cameron JL, Scudiere J, Hruban RH, Fishman EK, Ahuja N, et al. Surgical management of solid-pseudopapillary neoplasms of the pancreas (Franz or Hamoudi tumors): a single-institutional series. J Am Coll Surg. 2009;208:950–9.
32. Dong A, Wang Y, Dong H, Zhang J, Cheng C, Zuo C. FDG PET/CT findings of solid pseudopapillary tumor of the pancreas with CT and MRI correlation. Clin Nucl Med. 2013;38:e118–24.
33. Kang CM, Cho A, Kim H, Chung YE, Hwang HK, Choi SH, Lee WJ. Clinical correlations with 18FDG PET scan patterns in solid pseudopapillary tumors of the pancreas: Still a surgical enigma? Pancreatology. 2014;14:515–23.
34. Gaujoux S, Tang L, Klimstra D, Gonen M, Brennan MF, D'Angelica M, et al. The outcome of resected cystic pancreatic endocrine neoplasms: a case-matched analysis. Surgery. 2012;151:518–25.
35. Boninsegna L, Partelli S, D'Innocenzio MM, Capelli P, Scarpa A, Bassi C, et al. Pancreatic cystic endocrine tumors: a different morphological entity associated with a less aggressive behavior. Neuroendocrinology. 2010;92:246–51.
36. Bordeianou L, Vagefi PA, Sahani DV, Deshpande V, Rakhlin E, Warshaw AL, Fernández-del Castillo C. Cystic pancreatic endocrine neoplasm: a distinct tumor type? J Am Coll Surg. 2008;206:1154–8.
37. Pasquali C, Rubello D, Sperti C, Gasparoni P, Liessi G, Chierichetti F, et al. Neuroendocrine tumor imaging: can 18F-fluorodeoxyglucose positron emission tomography detect tumors with poor prognosis and aggressive behavior? World J Surg. 1998;22:588–92.
38. Pasquali C, Sperti C, Lunardi C, Scappin S, Chierichetti F, Liessi G, Pedrazzoli S. La tomografia ad emissione di positroni con fluorodesossiglucosio nei tumori neuroendocrini gastro-entero-pancreatici: ruolo diagnostico e implicazioni prognostiche. Suppl Tumori. 2005;4:S68–71.
39. Wild D, Bomanji JB, Benkert P, Maecke H, Ell PJ, Reubi JC, Caplin ME. Comparison of 68Ga-DOTANOC and 68Ga-DOTATATE PET/CT within patients with gastroenteropancreatic neuroendocrine tumors. J Nucl Med. 2013;54:364–72.
40. Choi MG, Kim SW, Han SS, Jang JY, Park YH. High incidence of extrapancreatic neoplasms in patients with intraductal papillary mucinous neoplasms. Arch Surg. 2006;141:51–6.
41. Marchegiani G, Malleo G, D'Haese JG, Wenzel P, Keskin M, Pugliese L, et al. Association between pancreatic IPMNs and extra-pancreatic malignancies. Clin Gastroenterol Hepatol. 2014. doi:10.1016/j.cgh.2014.11.029.
42. Beltrame V, Bissoli S, Chierichetti F, Milanetto AC, Morbin T, Pasquali C, Sperti C. FDG-PET incidental detection of second cancer during investigation for pancreatic diseases. JOP J Pancreas. 2011;12(Suppl):525.

When and How to Follow Patients with Cystic Tumors of the Pancreas

9

Giuseppe Malleo, Peter J. Allen, Claudio Bassi, and Roberto Salvia

9.1 Introduction

The natural history of pancreatic cystic neoplasms is poorly understood, because the vast majority of the data are retrospective and uncontrolled, and long-term follow-up is yet not available. Over the last decade, a selective approach to cystic neoplasms has been widely adopted in tertiary care centers, balancing the risk of malignancy with the risk of morbidity and mortality related to major pancreatic resections. Thanks to the better understanding of radiologic features and the publication of international guidelines, the initial management evolved toward fewer patients undergoing operative resection and fewer benign lesions being resected [1–3]. However, morphologic overlap between different families of cystic neoplasms does exist, and the diagnostic accuracy in patients who ultimately underwent resection has been shown to be unsatisfying [4, 5].

Patients managed nonoperatively are enrolled in radiologic surveillance protocols, with the aim of finding signs of possible progression to malignancy as early as possible. Surveillance protocols require periodic cross-sectional imaging and/or endoscopic ultrasound, at a high economic cost for the community. Furthermore, there is no ideal imaging modality to diagnose transformed pancreatic cystic neoplasms, and there is not general agreement on what is the optimum time frame to follow up for these lesions. Long-term results of surveillance protocols are started being reported in the literature, especially for lesions amenable of initial observation, such as serous cystic neoplasms (SCNs) and branch-duct intraductal papillary mucinous neoplasms (BD-IPMNs) [6–9].

In patients who undergo resection, either at the time of diagnosis or after observation, the chance of cure, the incidence of tumor recurrence, and disease-specific or overall survival depend on the cyst type and the presence of an invasive component, although long-term data are limited. This chapter describes the outcomes of

G. Malleo, MD (✉)
Unit of General and Pancreatic Surgery, G.B. Rossi Hospital, University of Verona Hospital Trust, P.Le L.A. Scuro 10, Verona 37134, Italy
e-mail: giuseppe.malleo@ospedaleuniverona.it

P.J. Allen, MD, FACS
Unit of Hepatopancreatic Surgery, Memorial Sloan Kettering Cancer Center, New York, NY, USA

Department of Surgery, Memorial Sloan Kettering Cancer Center, New York, NY, USA
e-mail: allenp@mskcc.org

C. Bassi, MD, FRCS, FACS
Unit of General and Pancreatic Surgery, University of Verona Hospital Trust, Verona, Italy

Department of Surgery and Oncology, G. B. Rossi Hospital, Verona University Hospital Trust, Verona, Italy
e-mail: claudio.bassi@univr.it

R. Salvia, MD, PhD
Unit of General and Pancreatic Surgery, University of Verona Hospital Trust, Verona, Italy

Department of Surgery, University of Verona – "GB Rossi" Hospital Trust, Verona, Italy
e-mail: roberto.salvia@univr.it

M. Del Chiaro et al. (eds.), *Cystic Tumors of the Pancreas*, DOI 10.1007/978-3-319-31882-0_9

primary surveillance of pancreatic cystic neoplasms, as well as the follow-up results after surgical resection.

9.2 Serous Cystic Neoplasms

The generally benign nature of SCN, combined with the high incidence of morbidity and the mortality rate associated with pancreatic resections, led to a management strategy weighed toward surveillance. A recent multicentric observational study of more than 2000 patients, conducted under the auspices of the International Association of Pancreatology (IAP), showed that the disease-specific mortality is lower than postoperative mortality [7]. These observations support the concept that SCN should be surveilled when the patient is asymptomatic and when a clear radiologic diagnosis is established. The safety of a periodic surveillance program and the generally slow growth rate of these lesions have been recently demonstrated by different authors [6, 10]. The optimal interval between follow-up imaging tests in pancreatic serous cystic neoplasms is yet unclear. Many institutions recommend imaging on a semiannual or annual basis for all the cystic neoplasms. According to the most recent data, cystic lesions presumed to be benign can be safely observed on a 2-year basis [11]. Clearly, surveillance can be tailored on the basis of cyst morphology (i.e., unclear discrimination between serous and mucinous lesions), patient's age, sex, and tumor location. In patients managed operatively, complete surgical resection ensures cure, and serous cystic neoplasms do not recur [12]. Therefore, a regular radiologic follow-up program is not necessary, thereby saving cost. Follow-up outpatient visits should be better focused on quality of life. Malignant SCNs (serous cystoadenocarcinomas) are exceptionally rare, with 27 cases being published. In the recent IAP multicentric analysis, only two cases were recorded [7]. Synchronous or metachronous liver metastases were the most frequent features associated with serous cystoadenocarcinomas. Mean survival was 36 months among the few cases with follow-up. The prognosis seems to be favorable also in patients with metastatic disease [13].

9.3 Mucinous Cystic Neoplasms

Mucinous cystic neoplasms (MCNs) have been associated with substantial risk of malignancy and generally require surgical resection, although small lesions (<4 cm) without mural nodules and eggshell calcifications, especially in elderly patients with comorbidities, may be observed. However, no data on patients with small MCN undergoing observation is available in the literature. Because most patients with MCN are middle-aged women with a long life expectancy, nonoperative management of low-risk lesions based on periodic imaging would require years of radiologic follow-up at high cost [14].

Radical resection of noninvasive neoplasms is associated with cure. These neoplasms do not recur and – as already pointed out for serous cystic neoplasms – outpatient follow-up should be focused on quality of life, rendering a regular radiologic post-resection surveillance probably unnecessary.

Minimally invasive MCNs (invasion limited to the ovarian stroma), but without tissue invasion, have an excellent prognosis. On occasion, undocumented foci of invasive carcinoma may exist within a presumably noninvasive proliferative MCN, and this stresses the importance of a careful histopathologic analysis of the entire lesion. In such cases, recurrence and metastases can be observed. In general, these patients should undergo a radiologic follow-up protocol, despite minimally invasive adenocarcinomas arising in MCN that are virtually cured by surgery, particularly if the neoplasms are completely examined histologically [15].

The 5-year survival of patients with invasive MCN (true cystadenocarcinoma) appears quite poor, ranging from 15 to 35 %, albeit still somewhat better than those for typical ductal adenocarcinoma of the pancreas. The extent of invasion is the most significant prognostic factor in malignant MCN. Some authors have suggested that patients with resected mucinous cystadenocarcinoma should be carefully followed on a 6-month basis with cross-sectional imaging, matching the interval to follow-up of ductal adenocarcinoma [16]. However, proof that surveillance imaging improves the prognosis compared with a strategy based on symptom recurrence is lacking.

9.4 Intraductal Papillary Mucinous Neoplasms (IPMNs)

9.4.1 Outcome of IPMN Managed Nonoperatively

The decision to follow an IPMN is based on the neoplasm type (main duct (MD)/mixed *versus* BD), patient age, family history, symptoms, comorbidities, perceived pancreatic cancer risk, and patient preference [1–3]. Initial follow-up is generally proposed only to patients with BD-IPMN devoid of malignant features on cross-sectional imaging, according to the current guidelines. Outcome metrics in patients initially managed nonoperatively are (1) morphologic progression and crossover to surgery, (2) development of a histologically proven invasive IPMN, and (3) development of a pancreatic ductal adenocarcinoma separate from the IPMN. The majority of papers focusing on this topic showed surveillance protocols to be relatively safe, although robust long-term data are lacking. In a cohort of 170 patients from the Memorial Sloan Kettering Cancer Center initially selected for surveillance, 97 underwent delayed resection because of endoscopic or radiologic changes and/or malignancy concern after a median follow-up period of 40 months. Of these, only 18 had an invasive IPMN on histopathology. Overall survival after delayed resection was 142 months for noninvasive disease and 126 months for invasive disease. Five patients initially selected for surveillance developed a pancreatic ductal adenocarcinoma in a region remote from the lesion being monitored, with a median time from diagnosis to resection of 20 months. In spite of an active surveillance program, no patient had stage I disease [8]. Another multi-institutional series from Japan analyzing 349 BD-IPMN patients who had no mural nodules at initial diagnosis (median follow-up of 3.7 years) showed that 62 patients (17.8 %) exhibited disease progression during follow-up. Twenty-two underwent surgery, but an invasive disease was found only in 9 patients. A pancreatic ductal adenocarcinoma developed in 7 patients (2.0 %). Of these, only 4 were resectable [17]. In a large series of 411 BD-IPMN patients from the Massachusetts General Hospital who were initially addressed to a surveillance protocol, 88 underwent delayed resection. No patient developed unresectable BD-IPMN carcinoma at a median follow-up of 60 months. Invasive cancer arising in BD-IPMN was found in 23 patients of the entire cohort (4 %), and an additional 21 patients (3.7 %) had or developed concurrent pancreatic ductal adenocarcinoma. Interestingly, 76 % of resected BD-IPMNs with carcinoma in situ and 95 % of resected BD-IPMNs with invasive cancer had high-risk stigmata or worrisome features according to the revised 2012 IAP guidelines. Caution was advised for larger lesions (>3 cm), even in the absence of worrisome features, because of an increased risk of harboring high-grade dysplasia [18]. In another large series of 569 Sendai-negative BD-IPMN patients enrolled in a surveillance program at the University of Verona (median follow-up of 56 months), the 5-year risk of pancreatic malignancies was 1.4 %, tenfold greater than expected according to the Italian tumor registries [9]. The pancreatic cancer incidence was lower than observed in Japanese studies. As an example, the 5-year incidence of pancreatic cancer in a series of 103 BD-IPMN patients conservatively followed up for ≥2 years at Kyoto University (median of 59 months) was 2.4% [19].

The Verona study also showed that the incidence of extrapancreatic malignancies during the follow-up period was not greater than the general population [9]. The concept that IPMN patients are not at risk of extrapancreatic carcinogenesis was also confirmed in a multicentric, European setting, indicating that a comprehensive cancer screening during the IPMN follow-up may not be warranted, as suggested by previous prevalence studies [20, 21].

Only two smaller series from France analyzed the results of patients with low-risk BD-IPMN with a minimum follow-up of 5 years. The former included 49 patients (mean follow-up period of 77 months). 77.5 % of patients remained free of symptoms. Five patients underwent delayed resection (mean time delay after diagnosis of 20 months). Pathologically, none of these patients had malignancy [22]. In the latter series, analyzing 53 patients (median follow-up of 84 months), crossover to surgery was necessary in three patients, none of whom had ultimately an invasive disease. However, an invasive advanced carcinoma occurred in two patients, both after 84 months from the diagnosis [23].

Interestingly, in small series of IPMNs meeting criteria for resection (Sendai positive) and not operated because of age and comorbidities, the outcome was relatively good (overall median disease-specific survival of 55 months), especially in the BD type. The authors proposed that a conservative approach in patients who are not surgically fit is also reasonable [24]. On the contrary, some authors claim that even Sendai-negative BD-IPMNs have a significant malignant potential (24.6 %) and propose a more liberal operative policy [25].

The debate on the optimal management of IPMN is still open, and there is little evidence in the literature to guide the frequency and type of surveillance for IPMN managed nonoperatively. Some authors propose that surveillance can be safely spaced to every 2 years or even discontinued after long-term stability in low-risk lesions. However, concern over the development of pancreatic ductal adenocarcinoma in the pancreas harboring IPMN prompts to continue active lifelong surveillance at short intervals [25]. Undoubtedly, surveillance results in significant utilization of cross-sectional imaging, endoscopic ultrasound, and economic investment.

9.4.2 Outcome After Resection of IPMN

The outcome after resection of IPMN depends on different factors including:

- Presence of an invasive component
- Histologic subtype
- Duct involvement
- Resection margin
- Lymph node status (in invasive IPMN)

The prognosis of patients with noninvasive IPMN is excellent, and the 5-year survival rate is reported to be >70 % in most series. Some series have even suggested a 5-year survival in excess of 90 % after resection. Conversely, the 5-year survival rate for invasive IPMN (carcinoma arising in the background of IPMN) ranges from 34 to 62 %. The outcome of invasive IPMN is therefore poor in comparison with noninvasive IPMN, but appears to be better than pancreatic ductal adenocarcinoma, which exhibits a 5-year survival rate ranging from 9 to 21 %. Whether this is due to a stage shift with earlier diagnosis of IPMN or due to a true less aggressive behavior of invasive IPMN remains controversial [26]. Disease recurrence may arise either in the pancreatic remnant or in peripancreatic or extrapancreatic sites.

Recent data indicates that invasive IPMN is a heterogeneous disease, because it can exhibit different histologic patterns, namely, colloid (colloid carcinoma), tubular (tubular adenocarcinoma), or oncocytic (oncocytic carcinoma). According to the reports by Furukawa et al. and by Mino-Kenudson et al., colloid carcinoma derives from intestinal-type IPMN and is associated with a particularly indolent behavior. In turn, intestinal IPMNs are mainly MD type. Tubular adenocarcinoma correlates with the gastric and the pancreatobiliary epithelial subtypes and is associated with a dismal prognosis, similar to that of pancreatic ductal adenocarcinoma. Gastric IPMNs are mainly BD type [26, 27]. Although gastric-type BD-IPMNs most often harbor low-grade dysplasia and absence of invasion, in the series by Mino-Kenudson et al., 15.6 % of surgically resected gastric-type IPMNs gave rise to tubular adenocarcinoma [26]. Oncocytic carcinoma derives from the uncommon oncocytic subtype and has a significantly better outcome than ductal adenocarcinoma [26, 27].

The clinical implications of surgical resection margin (frozen section of the pancreatic cut surface) are controversial, and the results in the literature are mixed on this topic [28]. In general, not all the studies found a strong correlation between margin status and risk of recurrence. There have been reports of invasive carcinomas in association with only mild or moderate dysplasia within the IPMN in the remnant pancreas [1]. A meta-analysis published in 2012 showed that the recurrence rate in patients with noninvasive IPMN was 3.72 % with negative margins and 9.56 % with positive margins. The same meta-analysis showed that recurrence after surgical resection of invasive IPMN occurred in 33.8 % of patients with negative margins and in 53.6 % of patients with positive margins [29]. In a recent paper by the Seoul National University Hospital group, 403 consecutive patients who underwent resection of IPMN were followed on average for 44 months. The overall recurrence rate was 10.7 %. Pathologic grade of dysplasia was associated with recurrence rate. IPMNs involving the main duct had a higher rate of recurrence. Multivariate analysis revealed that the degree of dysplasia was the most important predictor of recurrence. The overall 5-year disease-free survival rate was 78.9 % and was significantly lower in patients with high-grade dysplasia than in those with low- or intermediate-grade dysplasia. Importantly, of patients with benign or noninvasive IPMN, 5.4 % had recurrence including distant metastasis. The authors concluded that thorough postoperative surveillance is needed also for those with noninvasive IPMN, especially for those with HGD [30]. In another paper from the Massachusetts General Hospital analyzing 412 resected IPMNs, 17 % of patients experienced IPMN recurrence after a median follow-up of 58 months. Invasive component and a positive resection margin were predictors of recurrence. Invasive IPMN recurred in 45 % of cases, whereas noninvasive in only 9 %; patterns depended on IPMN subtypes and duct involvement. In particular, the risk of recurrence was greater in tubular than in colloid carcinomas. Furthermore, oncocytic type seems to have a peculiar biology, with recurrence taking place as far out as 11 years after removal of the primary tumor, and an excellent survival. Regarding the duct involvement, recurrence after resection of a benign BD-IPMN was uncommon and, when it occurred, it did so almost invariably as a noninvasive tumor. In addition, the risk of developing a new pancreatic ductal adenocarcinoma during follow-up after resection for IPMN was only 0.5 %. This low incidence is no different than the one expected in the American population, stratified by age group. Taken together, the extreme rarity of the occurrence of metachronous PDAC after the resection of IPMN, coupled with the recurrence pattern of BD type, suggests that in older individuals, follow-up after resection of a benign BD-IPMN could be avoided [31]. Lymph node status is another factor affecting long-term outcome in invasive IPMN [32]. The 5-year survival of patients with positive lymph nodes ranged from 20 to 30 %, while N0 patients lived much longer, in the range from 80 to 85 %. Lymph node ratio >0.2 has been shown to be associated with worse prognosis [32]. Data from the Surveillance, Epidemiology, and End Results (SEER) registry database suggests that increased lymph node counts were associated with improved survival in invasive IPMN patients. The cutoff value of lymph node count was 16 for this improvement [33]. Data from a meta-analysis demonstrated that nearly 77 % of lymph node-positive patients recurred, while disease recurrence occurred only 30.8 % of patients with negative lymph nodes [29].

9.5 Solid Pseudopapillary Neoplasms (SPNs)

Recent data indicates that the number of SPNs reported in the literature has seen a sevenfold increase since 2000, compared with previous studies. In a systematic review of 2285 patients who underwent pancreatic resection, follow-up details were available in 1952 patients. A tumor recurrence was observed in 86 patients (4.4 %); the median time to recurrence was 50.5 months

[34]. A retrospective multicenter study that included data from 351 patients who underwent surgical resection from January 1990 to December 2008 at 17 Korean medical institutions showed that only 9 patients (2.6 %) experienced tumor recurrence after the initial pancreatic SPT resection. On multivariate analysis, a tumor size larger than 8 cm, microscopic malignant features, and stage IV were significant prognostic factors for tumor recurrence. When combined with stage IV, the microscopic malignant features and the 2010 World Health Organization definition of solid pseudopapillary carcinoma more successfully differentiated future recurrence risk groups [35]. In another Korean study of 106 patients, after a median follow-up of 56.9 months from resection, two patients with high-grade malignant SPN had evidence of tumor recurrence in the lymph nodes and liver [36]. Taken together, these results indicate that more than 95 % of patients with solid pseudopapillary neoplasms limited to the pancreas are cured by complete surgical excision. Local invasion or resectable liver and lymph node metastases are not absolute contraindications for resection, and some patients with advanced tumors can survive for more than 10 years after the operation [37]. A careful follow-up is necessary, because recurrence of the disease in the liver or lymph nodes is possible, yet uncommon. The treatment of recurrent disease is anecdotal. In the few cases in which radiotherapy or chemotherapy was used, results were encouraging [38].

9.6 Final Remarks

The natural history of pancreatic cystic neoplasms is largely unknown in the long term, and data beyond 5 years are virtually lacking. Because it seems that survival is clearly favorable in comparison with pancreatic ductal adenocarcinoma, it will be of great importance to understand how these neoplasms behave, with respect to the time to progression, the risk of developing a new cyst or additional malignancy after resection (e.g., in IPMN), and the risk of disease-specific mortality. Accurate surveillance, either pre- or postoperatively, seems mandatory in the majority of cystic neoplasms, since most have the potential to become malignant or to recur. For those that become malignant, it may take perhaps as many as 10 years or more for that evolution. So early reports with limited length of follow-up are just the beginning and are not long enough to really capture the natural history of these neoplasms.

References

1. Tanaka M, Castillo CF, Adsay V, Chari ST, Falconi M, Jang J-Y, et al. International consensus guidelines 2012 for the management of IPMN and MCN of the pancreas. Pancreatology. 2012;12:183–97.
2. Del Chiaro M, Verbeke C, Salvia R, Klöppel G, Werner J, McKay C, et al. European experts consensus statement on cystic tumours of the pancreas. Dig Liver Dis. 2013;45:703–11.
3. Vege SS, Ziring B, Jain R, Moayyedi P, Clinical Guidelines Committee, American Gastroenterology Association. American gastroenterological association institute guideline on the diagnosis and management of asymptomatic neoplastic pancreatic cysts. Gastroenterology. 2015;148:819–22.
4. Salvia R, Malleo G, Marchegiani G, Pennacchio S, Paiella S, Paini M, et al. Pancreatic resections for cystic neoplasms: from the surgeon's presumption to the pathologist's reality. Surgery. 2012;152:S135–42.
5. Del Chiaro M, Segersvärd R, Pozzi Mucelli R, Rangelova E, Kartalis N, Ansorge C, et al. Comparison of preoperative conference-based diagnosis with histology of cystic tumors of the pancreas. Ann Surg Oncol. 2014;21:1539–44.
6. Malleo G, Bassi C, Rossini R, Manfredi R, Butturini G, Massignani M, et al. Growth pattern of serous cystic neoplasms of the pancreas: observational study with long-term magnetic resonance surveillance and recommendations for treatment. Gut. 2012;61:746–51.
7. Jais B, Rebours V, Malleo G, Salvia R, Fontana M, Maggino L, et al. Serous cystic neoplasm of the pancreas: a multinational study of 2622 patients under the auspices of the International Association of Pancreatology and European Pancreatic Club (European Study Group on Cystic Tumors of the Pancreas). Gut. 2016;65(2):305–12.
8. Lafemina J, Katabi N, Klimstra D, Correa-Gallego C, Gaujoux S, Kingham TP, et al. Malignant progression in IPMN: a cohort analysis of patients initially selected for resection or observation. Ann Surg Oncol. 2013;20:440–7.
9. Malleo G, Marchegiani G, Borin A, Capelli P, Accordini F, Butturini G, et al. Observational study of the incidence of pancreatic and extrapancreatic malignancies during surveillance of patients with

branch-duct intraductal papillary mucinous neoplasm. Ann Surg. 2015;261:984–90.
10. El-Hayek KM, Brown N, O'Rourke C, Falk G, Morris-Stiff G, Walsh RM. Rate of growth of pancreatic serous cystadenoma as an indication for resection. Surgery. 2013;154:794–800.
11. Das A, Wells CD, Nguyen CC. Incidental cystic neoplasms of pancreas: what is the optimal interval of imaging surveillance? Am J Gastroenterol. 2008;103:1657–62.
12. Sakorafas GH, Smyrniotis V, Reid-Lombardo KM, Sarr MG. Primary pancreatic cystic neoplasms revisited. Part I: serous cystic neoplasms. Surg Oncol. 2011;20(2):e84–92.
13. Wasel BA, Keough V, Huang W-Y, Molinari M. Histological percutaneous diagnosis of stage IV microcystic serous cystadenocarcinoma of the pancreas. BMJ Case Rep. 2013;2013.
14. Crippa S, Salvia R, Warshaw AL, Domínguez I, Bassi C, Falconi M, et al. Mucinous cystic neoplasm of the pancreas is not an aggressive entity: lessons from 163 resected patients. Ann Surg. 2008;247:571–9.
15. Lewis GH, Wang H, Bellizzi AM, Klein AP, Askin FB, Schwartz LE, et al. Prognosis of minimally invasive carcinoma arising in mucinous cystic neoplasms of the pancreas. Am J Surg Pathol. 2013;37:601–5.
16. Sakorafas GH, Smyrniotis V, Reid-Lombardo KM, Sarr MG. Primary pancreatic cystic neoplasms revisited: part II. Mucinous cystic neoplasms. Surg Oncol. 2011;20:e93–101.
17. Maguchi H, Tanno S, Mizuno N, Hanada K, Kobayashi G, Hatori T, et al. Natural history of branch duct intraductal papillary mucinous neoplasms of the pancreas. Pancreas. 2011;40:364–70.
18. Sahora K, Mino-Kenudson M, Brugge W, Thayer SP, Ferrone CR, Sahani D, et al. Branch duct intraductal papillary mucinous neoplasms: does cyst size change the tip of the scale? A critical analysis of the revised international consensus guidelines in a large single-institutional series. Ann Surg. 2013;258:466–75.
19. Sawai Y, Yamao K, Bhatia V, Chiba T, Mizuno N, Sawaki A, et al. Development of pancreatic cancers during long-term follow-up of side-branch intraductal papillary mucinous neoplasms. Endoscopy. 2010;42:1077–84.
20. Marchegiani G, Malleo G, D'Haese JG, Wenzel P, Keskin M, Pugliese L, et al. Association between pancreatic intraductal papillary mucinous neoplasms and extrapancreatic malignancies. Clin Gastroenterol Hepatol. 2015;13:1162–9.
21. Sugiyama M, Atomi Y. Extrapancreatic neoplasms occur with unusual frequency in patients with intraductal papillary mucinous tumors of the pancreas. Am J Gastroenterol. 1999;94:470–3.
22. Arlix AA, Bournet BB, Otal PP, Canevet GG, Thevenot AA, Kirzin SS, et al. Long-term clinical and imaging follow-up of nonoperated branch duct form of intraductal papillary mucinous neoplasms of the pancreas. Pancreas. 2012;41:295–301.
23. Khannoussi W, Vullierme MP, Rebours V, Maire F, Hentic O, Aubert A, et al. The long term risk of malignancy in patients with branch duct intraductal papillary mucinous neoplasms of the pancreas. Pancreatology. 2012;12:198–202.
24. Piciucchi M, Crippa S, Del Chiaro M, Valente R, Pezzilli R, Falconi M, et al. Outcomes of intraductal papillary mucinous neoplasm with "Sendai-positive" criteria for resection undergoing non-operative management. Dig Liver Dis. 2013;45:584–8.
25. Fritz S, Klauss M, Bergmann F, Hackert T, Hartwig W, Strobel O, et al. Small (sendai negative) branch-duct IPMNs. Ann Surg. 2012;256:313–20.
26. Mino-Kenudson M, Fernandez-Del CC, Baba Y, Valsangkar NP, Liss AS, Hsu M, et al. Prognosis of invasive intraductal papillary mucinous neoplasm depends on histological and precursor epithelial subtypes. Gut. 2011;60:1712–20.
27. Furukawa T, Hatori T, Fujita I, Yamamoto M, Kobayashi M, Ohike N, et al. Prognostic relevance of morphological types of intraductal papillary mucinous neoplasms of the pancreas. Gut. 2011;60:509–16.
28. He J, Cameron JL, Ahuja N, Makary MA, Hirose K, Choti MA, et al. Is it necessary to follow patients after resection of a benign pancreatic intraductal papillary mucinous neoplasm? J Am Coll Surg. 2013;216:657–65.
29. Leng KM, Wang ZD, Zhao JB, Cui Y-F, Zhong XY. Impact of pancreatic margin status and lymph node metastases on recurrence after resection for invasive and noninvasive intraductal papillary mucinous neoplasms of the pancreas: a meta-analysis. Dig Surg. 2012;29:213–25.
30. Kang MJ, Jang JY, Lee KB, Chang YR, Kwon W, Kim SW. Long-term prospective cohort study of patients undergoing pancreatectomy for intraductal papillary mucinous neoplasm of the pancreas: implications for postoperative surveillance. Ann Surg. 2014;260:356–63.
31. Marchegiani G, Mino-Kenudson M, Ferrone CR, Morales-Oyarvide V, Warshaw AL, Lillemoe KD, et al. Patterns of recurrence after resection of IPMN: who, when, and how? Ann Surg. 2015;262(6):1108–14 [Epub ahead of print].
32. Partelli S, Castillo CF-D, Bassi C, Mantovani W, Thayer SP, Crippa S, et al. Invasive intraductal papillary mucinous carcinomas of the pancreas. Ann Surg. 2010;251:477–82.
33. Wu W, Hong X, Tian R, You L, Dai M, Liao Q, et al. An increased total resected lymph node count benefits survival following pancreas invasive intraductal papillary mucinous neoplasms resection: an analysis using the surveillance, epidemiology, and end result registry database. PLoS One. 2014;9, e107962.
34. Law JK, Ahmed A, Singh VK, Akshintala VS, Olson MT, Raman SP, et al. A systematic review of solid-pseudopapillary neoplasms: are these rare lesions? Pancreas. 2014;43:331–7.

35. Kang CM, Choi SH, Kim SC, Lee WJ, Choi DW, Kim SW, Korean Pancreatic Surgery Club. Predicting recurrence of pancreatic solid pseudopapillary tumors after surgical resection: a multicenter analysis in Korea. Ann Surg. 2014;260:348–55.
36. Kim MJ, Choi DW, Choi SH, Heo JS, Sung JY. Surgical treatment of solid pseudopapillary neoplasms of the pancreas and risk factors for malignancy. Br J Surg. 2014;101:1266–71.
37. Sakorafas GH, Smyrniotis V, Reid-Lombardo KM, Sarr MG. Primary pancreatic cystic neoplasms of the pancreas revisited. Part IV: rare cystic neoplasms. Surg Oncol. 2012;21:153–63.
38. Papavramidis T, Papavramidis S. Solid pseudopapillary tumors of the pancreas: review of 718 patients reported in English literature. J Am Coll Surg. 2005;200:965–72.

The Standard Surgical Treatment of Cystic Tumors of the Pancreas

10

Richard D. Schulick and Marco Del Chiaro

10.1 Introduction

The prevalence of cystic tumors of the pancreas appears to be increasing in incidence over time, most likely due to the presence of more sophisticated imaging modalities, as well as the common use of high-definition imaging techniques (e.g., CT scan) for the diagnosis or follow-up of many different diseases and conditions in the general population. Today a prevalence of as high as 30 % of cystic neoplasms in the pancreas is reported by some studies in the general population [1, 2]. In parallel, the volume of pancreatic surgery performed for cystic neoplasm of the pancreas has increased over the years. In contrast to solid tumors of the pancreas, cystic lesions are much less classified as a "surgical disease." Cystic neoplasms of the pancreas, which are a subset of cystic lesions, are a relatively large group of pancreatic tumors as defined by the WHO in 2010 [3]. However, in the clinical practice, there are four more common cystic tumors of the pancreas: intraductal papillary mucinous neoplasms (IPMNs), mucinous cystic neoplasms (MCNs), serous cystic neoplasms (SCNs), and solid pseudopapillary neoplasms (SPNs). The relative distribution of these tumors is reported in Table 10.1.

Of note, some of those tumors can progress from benign to invasive cancer. In contrast, SCNs are almost, with extremely rare exception, always benign and do not require surgery if asymptomatic, not large, and not growing significantly.

For this reason, an accurate workup is important in order to clarify as much as possible the diagnosis and consequently engage the correct treatment. Unfortunately, recent studies show that the preoperative accuracy in defining the correct diagnosis is quite low and ranges from 60 to 70 % at the most experienced centers [4]. However, perhaps even if the rate of preoperative diagnostic errors is quite high, the clinical impact of these errors seems to be acceptable and less than 10 % [4].

Table 10.1 Distribution of cystic tumors of the pancreas

Tumor type	Distribution (%)
IPMN (intraductal papillary mucinous neoplasm)	48
SCN (serous cystic neoplasm)	20
MCN (mucinous cystic neoplasm)	18
SPN (solid pseudopapillary neoplasm)	6
Others	8

R.D. Schulick, MD, MBA, FACS (✉)
Department of Surgery, University of Colorado School of Medicine, 12631 E. 17th Avenue, C-305, Aurora, CO 80045, USA
e-mail: richard.schulick@ucdenver.edu

M. Del Chiaro, MD, PhD, FACS
Division of Surgery, Department of Clinical Science, Intervention and Technology (CLINTEC), Karolinska Institute at Center for Digestive Diseases, Karolinska University Hospital, K53, Stockholm 14186, Sweden
e-mail: marco.del.chiaro@ki.se; marco.del-chiaro@karolinska.se

M. Del Chiaro et al. (eds.), *Cystic Tumors of the Pancreas*, DOI 10.1007/978-3-319-31882-0_10

In this chapter we will describe the surgical indication for the treatment of the four most frequent cystic tumors of the pancreas.

10.2 Surgical Treatment of Intraductal Papillary Mucinous Tumors of the Pancreas (IPMN)

IPMNs of the pancreas are the most common cystic tumor of the pancreas. They can progress from adenoma to cancer analogous to the colonic polyps. For this reason, the correct treatment of IPMN of the pancreas can represent a large opportunity for the prevention or early treatment of pancreatic cancer. However, unlike colon polyps that are very accessible to surveillance and biopsy, resection of IPMN requires a pancreatectomy which is a high-risk procedure. The management of these suspected lesions should be done very carefully, and the indication for surgery should be restricted to those patients with a significant increased risk for cancer.

Morphologically IPMNs of the pancreas are classified into three different subtypes: main-duct, branch- duct, and mixed-duct types. From a clinical point of view, when the main duct is involved in the IPMN (main-duct and mixed-duct types), the risk for cancer is higher than when only the side braches are involved. The frequency of invasive cancer or high-grade dysplasia in the forms involving the main pancreatic duct ranges from 60 to 70 %, definitely higher than in the forms involving the branch ducts only where the frequency is around 25 %. The mixed-duct type of IPMN has an intermediate risk of invasive cancer or high-grade dysplasia [5]. Accordingly, the clinical management of these lesions is different.

10.2.1 Main-Duct and Mixed-Duct IPMN

Both the international and European guidelines for cystic tumors of the pancreas [5, 6] recommend a surgical resection for all the patients with IPMN involving the main pancreatic duct who are fit for surgery. In this case, a resection following the oncologic principles of pancreatic cancer surgery should be undertaken. However, there is a significant amount of controversy around the extent of resection, especially when the main-duct involvement is limited to a restricted part of the gland. Under these circumstances there is a significant temptation to perform a partial pancreatectomy (pancreaticoduodenectomy or distal pancreatectomy) (Fig. 10.1). If this is to be done, a frozen section of the resection margin is strongly recommended (see paragraph on frozen section on IPMN). This is done, even in the context that IPMN can be discontinuous and can be a field defect of the entire pancreas. Nonetheless, there are certain findings at the resection margin that may drive further resection (invasive cancer or high-grade dysplasia) in the right context when a more limited pancreatectomy was being considered.

Even in the case of complete dilatation of the main pancreatic duct (Fig. 10.2), the European guidelines recommend an initial pancreaticoduodenectomy and a frozen section of the transection margin before proceeding to a total pancreatectomy. The reason for this approach is that in some cases, the dilatation of the duct in the body and tail of the pancreas is not due to complete ductal involvement by IPMN, but secondary to ductal obstruction from mucus or a solid component of the IPMN in the head of the pancreas. Under these circumstances, consideration of less than total pancreatectomy may be considered (see paragraph on frozen section on IPMN). In fit patients who otherwise have longevity, and who have clear total main-duct involvement, diffuse solid nodules, or multifocal solid nodules, a total pancreatectomy should be planned and undertaken.

If a partial pancreatectomy is performed and the primary lesion is known to be an IPMN with invasive cancer (either from initial diagnostic biopsy or intraoperative frozen section), then completion of total pancreatectomy or stopping should be considered in the context of what is currently at the margin and the patient's

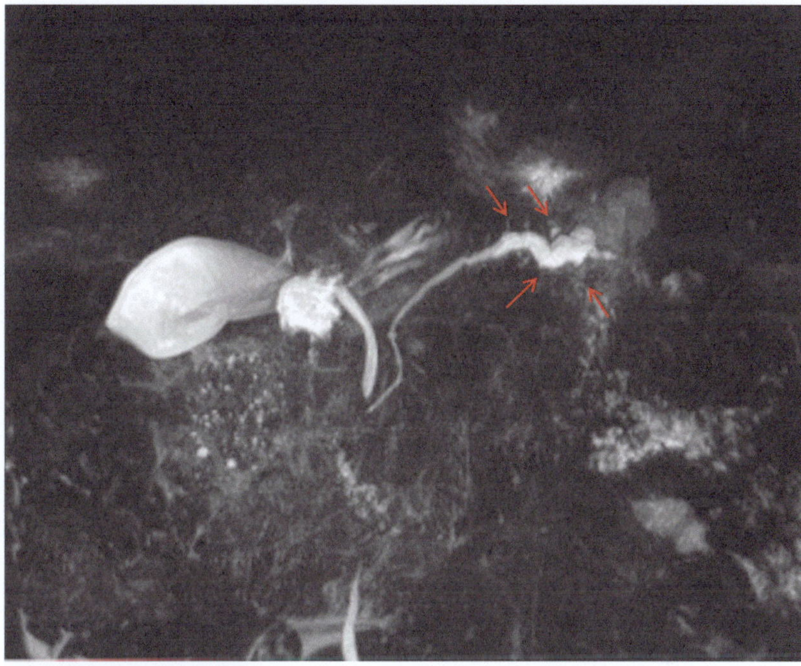

Fig. 10.1 MRCP of a mixed-type IPMN localized in the tail of the pancreas. The *arrows* show the dilatation of the main pancreatic duct and of the branch ducts

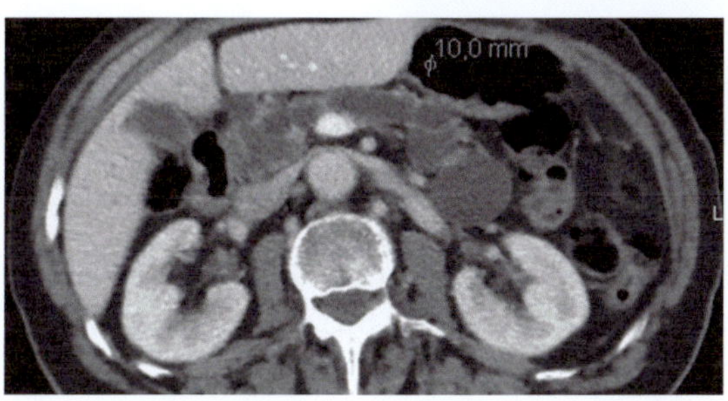

Fig. 10.2 Mixed-type IPMN completely involving the main pancreatic duct and with large branch-duct dilatation

prognosis [6]. For example, if a pancreaticoduodenectomy is performed and the uncinate margin is positive for cancer, the neck should not be further resected for high-grade dysplasia and perhaps even for invasive cancer. If a pancreaticoduodenectomy is performed for a known cancer in the head, and the uncinate and bile duct margins are negative for cancer, then most would further resect invasive cancer at the neck. Consideration of no further resection in this circumstance could be given for high-grade dysplasia at the neck, and certainly only a limited further resection (not total pancreatectomy) should be considered (Fig. 10.3).

10.2.2 Branch-Duct IPMN

The natural history of branch-duct IPMN seems to be different from those involving the main duct. The frequency of malignancy is lower, and only around 1 % of the patients, who are deemed to be low risk and under a surveillance program, develop pancreatic malignancy over time (at least over 10 years) [7]. For this reason, many of these patients are handled conservatively (see Chapter 10). However, resection is indicated in some circumstances in patients affected by branch-duct IPMN. Patients with symptoms that can be correlated to IPMN (jaundice, acute pancreatitis, abdominal pain) and radiological signs of malignancy (enlargement of the main pancreatic duct, mural nodules, rapid increase size) at presentation are often indicated for surgical resection (Table 10.2). The issue of size is controversial and has been strongly debated. Over the last 10 years, the diameter of a side-branch IPMN has been deemphasized, but there are data to both support this and to refute this trend. The European guidelines extended the limit for conservative management of BD-IPMN to four cm in diameter, in the absence of other risk factors or radiological signs of malignancy [6]. However, as stated by the

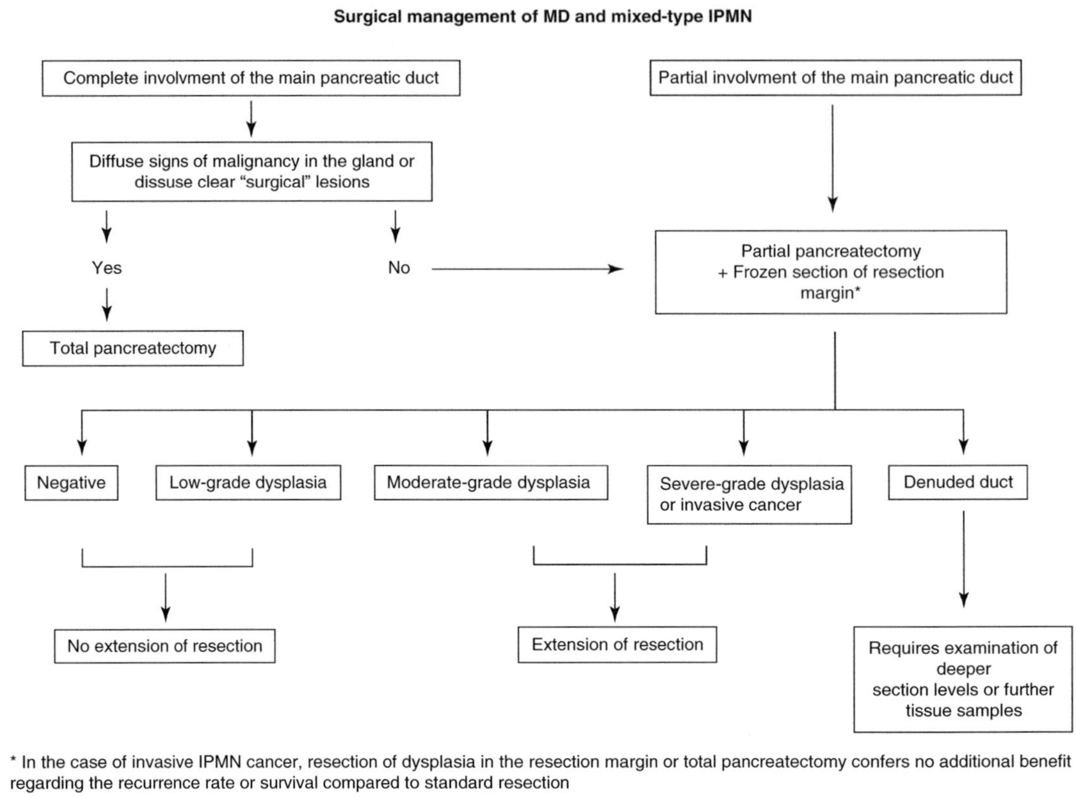

Fig. 10.3 Algorithm for surgical treatment of MD-IPMN and mixed-type IPMN

Table 10.2 Clinical and radiological criteria for resection according to European guidelines

Absolute indications
Symptoms related to IPMN (i.e., jaundice, diabetes, acute pancreatitis)
Mural nodules
Dilatation of the main pancreatic duct >6 mm
Relative indications
Rapidly increasing size
Elevated serum levels of CA 19-9

international guidelines [5], surgery can be considered an option for smaller lesions (>3 cm), even without radiological worrisome features or symptoms, in young patients fit for surgery.

In patients with branch-duct IPMN with either known or suspected malignancy, a conventional radical operation (pancreaticoduodenectomy or distal pancreatectomy with splenectomy) should be performed. Otherwise, consideration may be given to parenchyma-sparing procedures (central pancreatectomy or enucleation), as well as splenic preservation [5, 6]. Most consider branch-duct IPMN to be a field defect resulting in multifocal disease. Each cyst is thought to arise independently and thus should be treated autonomously. For this reason, even in patients with multiple lesions distributed through the pancreas, only the ones "at risk" should be surgically treated.

10.2.3 Role of Frozen Section in the Intraoperative Management of IPMN of the Pancreas

Frozen section of the resection margin is always indicated during surgery for IPMN of the pancreas, independent of the morphologic subtype.

According to the European guidelines for cystic tumors of the pancreas, additional resection of pancreatic parenchyma and further frozen section should be done in case there are invasive cancer and high-grade or moderate-grade dysplasia present at the margin. No additional resection is recommended for low-grade dysplasia. Many groups will not also chase a margin with moderate-grade dysplasia. A known cancer in the resected specimen or positive margins for cancer elsewhere will definitely lower or eliminate the need for further resection. Sometimes, the frozen section reveals a denuded duct which should not be considered a negative margin; therefore an additional resection and frozen section should be considered if it will affect management. All of these indications should be evaluated in the context of the patient's fitness (age), performance status, and compliance.

When a known cancer arising in an IPMN has been resected, the role of frozen section margin of the pancreatic neck/body margin is diminished. This is because the already resected cancer significantly drives the prognosis of the patient, not the remaining noncancerous side-branch or microscopic IPMNs. Even in cases where the frozen section margin has no IPMN or only low-grade dysplasia, this is no guarantee that the remnant gland does not harbor a malignancy or a lesion that will progress to malignancy. IPMN of the pancreas seems to be a disease that involves the entire gland and may harbor what are termed skip lesions. Today there are no validated methods that reliably detect these skip lesions pre- or intraoperatively, other than those that are used to bring the patient to the operating room for the index lesion(s). However, some promising results seem to come from the pre- or intraoperative use of pancreatic ductoscopy (Fig. 10.4) [8].

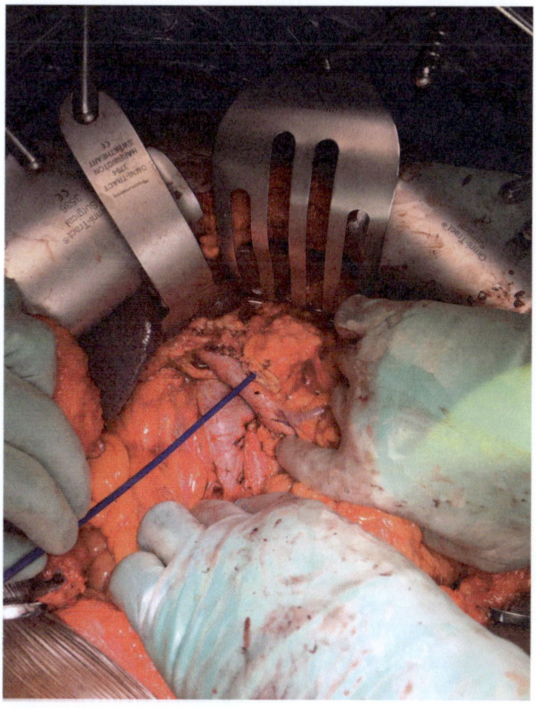

Fig. 10.4 Intraoperative use of pancreatoscopy in a patient who underwent pancreaticoduodenectomy for MD-IPMN

10.2.4 Treatment of Locally Advanced IPMN Cancer

Presently, there are no recommendations that exist regarding the treatment of locally advanced IPMN cancer. For this reason, the authors suggest using the currently accepted guidelines for "garden-variety" ductal adenocarcinoma [9]. Tumors with limited involvement of the superior mesenteric-portal vein (SMPV) and without involvement of the critical arterial structures can be resected upfront (Fig. 10.4). In contrast, borderline resectable tumors (resectable involvement of the SMPV and/or less than 50 % of the circumference of critical arterial structures) should be treated with neoadjuvant therapy and reevaluated for surgery after that.

10.2.5 Follow-Up After Resection

Data from the literature show that IPMN of the pancreas can recur (or persist) after surgery and can even progress. Overall, it is estimated that over 15 % of these patients over a 10–15-year period develop a recurrence that dictates the need for repeat resection (and unfortunately in some cases malignancy that cannot be resected) [10]. The goals of postoperative surveillance in patients surgically resected for IPMN of the pancreas include (a) progression of known remaining lesions, (b) development of new IPMN in the pancreas remnant, and (c) local recurrence or distant metastases in case of IPMN cancer.

The strategy for surveillance of resected (benign) IPMN is different in the European compared to the international guidelines. For malignant IPMN the follow-up of these patients can mirror that of patients surgically treated for non-IPMN ductal adenocarcinoma. For nonmalignant IPMN, the European guidelines recommend a yearly follow-up (to include cross-sectional imaging) in patients with or without known lesions remaining within the pancreas [6]. In the international guidelines the follow-up of these patients is personalized according with the marginal status and the histotype [5].

10.3 Surgical Treatment of Mucinous Cystic Neoplasms (MCNs)

MCN of the pancreas is a mucinous tumor typically found in females (90 %) and located in the body and tail (90 %) of the pancreas. Similar to IPMN, MCN has the ability to become malignant. In the case of highly suspected or known MCN, historically there has been a strong tendency toward surgical resection [11]. Between 12 and 20 % of resected MCNs are associated with invasive carcinoma. Data from the literature seem to indicate a more indolent biology of these lesions than IPMN. Even large lesions can remain benign even for a long period of time (Fig. 10.5).

When MCNs are small, they can be hard to distinguish from oligocystic SCN or branch-duct IPMN which are typically observed rather than resected. In order to prevent overtreatment of these lesions, the European guidelines on cystic tumors of the pancreas proposed a more conservative approach [6]. Today surgical resection is always indicated in patients with worrisome radiological features, with symptoms, or with a biopsy diagnostic of MCN. However, for lesions less than 4 cm in diameter, and which could be SCN or branch-duct IPMN, a surveillance strategy, as reported in Fig. 10.6, can be adopted.

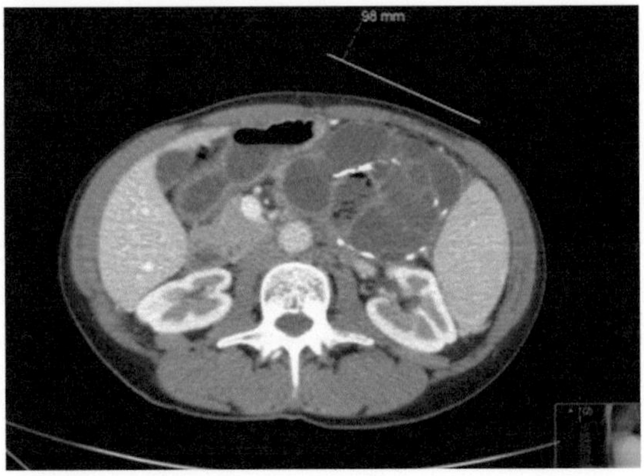

Fig. 10.5 MCN of the pancreas, 10 cm in diameter, with high-grade dysplasia at the histology

Frozen section of the cyst wall of an MCN can be falsely negative. There are regressive changes within MCNs and a significant part of the cyst inner wall can be denuded. This can cause an erroneous diagnosis of pseudocyst at the frozen section. For this reason an intraoperative frozen section of a part of the cyst wall in order to make a differential diagnosis with other cyst types can be erroneous. Finding ovarian stroma on the cyst wall is diagnostic of MCN.

In case of suspected malignant MCN, a standard resection for cancer should be performed. If there is very low or no suspicion of malignancy, spleen-preserving procedures or parenchyma-sparing procedures (enucleation, central pancreatectomy) can be used.

Following complete resection of benign MCN, follow-up for recurrence or malignancy is not necessary; it is a unifocal disease the great majority of the time. In case of malignant MCN, follow-up similar to ductal adenocarcinoma is recommended [6].

10.4 Surgical Treatment of Serous Cystic Neoplasms (SCNs)

SCN is considered a benign disease. There are very limited reports in literature of malignant SCN and authors disagree on the real existence of invasive forms of SCN. In a recent large multicenter series, the rate of malignant SCN was 0.001 % [12]. For this reason, a conservative

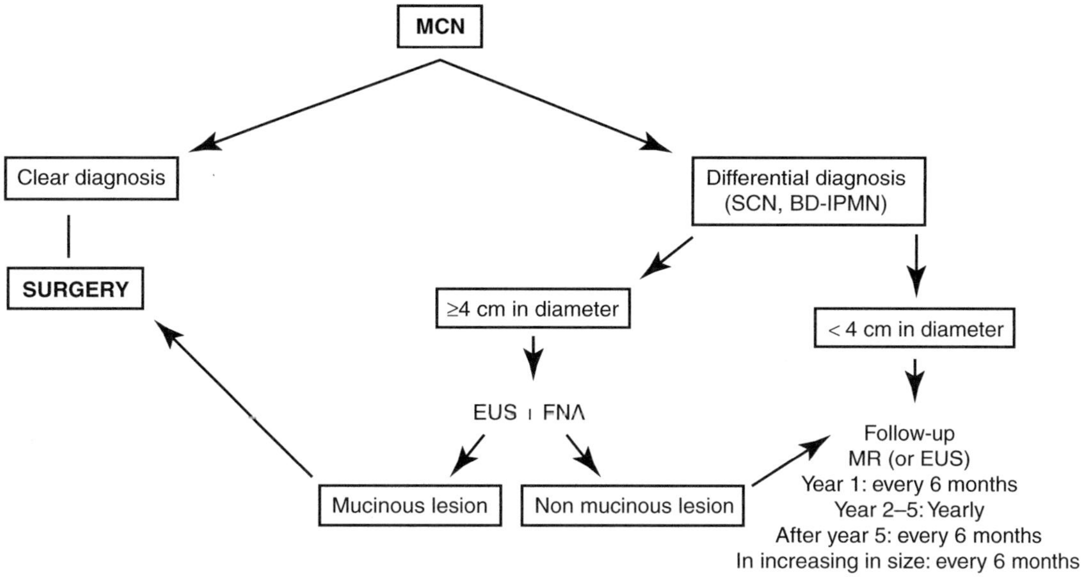

Fig. 10.6 Algorithm for the treatment of patients with suspected MCNs

approach is the treatment of choice in the great majority of patients with SCN.

SCNs are resected usually for one of two reasons: (a) they are misdiagnosed as potentially being one of the more dangerous cystic lesions of the pancreas (IPMN, MCN, or cystic neuroendocrine tumors) or (b) they are large and/or symptomatic. Oligocystic SCN is more often misdiagnosed as an IPMN or MCN, whereas microcystic SCN is more often misdiagnosed as a cystic neuroendocrine tumor [4]. Symptoms in patients with SCN are typically related to the growth of the tumors and mass effect, which can be manifested as jaundice, pain, and recurrent pancreatitis (Fig. 10.7). Absolute dimensions are not, today, considered an indication for resection. However, oligo-macrocystic lesions located in the head of the pancreas seem to have a higher rate of growth which is sometimes taken as a prognostic factor for later development of symptoms. In young and fit patients and with SCNs larger than 6 cm, a resection can be considered [6, 13, 14].

Pancreas- or parenchyma-sparing procedure should almost always be performed when it is possible. Standard oncologic resections should be performed for those very rare patients that have a known cancer or otherwise are highly suspected of harboring a cancer.

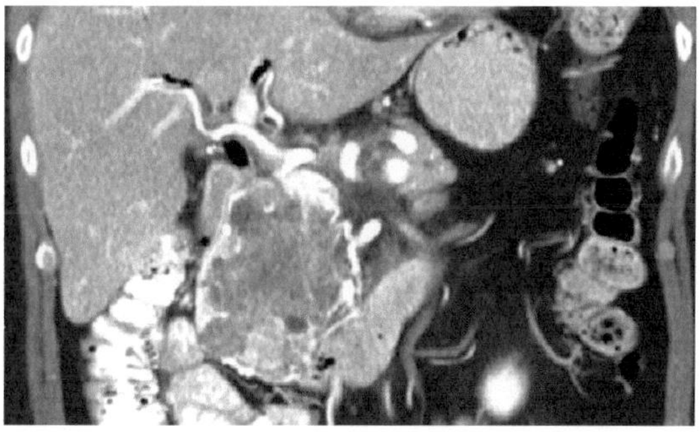

Fig. 10.7 Patient with large microcystic SCN in the head of the pancreas that is discovered because of jaundice

10.5 Surgical Treatment of Solid Pseudopapillary Neoplasms (SPNs)

SPNs are rare solid and cystic tumors of the pancreas. Because of their prevalence in younger patients, and their relatively good prognosis, they are important to consider in the differential. Generally, they affect young women in their second decade, but these tumors can be found also in pediatric age, as well as middle-aged women. This neoplasm has a low malignant potential and the prognosis after resection is excellent with a 5-year survival rate of 95 % [6, 14, 15]. These tumors rarely are symptomatic at a small size. Therefore, at the moment of clinical presentation, they are generally large and sometimes with invasion of surrounding structures (vessels or other organs) and rarely distant metastasis (mostly liver metastases). However, because of the relatively indolent behavior and the excellent prognosis, extended resections (including vascular structures, adjacent organs, and even simultaneous resection of distant metastases) are recommended with usually good long-term results. Even debulking surgery offers advantages in these patients compared with palliation, if patients are suitably selected [16, 17].

10.6 Summary

- The prevalence of cystic tumors of the pancreas appears to be increasing in incidence due to increased use of higher definition imaging.
- The volume of pancreatic surgery performed for cystic neoplasms is increasing.
- The four most common types of cystic neoplasms of the pancreas are:
  - Intraductal papillary mucinous neoplasm (IPMN)
  - Mucinous cystic neoplasm (MCN)
  - Serous cystic neoplasm (SCN)
  - Solid pseudopapillary neoplasm (SPN)
- Differentiation between these main four types, as well as their subtypes, and assessing their malignant potential are important to appropriately select which patients benefit from resection.

References

1. Zhang XM, Mitchell DG, Dohke M, et al. Pancreatic cysts: depiction on single-shot fast spin-echo MR images. Radiology. 2002;223:547–53.
2. Girometti R, Intini S, Brondani G, et al. Incidental pancreatic cysts on 3D turbo spin echo magnetic resonance cholangiopancreatography: prevalence and relation with clinical and imaging features. Abdom Imaging. 2011;36:196–205.
3. Bosman FT, Carneiro F, Hruban RH, Theise ND. WHO classification of tumours of the digestive system. 4th ed. Lyon: International Agency for Research on Cancer; 2010.
4. Del Chiaro M, Segersvärd R, Pozzi Mucelli R, et al. Comparison of preoperative conference-based diagnosis with histology of cystic tumors of the pancreas. Ann Surg Oncol. 2014;21(5):1539–44.
5. Tanaka M, Fernandez del Castillo C, Adsay V, et al. International consensus guidelines 2012 for the management of IPMN and MCN of the pancreas. Pancreatology. 2012;12:183–97.
6. Del Chiaro M, Verbeke C, Salvia R, et al. European experts consensus statement on cystic tumors of the pancreas. DLD. 2013;45:703–11.
7. Malleo G, Marchegiani G, Borin A, et al. Observational study of the incidence of pancreatic and extrapancreatic malignancies during surveillance of patients with branch-duct intraductal papillary mucinous neoplasm. Ann Surg. 2015;261(5):984–90. doi:10.1097/SLA.0000000000000884.
8. Arnelo U, Siiki A, Swahn F, et al. Single-operator pancreatoscopy is helpful in the evaluation of suspected intraductal papillary mucinous neoplasms (IPMN). Pancreatology. 2014;14(6):510–4.
9. Hartwiq W, Vollmer CM, Fingerhut A, et al. Extended pancreatectomy in pancreatic ductal adenocarcinoma: definition and consensus of the International Study Group for Pancreatic Surgery (ISGPS). Surgery. 2014;156(1):1–14.
10. He J, Cameron JL, Ahuja N, et al. Is it necessary to follow patients after resection of a benign pancreatic intraductal papillary mucinous neoplasm? J Am Coll Surg. 2013;216(4):657–65.
11. Tanaka M, Chari S, Adsay V, et al. International consensus guidelines for management of intraductal papillary mucinous neoplasms and mucinous cystic neoplasms of the pancreas. Pancreatology. 2006;6:17–32.
12. Jaïs B, Rebours V, Malleo G, et al. Pancreatic serous cystadenoma related mortality is almost nil. Pancreatology. 2014;14(3):S4.
13. Malleo G, Bassi C, Rossini R, et al. Growth pattern of serous cystic neoplasms of the pancreas: observational study with long-term magnetic resonance surveillance and recommendations for treatment. Gut. 2011;2011:22.
14. Sakorafas GH, Smyrniotis V, Reid-Lombardo KM, et al. Primary pancreatic cystic neoplasms of the pancreas revisited. Part IV: Rare cystic neoplasms. Surg Oncol. 2011;2011:2.
15. Tipton SG, Smyrk TC, Sarr MG, et al. Malignant potential of solid pseudopapillary neoplasm of the pancreas. Br J Surg. 2006;93:733–7.
16. Papavramidis T, Papavramidis S. Solid pseudopapillary tumors of the pancreas: review of 718 patients reported in English literature. J Am Coll Surg. 2005;200:965–72.
17. Lee JS, Han HJ, Choi SB, et al. Surgical outcomes of solid pseudopapillary neoplasm of the pancreas: a single institution's experience for the last ten years. Am Surg. 2012;78:216–9.

11 Parenchyma-Sparing Pancreatic Resections in Cystic Tumors of the Pancreas

Thilo Hackert and Markus W. Büchler

11.1 Background

Among cystic lesions of the pancreas which are frequent findings, three important cystic entities have to be differentiated, namely, serous cystic neoplasms (SCN), mucinous cystic neoplasms (MCN), and intraductal papillary mucinous neoplasms (IPMN). As autopsy findings suggest a frequency of cystic pancreatic lesions in elderly people of up to 25 %, these findings are increasingly seen in the clinical practice, and management is a growing topic many disciplines have to deal with [1, 2]. The important clinical impact of all cystic lesions in the pancreas is the malignant potential arising from some of them, which requires increasing efforts in recognizing and managing these changes correctly. SCN, which represent about 15 % of all cystic lesions, are uncomplicated lesions that are predominantly found in women (80–90 %) of 60 years and older [3]. SCN do not bear any relevant malignant potential and are therefore a rare entity in surgical patient collectives. In contrast, MCN represent a precursor of pancreatic cancer and show a malignant transformation via an adenoma-carcinoma sequence in up to 50 % of all cases [4–8]. From this point of view, they are often subjected to a formal resection, e.g., distal pancreatectomy. However, depending on the location and size, they may be suitable for parenchyma-sparing approaches as well, presuming no malignancy is confirmed in an intraoperative frozen section.

IPMN represent 35 % of all cystic pancreas lesions with an increasing frequency due to improved diagnostics and an increasing clinical attention. About 65 % of all IPMN are located in the pancreatic head and uncinate process, 24 % in the body, and 11 % in the tail of the gland [9, 10]. Main-duct IPMN, characterized by a dilation of the pancreatic duct of more than 5 mm, bear an estimated 70 % risk of malignant transformation, which implies the fact that the diagnosis of main-duct or mixed-type IPMN can be regarded as a general indication for a formal oncological resection and is rarely suitable for a parenchyma-sparing central pancreatectomy [11, 12] (Fig. 11.1).

In contrast, branch-duct IPMN (BD-IPMN) have to be regarded in a more differentiated way. As the overall risk of malignancy is lower than in main-duct and mixed-type IPMN, there is ongoing discussion about this risk with regard to size, growth tendency, and radiological features of potentially high-risk BD-IPMN. Regarding the indication for surgical treatment of BD-IPMN, there is an ongoing debate, especially with regard to lesions <3 cm in diameter and without "worrisome features" according to the Fukuoka guidelines that were published in 2012 as an

T. Hackert, MD • M.W. Büchler, MD (✉)
Department of Surgery, University of Heidelberg, Im Neuenheimer Feld 110, Heidelberg 69120, Germany
e-mail: thilo_hackert@med.uni-heidelberg.de; markus_buechler@med.uni-heidelberg.de

M. Del Chiaro et al. (eds.), *Cystic Tumors of the Pancreas*, DOI 10.1007/978-3-319-31882-0_11

update of the original 2006 Sendai consensus [11, 12]. In different larger series, the incidence of malignant branch-duct IPMN (including in situ and invasive carcinoma) was approximately 25 % among all IPMN below 3 cm without any reliable cutoff in diameter [13–18]. The existence of mural nodules as a guideline predictor of malignancy did not correlate with malignancy and neither did the existence of clinical symptoms [14, 15, 18]. These findings underline that size alone and currently established markers of potential malignancy are no reliable predictors and even small branch-duct IPMN have a relevant risk of malignancy. Individual decisions for resection under evaluation of all morphological and clinical factors (including imaging, tumor markers, symptoms, progression, and prior patient history) seem to offer the best approach at the moment. As the intention should be to prevent malignancy, the cystic pancreatic lesions, which are most suitable for parenchyma-sparing resections, especially enucleations, are branch-duct IPMN (BD-IPMN). As BD-IPMN can be localized throughout the entire pancreas, also central pancreatectomies are possible for lesions in the body of the gland (Fig. 11.2).

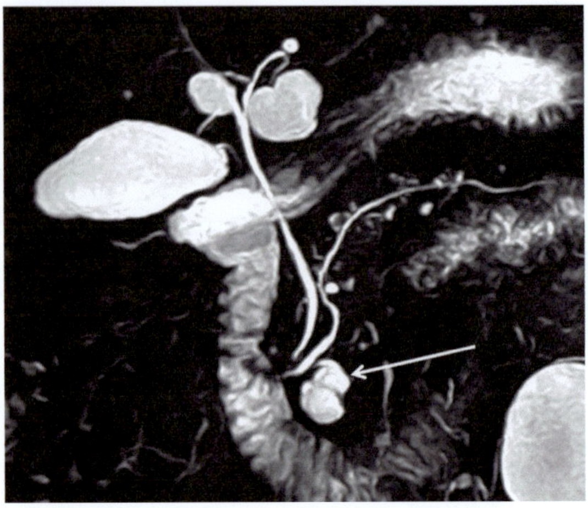

Fig. 11.1 MRCP scan showing a BD-IPMN located in the uncinate process (*white arrow*)

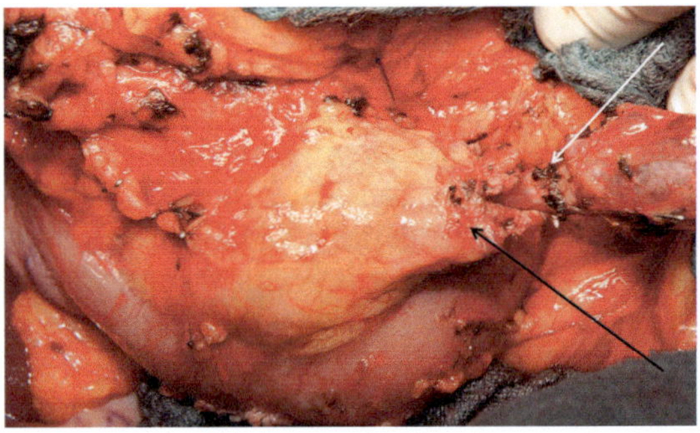

Fig. 11.2 Intraoperative finding of the same patient (Fig. 11.1). BD-IPMN (*white arrow*: connection to the pancreatic duct) during enucleation from the uncinate process (*black arrow*)

11.2 Surgical Technique of Enucleation

Enucleations for small cystic lesions, including especially branch-duct IPMN, offer a limited type of resection with the chance to preserve all healthy pancreatic tissue as only the altered tissue is removed [19–23]. They can safely and oncologically feasibly be performed if the benign character of the excised lesion is confirmed by intraoperative frozen section. In case of unexpected malignancy, a more extended resection should be chosen to meet the oncological requirements including a safety margin and lymphadenectomy. Although enucleations are usually performed for a single lesion, also two or even more cysts may be removed synchronously by this approach. A tumor size of 3 cm in diameter can be regarded as the limit for a safely performed enucleation. Tumors measuring more than 3 cm in size show malignant histological changes significantly more frequently, making a local surgical approach impossible. Besides, tissue trauma and wound surface following an enucleation reach a critical size for development of fistulas or other complications including bleeding or postoperative pancreatitis.

Successful enucleations are highly dependent on precise preoperative and/or intraoperative diagnosis of location of the cystic lesion. Especially in small cystic processes that are not located close below the pancreatic capsule, it can be challenging to identify them intraoperatively by palpating and inspecting the pancreas, even for experienced surgeons. Therefore, besides a high-quality preoperative MRI scan [24] which allows to limit the parts of the pancreas that have to be explored and gives a valid localization in the majority of the patients, the possibility of performing an intraoperative ultrasound always has to be provided regardless if enucleation is attempted via an open laparotomy or laparoscopically [25]. The sensitivity and specificity of this diagnostic tool are very high and allow an accurate localization in nearly all patients when combined with the experience of the surgeon performing the exploration [19, 20]. Furthermore, intraoperative ultrasound allows to rule out unrecognized multifocal lesions and is useful to visualize the cyst's connection to the pancreatic duct. After identifying the cystic lesion, enucleation in open surgery is performed by incising the pancreatic capsule and consecutive careful dissection along the cyst under clip ligation or stitching of vessels supplying the lesion. For stitching within the pancreatic tissue, thin atraumatic and non-resorbable suture material is preferable (e.g., 5-0 polypropylene). Careful bipolar coagulation or ultrasound dissection can be used in addition for an atraumatic preparation. Special attention needs to be paid to the connection to the pancreatic duct. This should not be missed and must be closed by clip or suture ligation to avoid high-volume enzyme leakage. In order to minimize the risk of parenchyma leaking, the pancreatic capsule can be closed above the resection site with single-stitch sutures. To date, there is no evidence for the efficacy of any additional sealant or glue application to prevent leakage. A simple possibility to cover the resection site is the use of a pedicled ligamentum teres hepatis flap which can – after mobilization from the abdominal wall – be brought to the site of resection in the pancreatic head or the proximal part of the pancreatic body without tension and fixed by suture [26].

Laparoscopically, enucleations for cystic lesions can be performed via a 4-trocar access as described for neuroendocrine pancreatic tumors [27, 28]. In the laparoscopic approach, a precise localization diagnosis is even more important as inspection and palpation of the pancreas are not possible as in open operations, which implies that laparoscopic ultrasound is required in many cases. The enucleation itself can be done by ultrasound dissection as well as by bipolar tissue sealing and cutting devices. Suturing of the pancreatic capsule can be done after removal of the specimen comparable to the open procedures; additional sealants may be used but their routine application is not supported by any evidence yet.

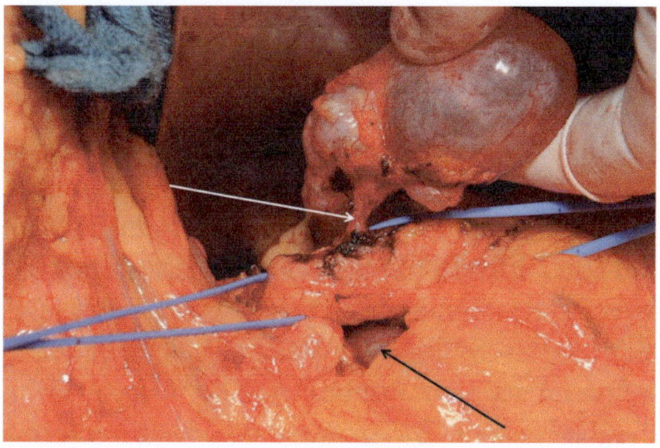

Fig. 11.3 Large BD-IPMN in the body of the pancreas. Although >3 cm in diameter, indication for enucleation due to the suitable location. Pancreatic body partly mobilized and lifted with blue tapes from the superior mesenteric vein (*black arrow*). Enucleation and identification of the connection to the main pancreatic duct (*white arrow*)

Drain placement is essential after enucleations, as currently fistula rates of 20–45 % are reported, most of them, however, clinically uncomplicated [19, 20]. In addition, the prophylactic use of octreotide seems to be recommendable in patients undergoing enucleations for cystic pancreatic lesions as the remaining pancreas is usually soft and healthy and the prophylactic use of somatostatin analogs can have a beneficial effect in prevention of postoperative fistulas in this setting [29] (Fig. 11.3).

11.3 Surgical Technique of Central Pancreatectomy

Central pancreatectomy is another limited resection approach for localized and benign cystic lesions located in the body of the gland. A segment between the level of the superior mesenteric vein/portal vein axis and the remaining tail of the gland can be resected under preservation of all healthy tissue [30–33]. Pancreatic transection can either be carried out proximally with a stapler or by scalpel and by scalpel toward the distal margin. The sharply cut margin toward the head is afterward primarily closed similar to the procedure during distal pancreatectomy. The distal stump of the pancreas is further mobilized from the splenic vein and artery, with ligation of small tributaries, over 2 cm lateral to the cut end. A transected jejunal loop is brought up transmesocolically, and a pancreaticojejunostomy is performed in a similar fashion as in pancreatoduodenectomy. Reconstruction is accomplished with a retrocolic Roux-en-Y loop of the jejunum. The already closed pancreatic head remnant can finally be covered with the same jejunal loop by sutures between the seromuscular layer of the jejunum and the capsule of the pancreas. Reconstruction is completed by an infracolic Roux-en-Y enteroenterostomy. Alternatively, a double anastomosis technique with two pancreaticojejunostomies is possible but prolongs operation time and does not necessarily offer any benefit compared to merely closing the cut margin toward the pancreatic head. Another possibility for reconstruction following central pancreatectomy is the creation of a pancreaticogastrostomy and simple closure of the cut margin toward the pancreatic head. However, this technique does not seem to be superior to pancreaticojejunostomy in terms of fistula rates or postoperative pancreatic function but might bear an increased risk for postoperative bleeding from the pancreatic stump as this is not covered in pancreaticogastrostomy. Although these bleeding events can often be handled endoscopically, they might contribute to other consecutive complications.

As in enucleations, drain placement toward the anastomosis and the cut margin is recommended at the end of the operation, and a prophylactic octreotide application seems reasonable based on the same basic considerations as described above. The most frequent complication of central pancreatectomy is the occurrence of postoperative pancreatic fistulas, which is observed in approximately 40 % of all patients. Comparable to enucleation, most of these fistulas are uncomplicated and do not cause consecutive complications under conservative management [30–33].

11.4 Complication Management and Postoperative Outcome

An important aspect in all types of pancreatic surgery is the management of potential postoperative complications. As mentioned before, postoperative pancreatic fistula is the most frequent and important complication in both enucleation and central pancreatectomy [34]. In large series of resected cystic pancreatic neoplasias in which all types of operations were performed, overall morbidity rates of approximately 35–50 % and mortality rates of 0–1 % are reported [35, 36]. When the parenchyma-sparing approaches of enucleation and central pancreatectomy are regarded, postoperative fistulas occur in up to 45 % of the patients. The majority of these fistulas is clinically harmless and can be treated by maintenance of the intraoperatively placed drainage without further morbidity. In case of delayed fistulas that become evident by clinical symptoms such as pain, fever, and elevated leukocyte count and C-reactive protein after drain removal, the therapy of choice is percutaneous drain insertion after diagnostic CT scan. If the drain can be placed sufficiently, no further complications have to be expected. A current meta-analysis comparing enucleations with standard resections included 22 observational studies. Operation time, blood loss, length of hospital stay, and postoperative endocrine and exocrine insufficiency were significantly lower after enucleation. Mortality, overall complications, reoperation rate, and delayed gastric emptying did not show significant differences. Although overall postoperative pancreatic fistula rate was significantly higher after enucleations, the elevated fistula rate did not have further consequences in terms of mortality or overall morbidity, which underlines that most of these fistulas are harmless [37].

In case of persistent leakage from the pancreatic duct, a diagnostic endoscopic retrograde pancreaticography is helpful, which can be performed approximately 14 days postoperatively if drain output does not decrease. This examination shows the site of leakage after enucleation and can often be used as a therapeutic tool as well, if transpapillary stenting is technically possible.

After central pancreatectomy, it may be useful to confirm a leakage from the cut margin at the pancreatic head and evaluate the possibility of transpapillary stent insertion as well. Although this intervention does not abolish leakage itself, the facilitated transpapillary drainage can help to accelerate closure of the fistula. A leakage from the pancreatic anastomosis toward the tail of the gland after central, however, cannot be treated endoscopically unless a pancreaticogastrostomy has been performed.

Other complications such as post-pancreatectomy hemorrhage or infected fluid collections are less frequently observed and can mainly be subjected to interventional radiological therapy as well. The overall reoperation rate in the reported series ranges between 5 and 8 %.

Parenchyma-sparing resections show excellent long-term outcome result with regard to endo- and exocrine pancreatic function when compared to formal standard resections which show long-term exocrine insufficiency rates with the need for enzyme and vitamin replacement of approximately 20 % after partial pancreatoduodenectomy and approximately 10 % after distal resections, respectively. Regarding endocrine function, a new-onset postoperative diabetes mellitus has to be expected in 10 % of all patients after partial pancreatoduodenectomy and up to 20 % after distal pancreatectomy [20]. In contrast, in patients undergoing enucleations or central pancreatectomies, no resection-related impairment of endocrine or exocrine pancreatic function has to be expected during long-term follow-up, and enzyme replacement or antidiabetic therapy is rarely necessary unless pancreatic function has already been compromised preoperatively. Furthermore, both procedures offer an excellent quality of life [22, 23, 30–33].

11.5 Prognosis

The prognosis of surgically resected benign cystic lesions is excellent. In SCN, recurrence is extremely rare and no further surveillance is required. Regarding mucinous neoplasias and especially IPMN, 10-year survival rates of >95 % for both main-duct and BD-IPMN can be expected [9, 10, 16]. A very important topic in the management of IPMN patients is the lifelong postoperative follow-up with annual imaging control of the pancreatic remnant. This is preferably performed by MRI or can alternatively be done by endosonographic ultrasound in experienced hands. In addition, regular endoscopic controls focused on colorectal adenomas and Barrett dysplasia of the esophagus are

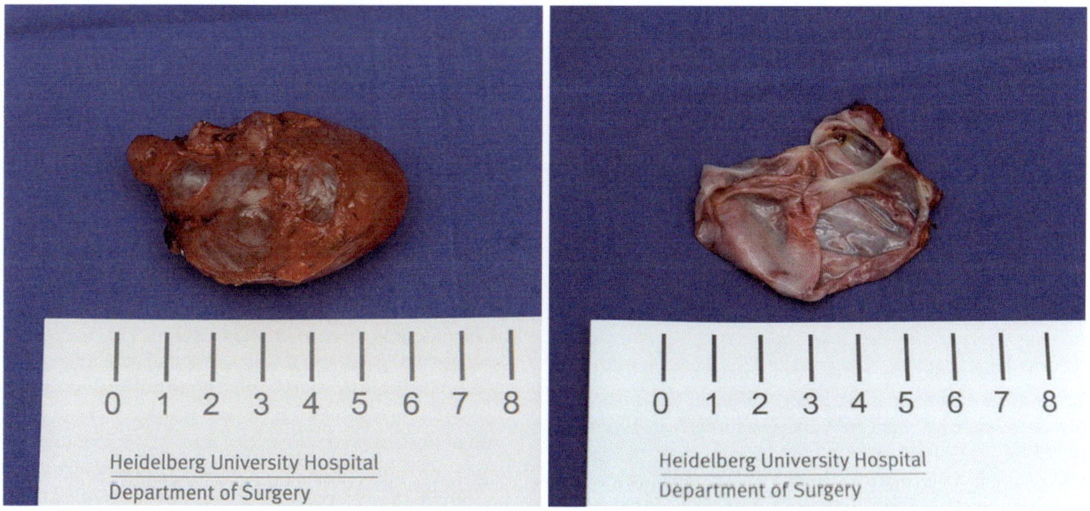

Fig. 11.4 Macroscopic aspect of the specimen (Fig. 11.3). Septated nodule, approximately Diameter approximately 5 cm, histologically borderline dysplasia

recommended as both pathologies are increasingly observed in IPMN patients [38, 39]. In case of IPMN recurrence, repeated resections should be performed to maintain the good prognosis and avoid malignancy. Overall prognosis even of IPMN-associated carcinomas is generally more favorable than the prognosis of pancreatic ductal adenocarcinoma (PDAC). In a study by Wasif et al. [40], 729 patients with IPMN-carcinomas were compared to 8082 PDAC patients. Overall survival in the collectives was 34 vs. 18 months. The most important factor influencing survival in this series was early resection. In tumor stages Tis and T1 of IPMN-associated carcinomas, 5- and 10-year survival rates were 70 % and 60 %, respectively. Another study including 132 IPMN-carcinoma patients vs. 1128 PDAC patients [41] demonstrated that this survival benefit decreases dramatically as soon as tumor stage exceeds T1 or if lymph node metastases are present, resulting in survival data as poor as they are found in PDAC patients. In this situation, even adjuvant therapy fails to improve survival [42], which underlines the importance of early resection to avoid progression to advanced tumor stages in IPMN patients (Fig. 11.4).

References

1. Kimura W, Nagai H, Kuroda A, Muto T, Esaki Y. Analysis of small cystic lesions of the pancreas. Int J Pancreatol. 1995;18(3):197–206.
2. Jani N, Bani Hani M, Schulick RD, Hruban RH, Cunningham SC. Diagnosis and management of cystic lesions of the pancreas. Diagn Ther Endosc. 2011;2011:478913. Epub 2011 Aug 22.
3. Matsumoto T, Hirano S, Yada K, Shibata K, Sasaki A, Kamimura T, Ohta M, Kitano S, Kashima K. Malignant serous cystic neoplasm of the pancreas: report of a case and review of the literature. J Clin Gastroenterol. 2005;39(3):253–6. Review.
4. Reddy RP, Smyrk TC, Zapiach M, Levy MJ, Pearson RK, Clain JE, Farnell MB, Sarr MG, Chari ST. Pancreatic mucinous cystic neoplasm defined by ovarian stroma: demographics, clinical features, and prevalence of cancer. Clin Gastroenterol Hepatol. 2004;2(11):1026–31.
5. Zamboni G, Scarpa A, Bogina G, Iacono C, Bassi C, Talamini G, Sessa F, Capella C, Solcia E, Rickaert F, Mariuzzi GM, Klöppel G. Mucinous cystic tumors of the pancreas: clinicopathological features, prognosis, and relationship to other mucinous cystic tumors. Am J Surg Pathol. 1999;23(4):410–22.
6. Goh BK, Tan YM, Chung YF, Chow PK, Cheow PC, Wong WK, Ooi LL. A review of mucinous cystic neoplasms of the pancreas defined by ovarian-type stroma: clinicopathological features of 344 patients. World J Surg. 2006;30:2236–45.
7. Izumo A, Yamaguchi K, Eguchi T, Nishiyama K, Yamamoto H, Yonemasu H, Yao T, Tanaka M, Tsuneyoshi M. Mucinous cystic tumor of the pancreas: immunohistochemical assessment of "ovarian-type stroma". Oncol Rep. 2003;10(3):515–25.
8. Thompson LD, Becker RC, Przygodzki RM, Adair CF, Heffess CS. Mucinous cystic neoplasm (mucinous cystadenocarcinoma of low-grade malignant potential) of the pancreas: a clinicopathologic study of 130 cases. Am J Surg Pathol. 1999;23(1):1–16.
9. D'Angelica M, Brennan MF, Suriawinata AA, Klimstra D, Conlon KC. Intraductal papillary mucinous neoplasms of the pancreas: an analysis of clinicopathologic features and outcome. Ann Surg. 2004;239(3):400–8.
10. Sohn TA, Yeo CJ, Cameron JL, Hruban RH, Fukushima N, Campbell KA, Lillemoe KD. Intraductal papillary mucinous neoplasms of the pancreas: an updated experience. Ann Surg. 2004;239(6):788–97; discussion 797–9.
11. Tanaka M, Chari S, Adsay V, Fernandez-del Castillo C, Falconi M, Shimizu M, Yamaguchi K, Yamao K, Matsuno S, International Association of Pancreatology. International consensus guidelines for management of intraductal papillary mucinous neoplasms and mucinous cystic neoplasms of the pancreas. Pancreatology. 2006;6(1–2):17–32. Review.
12. Tanaka M, Fernández-del Castillo C, Adsay V, Chari S, Falconi M, Jang JY, Kimura W, Levy P, Pitman MB, Schmidt CM, Shimizu M, Wolfgang CL, Yamaguchi K, Yamao K, International Association of Pancreatology. International consensus guidelines 2012 for the management of IPMN and MCN of the pancreas. Pancreatology. 2012;12:183–97.
13. Walsh RM, Vogt DP, Henderson JM, Hirose K, Mason T, Bencsath K, Hammel J, Brown N. Management of suspected pancreatic cystic neoplasms based on cyst size. Surgery. 2008;144:677–84.
14. Wong J, Weber J, Centeno BA, Vignesh S, Harris CL, Klapman JB, Hodul P. High-grade dysplasia and adenocarcinoma are frequent in side-branch intraductal papillary mucinous neoplasm measuring less than 3 cm on endoscopic ultrasound. J Gastrointest Surg. 2013;17:78–84.
15. Sahora K, Mino-Kenudson M, Brugge W, Thayer SP, Ferrone CR, Sahani D, Pitman MB, Warshaw AL, Lillemoe KD, Fernandez-del Castillo CF. Branch duct intraductal papillary mucinous neoplasms: does cyst size change the tip of the scale? A critical analysis of the revised international consensus guidelines in a large single-institutional series. Ann Surg. 2013;258:466–75.
16. Schmidt CM, White PB, Waters JA, Yiannoutsos CT, Cummings OW, Baker M, Howard TJ, Zyromski NJ, Nakeeb A, DeWitt JM, Akisik FM, Sherman S, Pitt HA, Lillemoe KD. Intraductal papillary mucinous neoplasms: predictors of malignant and invasive pathology. Ann Surg. 2007;246:644–51.

17. Jang JY, Kim SW, Lee SE, Yang SH, Lee KU, Lee YJ, Kim SC, Han DJ, Choi DW, Choi SH, Heo JS, Cho BH, Yu HC, Yoon DS, Lee WJ, Lee HE, Kang GH, Lee JM. Treatment guidelines for branch duct type intraductal papillary mucinous neoplasms of the pancreas: when can we operate or observe? Ann Surg Oncol. 2008;15:199–205.
18. Fritz S, Klauss M, Bergmann F, Hackert T, Hartwig W, Strobel O, Bundy BD, Büchler MW, Werner J. Small (Sendai negative) branch-duct IPMNs: not harmless. Ann Surg. 2012;256:313–20.
19. Crippa S, Bassi C, Salvia R, Falconi M, Butturini G, Pederzoli P. Enucleation of pancreatic neoplasms. Br J Surg. 2007;94:1254–9.
20. Hackert T, Hinz U, Fritz S, Strobel O, Schneider L, Hartwig W, Büchler MW, Werner J. Enucleation in pancreatic surgery: indications, technique, and outcome compared to standard pancreatic resections. Langenbecks Arch Surg. 2011;396:1197–203.
21. Del Chiaro M, Albiin N, Segersvärd R. Enucleation of branch duct-IPMN in a transplant patient. Pancreatology. 2013;13(3):312–3.
22. Sauvanet A, Gaujoux S, Blanc B, Couvelard A, Dokmak S, Vullierme MP, Ruszniewski P, Belghiti J, Lévy P. Parenchyma-sparing pancreatectomy for presumed noninvasive intraductal papillary mucinous neoplasms of the pancreas. Ann Surg. 2014;260(2):364–71.
23. Turrini O, Schmidt CM, Pitt HA, Guiramand J, Aguilar-Saavedra JR, Aboudi S, Lillemoe KD, Delpero JR. Side-branch intraductal papillary mucinous neoplasms of the pancreatic head/uncinate: resection or enucleation? HPB (Oxford). 2011;13:126–31.
24. Fatima Z, Ichikawa T, Motosugi U, Muhi A, Sano K, Sou H, Haradome H, Kiryu S, Araki T. Magnetic resonance diffusion-weighted imaging in the characterization of pancreatic mucinous cystic lesions. Clin Radiol. 2011;66(2):108–11. Epub 2010 Nov 18.
25. Shin LK, Brant-Zawadzki G, Kamaya A, Jeffrey RB. Intraoperative ultrasound of the pancreas. Ultrasound Q. 2009;25(1):39–48.
26. Hackert T, Lozanovski VJ, Werner J, Büchler MW, Schemmer P. Teres hepatis ligament flap plasty to prevent pancreatic fistula after tumor enucleation. J Am Coll Surg. 2013;217(4):e29–34.
27. Al-Kurd A, Chapchay K, Grozinsky-Glasberg S, Mazeh H. Laparoscopic resection of pancreatic neuroendocrine tumors. World J Gastroenterol. 2014;20(17):4908–16.
28. Langer P, Fendrich V, Bartsch DK. Minimally invasive resection of neuroendocrine pancreatic tumors. Chirurg. 2009;80(2):105–12.
29. Gurusamy KS, Koti R, Fusai G, Davidson BR. Somatostatin analogues for pancreatic surgery. Cochrane Database Syst Rev. 2013;(4):CD008370.
30. Goudard Y, Gaujoux S, Dokmak S, Cros J, Couvelard A, Palazzo M, Ronot M, Vullierme MP, Ruszniewski P, Belghiti J, Sauvanet A. Reappraisal of central pancreatectomy a 12-year single-center experience. JAMA Surg. 2014;149:356–63.
31. Müller MW, Friess H, Kleeff J, Hinz U, Wente MN, Paramythiotis D, Berberat PO, Ceyhan GO, Büchler MW. Middle segmental pancreatic resection: an option to treat benign pancreatic body lesions. Ann Surg. 2006;244:909–18.
32. Kang CM, Lee JH, Lee WJ. Minimally invasive central pancreatectomy: current status and future directions. J Hepatobiliary Pancreat Sci. 2014;21(12):831–40.
33. Song KB, Kim SC, Park KM, Hwang DW, Lee JH, Lee DJ, Lee JW, Jun ES, Shin SH, Kim HE, Lee YJ. Laparoscopic central pancreatectomy for benign or low-grade malignant lesions in the pancreatic neck and proximal body. Surg Endosc. 2015;29:937–46.
34. Hackert T, Werner J, Büchler MW. Postoperative pancreatic fistula. Surgeon. 2011;9:211–7.
35. Schnelldorfer T, Sarr MG, Nagorney DM, Zhang L, Smyrk TC, Qin R, Chari ST, Farnell MB. Experience with 208 resections for intraductal papillary mucinous neoplasm of the pancreas. Arch Surg. 2008;143:639–46.
36. Fritz S, Klauss M, Bergmann F, Strobel O, Schneider L, Werner J, Hackert T, Büchler MW. Pancreatic main-duct involvement in branch-duct IPMNs: an underestimated risk. Ann Surg. 2014;260(5):848–56.
37. Hüttner FJ, Koessler-Ebs J, Hackert T, Ulrich A, Büchler MW, Diener MK. Meta-analysis of surgical outcome after enucleation versus standard resection for pancreatic neoplasms. Br J Surg. 2015;102:1026–36.
38. Larghi A, Panic N, Capurso G, Leoncini E, Arzani D, Salvia R, Del Chiaro M, Frulloni L, Arcidiacono PG, Zerbi A, Manta R, Fabbri C, Ventrucci M, Tarantino I, Piciucchi M, Carnuccio A, Boggi U, Costamagna G, Delle Fave G, Pezzilli R, Bassi C, Bulajic M, Ricciardi W, Boccia S. Prevalence and risk factors of extrapancreatic malignancies in a large cohort of patients with intraductal papillary mucinous neoplasm (IPMN) of the pancreas. Ann Oncol. 2013;24(7):1907–11.
39. Reid-Lombardo KM, Mathis KL, Wood CM, Harmsen WS, Sarr MG. Frequency of extrapancreatic neoplasms in intraductal papillary mucinous neoplasm of the pancreas: implications for management. Ann Surg. 2010;251:64–9.
40. Wasif N, Bentrem DJ, Farrell JJ, Ko CY, Hines OJ, Reber HA, Tomlinson JS. Invasive intraductal papillary mucinous neoplasm versus sporadic pancreatic adenocarcinoma: a stage-matched comparison of outcomes. Cancer. 2010;116:3369–77.
41. Poultsides GA, Reddy S, Cameron JL, Hruban RH, Pawlik TM, Ahuja N, Jain A, Edil BH, Iacobuzio-Donahue CA, Schulick RD, Wolfgang CL. Histopathologic basis for the favorable survival after resection of intraductal papillary mucinous neoplasm-associated invasive adenocarcinoma of the pancreas. Ann Surg. 2010;251:470–6.
42. Turrini O, Waters JA, Schnelldorfer T, Lillemoe KD, Yiannoutsos CT, Farnell MB, Sarr MG, Schmidt CM. Invasive intraductal papillary mucinous neoplasm: predictors of survival and role of adjuvant therapy. HPB (Oxford). 2010;12:447–55.

12 Minimally Invasive Pancreatic Surgery for Cystic Tumors of the Pancreas

Camille L. Stewart and Barish H. Edil

12.1 Patient Selection

Patient selection is one of the most important variables for achieving success with minimally invasive pancreatic surgery, but few reports specifically comment on how patients are selected beyond qualifying for operative intervention. The ideal patient for minimally invasive pancreatic surgery has a low BMI (<30), few or no comorbidities, few or no previous abdominal surgeries, and no involvement of the pancreatic mass with the adjacent major vasculature. The literature on laparoscopic distal pancreatectomy and pancreaticoduodenectomy mirrors this judgment. Average BMIs range from 22 to 28 [1–6], and the majority of patients are American Society of Anesthesiologists (ASA) classes 2–3 or have Eastern Cooperative Oncology Group (ECOG) performance levels of 0–1 preoperatively [2, 4], equating to no activity restrictions or only restrictions with strenuous activity [7]. Others report limiting the laparoscopic approach to patients with smaller tumors (<3 cm) that are pathologically benign [8] or well to moderate grade differentiation [9, 10]. Asbun and Stauffer [2] report dissuading patients from pursuing a minimally invasive approach when a hostile abdomen is anticipated due to multiple previous abdominal surgeries or history of severe pancreatitis. As surgeons gain more experience, however, criteria for laparoscopic pancreatic surgery can be broadened. In our practice, a minimally invasive approach is offered to all patients, regardless of pathology, when adjacent structures are not involved; thus almost all cystic neoplasms are considered for laparoscopy. When tumors are small and we are planning a laparoscopic approach, we often have them preoperatively inked during endoscopic ultrasound [11]. This facilitates identification of the tumor, since palpation of the mass cannot be performed prior to resection.

12.2 General Laparoscopic Approach

We place the patient supine with arms extended, but patient positioning varies by institution. Lithotomy position can be used to allow the surgeon or assistant to stand between the patient's legs [12–15], and some use a right lateral approach for distal pancreatectomy [6]. Once pneumoperitoneum is achieved, we use 5 trocars to initiate any laparoscopic pancreatic surgery. This includes three 12 mm ports (umbilicus and bilateral midclavicular) and two 5 mm ports (bilateral anterior axillary). Most authors describe using 4–6 trocars in a similar fashion [1, 12], with an optional port

C.L. Stewart, MD • B.H. Edil, MD, FACS (✉)
Section of Surgical of Oncology, University of Colorado, 1165 Aurora Ct, Aurora, CO 80045, USA

Department of Surgery, University of Colorado Hospital, Aurora, CO, USA
e-mail: barish.edil@ucdenver.edu

M. Del Chiaro et al. (eds.), *Cystic Tumors of the Pancreas*, DOI 10.1007/978-3-319-31882-0_12

for liver retraction. The lesser sac is then entered by dividing the gastrocolic omentum up to the gastrosplenic ligament. This requires ligation of the short gastric vessels, which can be done with endosonic shears (our preference), electrothermal bipolar vessel sealer, or staplers, with reinforcement using titanium clips. We prefer to stay close to the greater curvature of the stomach to prevent the omentum from draping into our operative field. Once this is complete, the stomach can be retracted cephalad to expose the anterior pancreas.

12.3 Minimally Invasive Distal Pancreatectomy

Minimally invasive distal pancreatectomy is considered within the standard of care for benign and malignant pancreatic tail lesions [16, 17] and thus is often used for the treatment of cystic pancreatic neoplasms [6, 18, 19]. In the United States, the frequency of minimally invasive distal pancreatectomy is increasing, but remains the minority (<10%) of cases [20]. Initial reports of this approach began to surface in the mid-1990s, and to date, there are several studies that have documented the safety and efficacy of this procedure [15, 17, 21], with mortality reported at <1% [22]. Conversion to open rate ranges between 0 and 32% and averages around 12% [15, 22, 23]. Most often conversion is performed secondary to poor exposure, failure to progress, proximity of the mass to major vessels, or bleeding [9, 15, 18]. Males and those with more visceral fat are more likely to require conversion [15]. Centers with higher than average conversion rates attribute this to a lower threshold for conversion and a desire to maintain oncologic surgical principles [15]. Mean operative times typically range from 2.5 to 4.5 h [22], with a decrease in operative time with additional experience [6, 15]. Lee et al. [15] reported an average operative time of 3.5 h for the first 60 patients, which decreased to 3.0 h with the following 71 patients, but no difference in the conversion to open rate. Similarly, Song et al. [6] reported that over the course of their 5-year experience with 359 laparoscopic distal pancreatectomies, their operative times declined, with most cases at the end of their series taking <3 h. They also reported a dramatic decrease in their rate of pancreatic fistula formation, from 38 to 4%. Average complication rates are 23%, most often pancreatic fistula [22], with higher complication rates associated with longer resections of pancreas and BMI >27 [18].

Splenic preservation may be accomplished when performing distal pancreatectomy for cystic pancreatic tumors since extensive lymphadenectomy is usually not required. Kang et al. [19] compared minimally invasive spleen-preserving surgery to pancreaticosplenectomy and found that rates of splenic vein thrombosis and pancreatic leak were higher in the pancreaticosplenectomy group. They concluded that minimally invasive distal pancreatectomy with spleen preservation should be performed whenever possible. Worhunsky et al. [24] published a series comparing techniques of splenic preservation, either by splenic artery and vein conservation or by the Warshaw technique, in which the splenic artery and vein are sacrificed, and splenic perfusion depends on the short gastric vessels. Risks of the Warshaw technique include splenic infarction, sinistral portal hypertension, and gastric varices, but these complications are rarely observed [25]. Patients in this series with splenic preservation via the Warshaw technique tended to have more pancreas transected and longer operative times, but otherwise had similar outcomes to the vessel-preserving group. Another series of laparoscopic distal pancreatectomies that included a subset with the Warshaw technique reported transient splenic ischemia in nearly half of the patients, but this universally resolved [6]. Thus, while spleen preservation is recommended, the technique of splenic preservation should likely be determined based on the ease of the approach.

12.3.1 Operative Technique for Laparoscopic Distal Pancreatectomy

We perform this surgery using a total laparoscopic approach, generally with splenic artery and vein preservation when possible [26]. Five ports are placed into the abdomen and the lesser sac is entered. The greater curvature of the stomach is mobilized, as described above, to visualize the anterior pancreas and identify the area of inking if this has been performed preoperatively. Our dissection then begins at the inferior border of the pancreas using ultrasonic shears. When the inferior border is sufficiently mobilized, we then dissect out the dorsum of the pancreas. Blunt dissection is used to identify a filmy avascular plane, which is taken down again with ultrasonic shears. This is carried around the pancreatic tail, taking care to avoid the splenic hilum. Next, a tunnel is created between the dorsum of the pancreas and the parallel-coursing splenic vasculature. This window must be large enough to accommodate the end of an endo-GIA stapler. We use a medium-thick staple height load to transect the pancreatic neck, ensuring that the tumor is in the distal specimen. The remaining attachments of the distal pancreas are then dissected free from the splenic vasculature and hilum. An endoscopic bag is deployed to retrieve the specimen, which is removed through the umbilical port by extending this incision 10–15 mm. The specimen is sent to the pathology department for frozen section to confirm that the tumor is within the pancreatic specimen and that our margins are negative. We leave a drain by the cut edge of the pancreas, which is later used to test for a pancreatic leak once a regular diet is resumed. The abdomen is desufflated, the ports are closed, and the patient is awoken from anesthesia. Patients are then usually managed on the general surgery ward postoperatively.

12.3.2 Alternative Techniques for Minimally Invasive Distal Pancreatectomy

Since minimally invasive distal pancreatectomy requires a significant amount of experience to undertake, several authors have described methods to simplify this procedure and shorten the learning curve. An epigastric hand port may be used as minimally invasive pancreatic surgical experience is accrued. This 5–7 cm epigastric incision offers several advantages, including the ability to palpate major structures, easier retraction, facilitating blunt dissection, and permitting extracorporeal dissection of vascular structures [27, 28]. Sartori et al. [29] suggest using an electrothermal bipolar vessel sealer to transect the pancreas to help prevent pancreatic leak. Suzuki et al. [30] reported using a "lesser curvature" approach, in which the lesser sac is entered with the stomach retracted caudad, permitting dissection of the pancreas adjacent to the lesser curvature of the stomach instead. This is done to prevent the stomach from obscuring the view of the distal pancreas and spleen. In the same report, the authors also describe clamping the splenic artery early after its identification to decrease blood loss and facilitate removal of the spleen, by causing it to shrink. If a spleen-sparing procedure is planned, many believe that the Warshaw procedure [25] is technically easier than splenic vessel preservation, with similar overall results (see above). Centers that perform total robotic distal pancreatectomies claim they carry the same benefits of laparoscopic surgery, with the added benefits of improved view and increased dexterity [15]. Giulianotti et al. [31] write that the robotic platform facilitates splenic vascular dissection, permitting splenic preservation. However, these procedures tend to have longer operative times compared to their laparoscopic and open counterparts [15].

Yao et al. [8] and Huagvik et al. [32] both reported their experiences performing single-incision laparoscopic distal pancreatectomy and compared their results to traditional multiport laparoscopic distal pancreatectomy. In this approach, a 2.5–3 cm periumbilical incision is created, through which a multi-instrument port is inserted. The procedure is completed using a 10 mm lens and 2–3 working ports in a similar manner to a conventional multiport laparoscopic distal pancreatectomy. Both series reported equivalent outcomes in the single-incision and multiport laparoscopic patients, with the exception of shorter operative times and lower estimated blood loss in the single-incision group.

12.3.3 Comparison to Open Distal Pancreatectomy

Several studies exist comparing minimally invasive distal pancreatectomy to open pancreatectomy, but all are retrospective or nonrandomized, thereby introducing selection bias. In a high-volume single-institution series, Lee et al. [15] compared 131 laparoscopic distal pancreatectomies and 37 robotic procedures to 637 open surgeries. Patients in the laparoscopic and robotic groups were younger, fewer were being treated for adenocarcinoma, and fewer required adjacent organ resection. Estimated blood loss was lower, and there were fewer minor complications in the laparoscopic and robotic groups compared to the open group. Oncologic outcomes and mortality were found to be similar for all surgical modalities. In a similar but smaller series, Waters et al. [9] reported shorter hospitalization in the robotic group, but no difference in complication rates for all operative approaches. Robotic surgeries had significantly higher surgical costs, but this was evened out by the decrease in length of stay, making total costs similar for all operative approaches. Another study out of the United Kingdom had similar findings with their cost analysis comparing laparoscopic to open distal pancreatectomies [33].

An analysis of the US Nationwide Inpatient Sample retrospectively compared 382 minimally invasive distal pancreatectomies to 8,575 open distal pancreatectomies over a 12-year study period [20]. Patients in the minimally invasive group had shorter lengths of hospitalization and fewer immediate postoperative complications (specifically bleeding and infectious complications). Total charges and mortality were again similar between groups. It should be noted, however, that significantly fewer patients with pancreatitis had a minimally invasive approach and that these patients were found to have worse outcomes overall, potentially skewing the results. Similarly, a meta-analysis of 19 studies comparing laparoscopic to open distal pancreatectomy through 2010 reported several metrics that were improved for the laparoscopic group, including estimated blood loss, blood transfusion rate, wound infection rate, and length of hospitalization. Unfortunately, significant heterogeneity between studies and the absence of any prospective randomized studies limited their conclusions [23].

12.4 Minimally Invasive Pancreaticoduodenectomy

Despite the original description of this procedure 20 years ago [34], the acceptance of total laparoscopic pancreaticoduodenectomy has been slow, likely owing to the technical difficulty of the procedure. There are few reports describing laparoscopic pancreaticoduodenectomy in the United States; however, several centers (ours included) are performing them. The first reports of series greater than 30 patients in the late 2000s demonstrated that this could be done safely with low mortality and reasonable complication rates [1, 10, 13]. Average mortality for this procedure is reported at 1.8 % [22]. Conversion to open rate is reported between 5 and 15 % [1–3, 35], with this rate generally declining as operative experience accrues [3, 36]. Reasons for conversion to open most often are bleeding and failure to progress. Operative times, especially initially, can be quite long and may take upward of 13.5 h [3], but this also declines with increasing experience [3, 36]. In our practice, these operations typically require 4–6 h. Speicher et al. [36] reported that operative times significantly decreased after their first 10 patients and that after completing 50 minimally invasive pancreaticoduodenectomies, operative times for these cases were consistently lower compared to their open pancreaticoduodenectomies. Kim et al. [3] similarly reported that operative times on their first 100 patients steadily and significantly declined, from an average of 9.8 h initially down to 6.6 h for their more recent patients. They also described a significant decline in complications, specifically pancreatic fistula, need for blood transfusions, and length of hospitalization. Average complication rates are 38 % and most often are biliary or pancreatic fistulas [22].

12.4.1 Operative Technique for Total Laparoscopic Pancreaticoduodenectomy

The operative technique used at our institution is also a totally laparoscopic approach, which we have shown can be done in an efficient and safe manner [37]. The steps of this operation are different than the classic open pancreaticoduodenectomy; however, the oncologic measures taken in the operation are the same. Upon entering the abdomen and ruling out metastatic disease, the falciform ligament is taken down and used to retract the liver cephalad, giving exposure of the portal hilum. The lesser sac is then entered, identifying the gastroduodenal artery, common hepatic artery, and proper hepatic artery. The gastroduodenal artery is test occluded with a laparoscopic vascular clamp to confirm the pulse in the proper hepatic artery. The gastroduodenal artery is then ligated with a 3 0 silk suture and locking plastic endoclips. Next, the portal vein is identified posteriorly, allowing us to estimate the location of the superior mesenteric vein. Similar to the technique used in the laparoscopic distal pancreatectomy, dissection along the lower edge of the pancreas permits the creation of a tunnel underneath the pancreas neck. We find that the visualization of this tunnel is superior to the open technique. At this point the pancreas neck is transected with hook cautery after the pancreaticoduodenal arteries are controlled with an energy device.

Next, the pylorus of the stomach is identified and proximal to the pylorus the stomach is transected again using a laproscopic endo-GIA stapler. The gallbladder is removed, a bulldog is placed on the proximal common bile duct, and the common bile duct is divided. A Kocher maneuver is then performed to mobilize the first and second portion of the duodenum and the head of the pancreas. This is followed by mobilization of the proximal jejunum to the extent that it can rest adjacent to the body of the stomach without tension once pulled up through the ligament of Treitz. The duodenal-jejunal junction is then transected with another endo-GIA stapler. The uncinate process remains where visualization of the SMA allows for dissection with energy device to remove the final attachments. The specimen is removed in a bag through the umbilical port.

Reconstruction is performed in a similar fashion to the open pancreaticoduodenectomy. We start by inserting a pediatric feeding tube to stent open the pancreatic duct and create a duct. The pancreatic edge is then approximated to the jejunum in an end to side fashion using absorbable barbed locking suture is used for the posterior and anterior outer layer while 4-0 polydioxanone suture is used for the duct to mucosa anastomosis around the stent for the inner layer. This is done completely intracorporally. Interrupted 4-0 vicryl suture are also used to create the hepaticojejunostomy. Another pediatric feeding tube is inserted to stent open this anastomosis prior to the last few anterior stitches. The Roux limb of the jejunum is approximated to the stomach using an articulating endoscopic suturing device and interrupted 2-0 silk suture. A stapled antecolic gastrojejunostomy is performed, and the entrance for the stapler is closed again using the articulating endoscopic suturing device and interrupted 2-0 silk suture, completing the operation. The specimen is sent to the pathology department for frozen section to confirm that the tumor is within the pancreatic specimen and that our margins are negative. Our practice is to leave two drains at the end of the operation adjacent to the pancreatic and hepatic anastomoses. The abdomen is then desufflated, the ports are closed, and the patient is awoken from anesthesia. Patients are then generally transferred to the surgical intensive care unit for monitoring overnight and then transferred to the ward on postoperative day one.

12.4.2 Alternative Techniques for Minimally Invasive Pancreaticoduodenectomy

Many aspects of a total laparoscopic pancreaticoduodenectomy are challenging and require significant laparoscopic expertise. To overcome these challenges, several authors have published techniques to simplify this procedure. Some institutions [36] use two attending-level surgeons for these cases. Several authors also report performing parts of the vascular dissection and the reconstructive portion of the procedure extracorporeally through a minilaparotomy incision [38–40]. Wang et al. [39] reported that using a minilaparotomy to perform the anastomoses allowed patients to derive the benefits of a laparoscopic surgery, including decreased estimated blood loss and length of hospitalization while decreasing the technical demands of the procedure. Kim et al. [3] and Speicher et al. [36] both used a minilaparotomy to execute the reconstructive phase of the surgery as a learning bridge to total laparoscopic pancreaticoduodenectomy as they developed their minimally invasive pancreatic surgery programs.

There have also been many maneuvers described for total laparoscopic pancreaticoduodenectomy to facilitate dissection and reconstruction. Kuroki et al. [12] described a "pancreas-hanging maneuver" to facilitate dissection of the vascular structures. In this maneuver, they dissect out the entire specimen, leaving the pancreatic head and uncinate process attachments as the final steps of the procedure. They then use a Penrose drain tightened around the pancreatic head to provide gentle traction, exposing the plane of interest. Ogiso et al. [41] report using a retropancreatic dissection to expose the posterolateral aspect of the superior mesenteric artery, to improve identification of aberrant right and common hepatic arteries. Keck et al. [42] described using a pancreaticogastrostomy for the pancreaticoenterostomy because they think it is easier to execute laparoscopically. Nakamura et al. [40] recommend using an endoscopic linear stapler for pancreatic transection, specifically when performing a laparoscopic operation for IPMN, to stop extravasation of pancreatic juices after resection and to limit bleeding from the pancreatic parenchyma. They then remove the staples just around the main pancreatic duct when reconstruction is begun extracorporeally through a minilaparotomy.

Some authors believe that robotic surgical systems can be used to ease technical demands of laparoscopic surgery [31]. Giulianotti et al. [31] write that this platform improves visualization and instrument motion, allowing ligation of small vessel branches to avoid bleeding, which is more difficult to control in laparoscopic and open surgery. Gumbs et al. [22] report using a robotic laparoscope holder, which is controlled by foot pedal or voice activation. Chalikonda et al. [5] perform the pancreaticoduodenectomy laparoscopically and then use a robotic platform to perform the pancreaticojejunostomy and hepaticojejunostomy. A meta-analysis comparing total laparoscopic to robot-assisted pancreaticoduodenectomy, however, showed a higher EBL, more frequent conversion to open procedure, higher fistula rate, and longer hospitalization in the robot-assisted group [43].

12.4.3 Comparison to Open Pancreaticoduodenectomy

Like the reports for distal pancreatectomy, those comparing minimally invasive pancreaticoduodenectomy to an open approach must be interpreted with caution since all studies thus far are retrospective. A series by Asbun and Stauffer [2] compared 53 laparoscopic pancreaticoduodenectomies to 215 open surgeries and found that the laparoscopic group had lower estimated blood loss, fewer blood transfusions, and shorter ICU (1 versus 3 days) as well as total length of hospitalization (8 versus 12 days). Oncologic outcomes were similar, as were 3-month morbidity and mortality rates. While the authors did not describe any major differences between the two groups, the significant difference in estimated blood loss (200 mL versus 1000 mL) suggests that the retrospective nature of the study may have introduced selection bias. Later, Croome et al. [4] compared results from 108 patients who had laparoscopic pancreaticoduodenectomies to 214 patients who had open procedures, all for pancreatic ductal adenocarcinoma. They again reported lower estimated blood loss, lower rates of intraoperative transfusion, and shorter length of hospitalization (6 versus 9 days), as well as lower frequency of delayed gastric emptying in the laparoscopic group. They also showed equivalent mean operative times, rates of severe complications, and oncologic outcomes. Laparoscopic robot-assisted pancreaticoduodenectomy was compared to open procedure in 30 patients each by Chalikonda et al. [5]. They report longer operative times in the laparoscopic group, but similar estimated blood loss, morbidity, and mortality to the open group. The laparoscopic robot-assisted group also had a shorter hospital length of stay (10 versus 13 days). Again, the retrospective nature of this analysis must be noted, given that 4 of the patients in the open group ultimately had positive margins, compared to no patients in the minimally invasive group, suggesting selection bias. A recent meta-analysis of 11 studies comparing open to minimally invasive pancreaticoduodenectomy echoed the results of these individual studies, reporting that the minimally invasive procedures were associated with lower estimated blood loss, decreased wound infection rate, and a shorter hospital stay, with no difference in overall complications, surgical margins, lymph nodes retrieved, reoperation, or mortality [44]. It has also been reported that quality of life, specifically functional status, was improved in patients after laparoscopic pancreaticoduodenectomy in the first 6 months after surgery, despite having similar fistula and readmission rates to the open comparison group [45]. Mesleh et al. [46] also compared cost of laparoscopic pancreaticoduodenectomy to open surgery and found that, while the surgical costs were greater, the total cost for hospitalization was similar.

Borderline resectable pancreatic tumors are masses that involve major adjacent vasculature. These tumors can sometimes be treated at high-volume centers by pancreaticoduodenectomy with concomitant venous resection, often after a course of neoadjuvant therapy. This was previously thought to be an absolute contraindication to minimally invasive pancreaticoduodenectomy; however, Kendrick and Sclabas first reported performing major venous resection during total laparoscopic pancreaticoduodenectomy in 2011 [47]. Nearly all dissection was performed prior to venous transection, leaving this as the final step in the procedure. All but one patient in their first series had a tangential venous resection. This was followed by another series in 2014 [35], comparing 31 patients with total laparoscopic pancreaticoduodenectomy including vascular resection to 58 patients with an open approach. Tangential resection was used more often in the laparoscopic group compared to the open group, and there was a 13 % conversion to open rate. They report, however, similar operative times, similar rates of vascular patency postoperatively, and lower estimated blood loss in the laparoscopic group, with no difference in complication or mortality rate. Thus, in appropriately selected patients, vascular resection during total laparoscopic pancreaticoduodenectomy can be done safely and effectively. The authors, not surprisingly, caution that this technique should only be attempted by surgeons with extensive experience performing laparoscopic pancreaticoduodenectomy.

Port-site recurrence is a theoretical risk for all minimally invasive surgeries involving malignancy. To date, there has only been one report of port-site recurrence after minimally invasive pancreaticoduodenectomy for T3N1M0 pancreatic adenocarcinoma [48]. The resection was R0, and the authors report using a wound protector at the site of specimen retrieval and deny tumor spillage. As the number of minimally invasive pancreaticoduodenectomies reported in the literature increases, it will become possible to determine what the true rate of port-site recurrence is.

12.5 Laparoscopic Pancreas-Preserving and Natural Orifice Resections

Pancreatic enucleations and central pancreatic resections can be performed when benign or low-grade malignant lesions are detected and there is a desire for maximal parenchymal preservation [49]. These lesions, frequently neuroendocrine or cystic pancreatic neoplasms, are more often being detected as imaging techniques improve, and patients are often considered ideal candidates for minimally invasive approaches. Choice of enucleation or central resection is based on the location of the lesion relative to the main pancreatic duct. Lesions in the pancreatic neck or body that are adjacent to or involving the main pancreatic duct are better suited for central resection, because the risk of pancreatic duct injury during enucleation is high. One limitation of minimally invasive pancreas-sparing resection is that tactile feedback is lost, but is needed to select the appropriate procedure and determine how much tissue can be spared. Intraoperative laparoscopic ultrasound is thus often required to overcome these limitations [49].

Few reports exist of these pancreatic-sparing minimally invasive procedures, but those in existence generally show they are technically feasible and are safe [49, 50]. Song et al. [51] reported a comparison series of patients who underwent laparoscopic or open central pancreatectomy for removal of benign and low-grade malignant pancreatic lesions. While operative times were longer for the laparoscopic patients compared to their open counterparts, likely because of the additional time for intracorporeal distal pancreaticojejunostomy, these patients had shorter hospitalizations (14 versus 22 days) and similar rates of complications. In this same study, additional comparison was made between laparoscopic central pancreatectomy and laparoscopic extended distal pancreatectomy. The patients with an extended distal pancreatectomy had shorter operative times, shorter hospitalizations (9 versus 14 days), and fewer overall complications compared to the central pancreatectomy patients. These benefits were balanced by a higher frequency of new-onset diabetes (31 % versus 8 %). To prevent new-onset diabetes, another group described performing auto-islet transplantation after laparoscopic distal pancreatectomy for larger pancreatic neck and body cystic tumors [52]. After percutaneous portal vein islet reinfusion on postoperative day one, one patient out of three developed partial portal vein thrombosis. All three patients, however, continued to be insulin-free several months after surgery. Interestingly, there is also a report of successful uncomplicated laparoscopic central pancreatectomy in a 13-year-old child for a solid pseudopapillary pancreatic tumor [53], suggesting that these minimally invasive pancreas-sparing techniques can be considered in younger patients.

As the limits of our technical ability continue to be pushed, some have begun investigation of natural orifice pancreatic resections. Thakkar et al. [54] demonstrated the feasibility of this methodology using a snake robot and a transrectal approach in a porcine model. Recognizing the limitations that exist with natural orifice surgery, the authors conclude that their research may serve as a stepping stone to future novel approaches to limit morbidity in pancreatic surgery.

Conclusions

Minimally invasive techniques are lauded for their association with improved patient comfort and a variety of other benefits, but must prove equal or better than the open approach with regard to outcomes if they are to be widely accepted. With pancreatic surgery this may be even more important given the additional technical demands. Surgeons across the United States and the world are performing laparoscopic and robotic pancreatic surgery for cystic tumors and have shown that these procedures are safe and effective alternatives to their open counterparts. The retrospective and non-randomized nature of all comparison studies to date permits selection bias, however, making true superiority over open surgery difficult to determine at this time. Since a randomized study is unlikely in the near future, further studies can be strengthened by better defining selection criteria for candidates of minimally invasive pancreatic surgery.

References

1. Kendrick ML, Cusati D. Total laparoscopic pancreaticoduodenectomy: feasibility and outcome in an early experience. Arch Surg. 2010;145:19–23. doi:10.1001/archsurg.2009.243.
2. Asbun HJ, Stauffer JA. Laparoscopic vs open pancreaticoduodenectomy: overall outcomes and severity of complications using the accordion severity grading system. J Am Coll Surg. 2012;215:810–9. doi:10.1016/j.jamcollsurg.2012.08.006.
3. Kim SC, Song KB, Jung YS, Kim YH, Park DH, Lee SS, et al. Short-term clinical outcomes for 100 consecutive cases of laparoscopic pylorus-preserving pancreatoduodenectomy: improvement with surgical experience. Surg Endosc. 2013;27:95–103. doi:10.1007/s00464-012-2427-9.
4. Croome KP, Farnell MB, Que FG, Reid-Lombardo KM, Truty MJ, Nagorney DM, et al. Total laparoscopic pancreaticoduodenectomy for pancreatic ductal adenocarcinoma: oncologic advantages over open approaches? Ann Surg. 2014;260:633–40. doi:10.1097/SLA.0000000000000937.

5. Chalikonda S, Aguilar-Saavedra JR, Walsh RM. Laparoscopic robotic-assisted pancreaticoduodenectomy: a case-matched comparison with open resection. Surg Endosc. 2012;26:2397–402. doi:10.1007/s00464-012-2207-6.
6. Song KB, Kim SC, Park JB, Kim YH, Jung YS, Kim MH, et al. Sing-center experience of laparoscopic left pancreatic resection in 359 consecutive patients: changing the surgical paradigm of left pancreatic resection. Surg Endosc. 2011;25:3364–72. doi:10.1007/s00464-011-1727-9.
7. Oken MM, Creech RH, Tormey DC, Horton J, David TE, McFadden ET, et al. Toxicity and response criteria of the Eastern Cooperative Oncology Group. Am J Clin Oncol. 1982;5:649–55.
8. Yao D, Wu S, Li Y, Chen Y, Yu X, Han J. Transumbilical single-incision laparoscopic distal pancreatectomy: preliminary experience and comparison to conventional multi-port laparoscopic surgery. BMC Surg. 2014;14:105. doi:10.1186/1471-2482-14-105.
9. Waters JA, Canal DF, Wiebke EA, Dumas RP, Beane JD, Aguilar-Saavedra JR, et al. Robotic distal pancreatectomy: cost effective? Surgery. 2010;148:814–23. doi:10.1016/j.surg.2010.07.027.
10. Palanivelu C, Jani K, Senthilnathan P, Parthasarathi R, Rajapandian S, Madhankumar MV. Laparoscopic pancreaticoduodenectomy: technique and outcomes. J Am Coll Surg. 2007;205:222–30.
11. Lennon AM, Newman N, Makary MA, Edil BH, Shin EJ, Khashab MA, et al. EUS-guided tattooing before laparoscopic distal pancreatic resection (with video). Gastrointest Endosc. 2010;72:1089–94. doi:10.1016/j.gie.2010.07.023.
12. Kuroki T, Tajima Y, Kitasato A, Adachi T, Kanematsu T. Pancreas-hanging maneuver in laparoscopic pancreaticoduodenectomy: a new technique for the safe resection of the pancreas head. Surg Endosc. 2010;24:1781–3. doi:10.1007/s00464-009-0814-7.
13. Palanivelu C, Rajan PS, Rangarajan M, Vaithiswaran V, Senthilnathan P, Parthasarathi R, et al. Evolution in techniques of laparoscopic pancreaticoduodenectomy: a decade long experience from a tertiary center. J Hepatobiliary Pancreat Surg. 2009;16:731–40. doi:10.1007/s00534-009-0157-8.
14. Dulucq JL, Wintringer P, Mahajna A. Laparoscopic pancreaticoduodenectomy for benign and malignant diseases. Surg Endosc. 2006;20:1045–50.
15. Lee SY, Allen PJ, Sadot E, D'Angelica MI, DeMatteo RP, Fong Y, et al. Distal pancreatectomy: a single institution's experience in open, laparoscopic, and robotic approaches. J Am Coll Surg. 2015;220:18–27. doi:10.1016/j.jamcollsurg.2014.10.004.
16. Song KB, Kim SC, Park KM, H Nakamura DW, Lee JH, Lee DJ, et al. Laparoscopic central pancreatectomy for benign or low-grade malignant lesions in the pancreatic neck and proximal body. Surg Endosc. 2015;29(4):937–46.
17. Iacobone M, Citton M, Nitti D. Laparoscopic distal pancreatectomy: up-to-date and literature review. World J Gastroenterol. 2012;18:5329–37. doi:10.3748/wjg.v18.i38.5329.
18. Weber SM, Cho CS, Merchant N, Pinchot S, Rettammel R, Nakeeb A, et al. Laparoscopic left pancreatectomy: complication risk score correlates with morbidity and risk for pancreatic fistula. Ann Surg Oncol. 2009;16:2825–33. doi:10.1245/s10434-009-0597-z.
19. Kang CM, Chung YE, Jung MJ, Hwang HK, Choi SH, Lee WJ. Splenic vein thrombosis and pancreatic fistula after minimally invasive distal pancreatectomy. BJS. 2014;101:114–9. doi:10.1002/bjs.9366.
20. Tran Cao HS, Lopez N, Chang DC, Lowy AM, Bouvet M, Baumgartner JM, et al. Improved perioperative outcomes with minimally invasive distal pancreatectomy: results from a population-based analysis. JAMA Surg. 2014;149:237–43. doi:10.1001/jamasurg.2013.3202.
21. Mabrut JY, Fernandez-Cruz L, Azagra JS, Bassi C, Delvaux G, Weerts J, et al. Laparoscopic pancreatic resection: results of a multicenter European study of 127 patients. Surgery. 2005;137:597–605.
22. Gumbs AA, Croner R, Rodriguez A, Zuker N, Perrakis A, Gayet B. 200 Consecutive laparoscopic pancreatic resections performed with a robotically controlled laparoscope holder. Surg Endosc. 2013;27:3781–91. doi:10.1007/s00464-013-2969-5.
23. Sui CJ, Li B, Yang JM, Wang SJ, Zhou YM. Laparoscopic versus open distal pancreatectomy: a meta-analysis. Asian J Surg. 2012;351:1–8. doi:10.1016/j.asjsur.2012.04.001.
24. Worhunsky DJ, Zak Y, Dua MM, Poultsides GA, Norton JA, Visser BC. Laparoscopic spleen-preserving distal pancreatectomy: the technique must suit the lesion. J Gastrointest Surg. 2014;18:1445–51. doi:10.1007/s11605-014-2561-x.
25. Ferrone CR, Konstantinidis IT, Sahani DV, Wargo JA, Fernandez-del Castillo C, Warshaw AL. Twenty-three years of the Warshaw operation for distal pancreatectomy with preservation of the spleen. Ann Surg. 2011;253:1136–9. doi:10.1097/SLA.0b013e318212c1e2.
26. Stewart CL, Raeburn C, Edil BH. Laparoscopic distal pancreatectomy for an ACTH secreting pancreatic neuroendocrine tumor. VideoEndocrinology. 2015;2:4. doi:10.1089/ve.2015.0049.
27. D'Angelica M, Are C, Jarnagin W, DeGregoris G, Coit D, Jaques D, et al. Initial experience with hand-assisted laparoscopic distal pancreatectomy. Surg Endosc. 2006;20:142–8.
28. Abe N, Mori T, Sugiyama M. Tips on laparoscopic distal pancreatectomy. J Hepatobiliary Pancreat Sci. 2014;21:e41–7. doi:10.1002/jhbp.95.
29. Sartori CA, Baiocchi GL. Transecting the pancreas neck with electrothermal bipolar vessel sealer (Ligasure) in laparoscopic left pancreatectomy. Surg Laparosc Endosc Percutan Tech. 2009;19:e175–6. doi:10.1097/SLE.0b013e3181b8fb3c.
30. Suzuki O, Nakamura F, Ambo Y, Nakamura T, Kishida A, Kashimura N. Lesser curvature approach in laparoscopic distal pancreatectomy. Surg Laparosc Endosc Percutan Tech. 2013;232:e57–60. doi:10.1097/SLE.0b013e31828a0b3f.
31. Giulianotti PC, Sbrana F, Bianco FM, Elli EF, Shah G, Addeo P, et al. Robot-assisted laparoscopic pancreatic

surgery: single-surgeon experience. Surg Endosc. 2010;24:1646–57. doi:10.1007/s00464-009-0825-4.
32. Haugvik SP, Rosok BI, Waage A, Mathisen O, Edwin B. Single-incision versus conventional laparoscopic distal pancreatectomy: a single-institution case–control study. Langenbecks Arch Surg. 2013;398:1091–6. doi:10.1007/s00423-013-1133-y.
33. Abu Hilal M, Hamdan M, Di Fabio F, Pearce NW, Johnson CD. Laparoscopic versus open distal pancreatectomy: a clinical and cost-effectiveness study. Surg Endosc. 2012;26:1670–4. doi:10.1007/s00464-011-2090-6.
34. Gagner M, Pomp A. Laparoscopic pylorus-preserving pancreaticoduodenectomy. Surg Endosc. 1994;8:408–10.
35. Croome KP, Farnell MB, Que FG, Reid-Lombardo KM, Truty MJ, Nagorney DM, et al. Pancreaticoduodenectomy with major vascular resection: a comparison of laparoscopic versus open approaches. J Gastrointest Surg. 2014. doi:10.1007/s11605-014-2644-8.
36. Speicher PJ, Nussbaum DP, White RR, Zani S, Mosca PJ, Blazer III DG, et al. Defining the learning curve for team-based laparoscopic pancreaticoduodenectomy. Ann Surg Oncol. 2014;21:4014–9. doi:10.1245/s10434-014-3839-7.
37. Paniccia A, Schulick RD, Edil BH. Total laparoscopic pancreaticoduodenectomy: a single-institutional experience. Ann Surg Oncol. 2015. 22(13): 4380–1.
38. Suzuki O, Kondo S, Hirano S, Tanaka E, Kato K, Tsuchikawa T, et al. Laparoscopic pancreaticoduodenectomy combined with minilaparotomy. Surg Today. 2012;42:509–13. doi:10.1007/s00595-011-0064-x.
39. Wang Y, Bergman S, Piedimonte S, Vanounou T. Bridging the gap between open and minimally invasive pancreaticoduodenectomy: the hybrid approach. Can J Surg. 2014;57:263–70.
40. Nakamura Y, Matsumoto S, Yoshioka M, Shimizu T, Yamahatsu K, Uchida E. Successful laparoscopic pancreaticoduodenectomy for intraductal papillary mucinous neoplasm: a case report and a reliable technique for pancreaticojejunostomy. J Nippon Med Sch. 2012;793:218–22.
41. Ogiso S, Conrad C, Araki K, Basso V, Bayet B. Posterior approach for laparoscopic pancreaticoduodenectomy to prevent replaced hepatic artery injury. Ann Surg Oncol. 2013;20:3120. doi:10.1245/s10434-013-3058-7.
42. Keck T, Kusters S, Wellner UF, Hopt UT, Karcz KW. Total laparoscopic partial pancreatoduodenectomy and reconstruction via laparoscopic pancreatogastrostomy. Langenbecks Arch Surg. 2012;397:1009–12. doi:10.1007/s00423-012-0964-2.
43. Orti-Rodriguez RJ, Rahman SH. A comparative review between laparoscopic and robotic pancreaticoduodenectomies. Surg Laparosc Endosc Percutan Tech. 2014;24:103–8. doi:10.1097/SLE.0b013e3182a2f0ad.
44. Qin H, Qui J, Zhao Y, Pan G, Zeng Y. Does minimally-invasive pancreaticoduodenectomy have advantages over its open method? A meta- analysis of retrospective studies. PLoS One. 2014;9, e104274. doi:10.1371/journal.pone.0104274.
45. Langan RC, Graham JA, Chin AB, Rubinstein AJ, Oza K, Nusbaum JA, et al. Laparoscopic-assisted versus open pancreaticoduodenectomy: early favorable physical quality-of-life measures. Surgery. 2014;156: 379–84. doi:10.1016/j.surg.2014.03.018.
46. Mesleh MG, Stauffer JA, Bowers SP, Asbun HJ. Cost analysis of open and laparoscopic pancreaticoduodenectomy: a single institution comparison. Surg Endosc. 2013;27:4518–23. doi:10.1007/s00464-013-3101-6.
47. Kendrick ML, Sclabas GM. Major venous resection during total laparoscopic pancreaticoduodenectomy. HPB. 2011;13:454–8. doi:10.1111/j.1477-2574.2011.00323.x.
48. Young S, Abbitt P, Hughes SJ. Port-site recurrence of pancreatic adenocarcinoma following laparoscopic pancreaticoduodenectomy. J Gastrointest Surg. 2012; 16:2294–6. doi:10.1007/s11605-012-2050-z.
49. Kuroki T, Eguchi S. Laparoscopic parenchyma-sparing pancreatectomy. J Hepatobiliary Pancreat Sci. 2014;21:323–7. doi:10.1002/jhbp.29.
50. DiNorcia J, Lee MK, Reavey PL, Genkinger JM, Lee JA, Schrope BA, et al. One hundred and thirty resections for pancreatic neuroendocrine tumor: evaluating the impact of minimally invasive and parenchyma-sparing techniques. J Gastrointest Surg. 2010;14:1536–46. doi:10.1007/s11605-010-1319-3.
51. Song KB, Kim SC, Park KM, Hwang DW, Lee JH, Lee DJ, et al. Laparoscopic central pancreatectomy for benign or low-grade malignant lesions in the pancreatic neck and proximal body. Surg Endosc. 2015;29:937–46. doi:10.1007/s00464-014-3756-7.
52. Balzano G, Carvello M, Piemonti L, Nano R, Ariotti R, Mercalli A, et al. Combined laparoscopic spleen-preserving distal pancreatectomy and islet autotransplantation for benign pancreatic neoplasm. World J Gastroenterol. 2014;20:4030–6. doi:10.3748/wjg.v20.i14.4030.
53. Sokolov YY, Stronogin SV, Donskoy DV, Povarnin OY, Vilesov AV. Laparoscopic pancreatic resections for solid pseudopapillary tumor in children. Eur J Pediatr Surg. 2009;19:399–401. doi:10.1055/s-0029-1237356.
54. Thakkar S, Awad M, Gurram KC, Tully S, Wright C, Sanan S, et al. A novel, new robotic platform for natural orifice distal pancreatectomy. Surg Innov. 2015. 22(3):274–82.

13 EUS-Guided Injection for Pancreatic Cyst Ablation

William R. Brugge

13.1 Background for Cyst Ablation

Pancreatic cystic neoplasms (PCNs) consist of a range of pancreatic tumors that have different morphological, histological, and clinical characteristics. The number of patients with PCNs has increased over the years as a result of improved imaging. PCNs range from benign lesions with a very low potential for malignancy to those with aggressive behavior. The management of PCNs may be challenging since surgery or long-term follow-up is needed in most of the patients. An advanced age may further complicate the surgical treatment in some of these patients with high morbidity and mortality risk. Therefore, safe and effective minimally invasive interventions as alternative options to surgical resection are warranted.

EUS guided pancreatic cyst ablation is based on the principle that injection of a cytotoxic agent into a pancreatic cystic lesion will result in ablation of the cyst epithelium [1]. The close contact between the injected agent and the epithelium may result in both immediate and delayed tissue necroses. The cytotoxic agent remains within the cyst cavity without extravasation into the parenchyma. Ethanol has been used most commonly in clinical studies as a primary ablation agent for the lining epithelium of the cyst and to reduce the influx of fluid [2].

W.R. Brugge, MD
Department of Gastroenterology, Massachusetts General Hospital, Boston, MA, USA
e-mail: wbrugge@partners.org

13.2 Technique of the Procedure

EUS-guided ethanol lavage of pancreatic cystic lesions is based on endoscopic techniques of FNA of the pancreas [3]. After prophylactic antibiotics are administered, a linear echoendoscope positioned in the duodenum, gastric body, or fundus provides access to pancreatic head, body, or tail, respectively, and guides the use of FNA. The injection of ablative agents into a cystic lesion requires the complete or partial evacuation of the fluid contents of the cyst. Although it may be difficult to aspirate the highly viscous fluid of mucinous cysts, it is necessary to provide room for the injected ablative agent. The collection of cyst fluid also provides diagnostic material for cytology and biochemical analysis. This principle of cyst injection therapy, coupled with a dead space of approximately 0.8 mL in the aspiration needle, limits target cysts to more than 10 mm in diameter. Once the needle is in place within the lumen of the cyst, the ablative agent is injected under real-time monitoring. Clouds of aerated liquid are readily observed with EUS, and the distribution can be easily determined during the procedure (Figs. 13.1 and 13.2). In many cases, ablative therapy is provided with a lavage of the liquid, such as ethanol, in and out of the cyst over several

M. Del Chiaro et al. (eds.), *Cystic Tumors of the Pancreas*, DOI 10.1007/978-3-319-31882-0_13

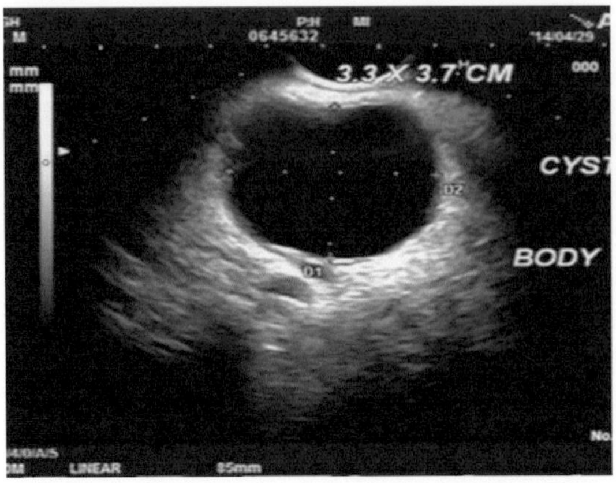

Fig. 13.1 EUS of a cystic neoplasm of the pancreas before injection therapy

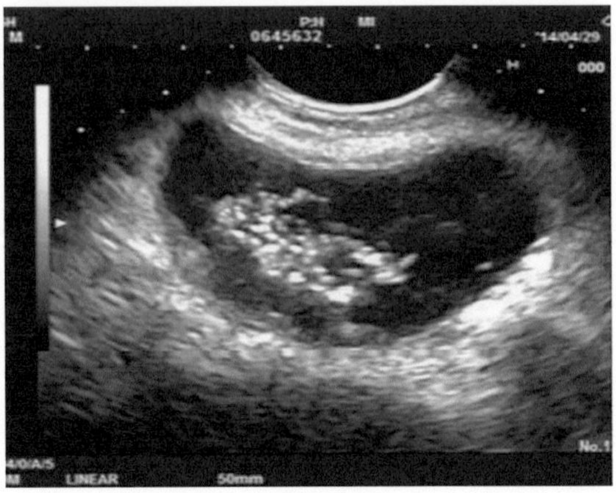

Fig. 13.2 EUS of a cystic neoplasm of the pancreas after injection of taxol

minutes. The injected ethanol is evacuated at the end of the lavage. A second ablative agent such as paclitaxel may be injected and left in the cyst cavity. The total injection volume should not exceed the volume of aspirated fluid. Unilocular cysts with a diameter of 1–2 cm are easily treated in one or two sessions. Larger and more complex lesions may require multiple lavage sessions [4] (DiMaio). The end point of ethanol lavage is elimination of the cyst as evidenced by cross-sectional imaging.

13.3 Outcomes of the Clinical Studies

EUS-guided ethanol injection into pancreatic cystic lesions was originally described using a variety of low concentrations of ethanol [3]. In the initial studies, the safety of cyst injection therapy was established first using saline solution, followed by highly diluted ethanol. There was no evidence of clinical pancreatitis with injection of ethanol using concentrations up to 80 %. Eight of 23 patients (35 %) with follow-up had complete resolution in 12 months. All septated cysts persisted despite ethanol ablation therapy. There was no significant difference in cyst resolution according to the ethanol concentration. Small numbers of lavaged cystic lesions were resected, and there was evidence of epithelial ablation with pancreatitis [3]. In a randomized, prospective, multicenter trial, ethanol lavage was found to provide greater rates of complete ablation as compared with saline lavage [5]. The overall CT-defined rate of complete pancreatic cyst ablation was 33.3 %, in 12 of 36 cysts lavaged with ethanol. The histology of four resected cysts demonstrated epithelial ablation ranging from 0 % (saline solution alone) to 50–100 % (one or two ethanol lavages). Although one patient developed transient pancreatitis, approximately 20 % of patients from both groups (ethanol and saline) experienced some abdominal pain the day after lavage. Twelve patients with pancreatic cysts that had previously resolved after ethanol lavage were followed up to determine long-term results. The median follow-up was 26 months (range 13–39) after initial resolution, and no evidence of cyst recurrence was shown in any patient [6]. Paclitaxel is a chemotherapeutic agent inhibiting cell processes which are dependent on microtubules. It can exert a durable effect on the epithelium within the cyst cavity with a low risk of leakage since it is hydrophobic and viscous in nature. Ethanol lavage has been coupled with paclitaxel injection in a large series with a variety of pancreatic cystic lesions [7]. It was hypothesized that the epithelial distortion by ethanol could allow the diffusion of paclitaxel in the injured epithelium. The combination of ethanol and paclitaxel injection resulted in elimination of the cysts, as determined by CT scanning, in 29/47 (62 %) of patients, in a median follow-up period of 21.7 months. On univariate analysis, EUS diameter and original cyst volume predicted resolution. However, the high viscosity of paclitaxel made injection into the cyst difficult. In contrast, ethanol is easily injected and aspirated from the cyst and at times reduces the cyst fluid viscosity, thus aiding in cyst evacuation. The combination of ethanol and paclitaxel is also capable of ablating septated cystic lesions, a much more difficult target for EUS injection therapy [8]. Complete resolution was achieved in six of ten patients with septated cysts after ethanol lavage and paclitaxel injection. Presumably, the surface area of a septated cyst is quite large, and it is difficult to be certain that the cytotoxic injectant comes in contact with all of the epithelium. The effectiveness of two EUS-guided ethanol lavage sessions for suspected branch-duct intraductal papillary mucinous neoplasms was evaluated in 13 patients [4]. Complete resolution of the cystic lesion was not seen by imaging in any patient after the first session but occurred in 5 (38 %) of 13 patients after second EUS treatments.

Results of EUS-guided cyst injection trials are summarized in Table 47–2. These preliminary studies showed the feasibility and safety of EUS-guided alcohol and paclitaxel injection into PCNs. It inhibits or slows the growth of the cyst, and complete ablation is possible in some cases. The results of median follow-up up to 2 years are encouraging, but the longer term effect of ethanol and paclitaxel injection is not clear. Most of the studies did not include a control group. Cyst type or the diagnosis could not be identified in some cases based only on imaging findings. The technical detail of the procedure, proposed indications, and most suitable cyst types are not standardized yet. Therefore, until some of these issues are resolved, the indication should be limited to selected patients such as those at high risk for surgery, and it should be used with caution in routine practice. International consensus guidelines for the management of mucinous cysts of the pancreas don't recommend EUS-guided cyst ablation of mucinous cysts outside of a closely monitored research protocol [9].

References

1. Brugge WR. EUS-guided tumor ablation with heat, cold, microwave, or radiofrequency: will there be a winner? Gastrointest Endosc. 2009;69(2 Suppl):S212–6.
2. Matthes K, Mino-Kenudson M, Sahani DV, et al. Concentration-dependent ablation of pancreatic tissue by EUS-guided ethanol injection. Gastrointest Endosc. 2007;65(2):272–7.
3. Gan SI, Thompson CC, Lauwers GY, et al. Ethanol lavage of pancreatic cystic lesions: initial pilot study. Gastrointest Endosc. 2005;61(6):746–52.
4. DiMaio CJ, DeWitt JM, Brugge WR. Ablation of pancreatic cystic lesions: the use of multiple endoscopic ultrasound-guided ethanol lavage sessions. Pancreas. 2011;40(5):664–8.
5. DeWitt J, McGreevy K, Schmidt CM, et al. EUS-guided ethanol versus saline solution lavage for pancreatic cysts: a randomized, double-blind study. Gastrointest Endosc. 2009;70(4):710–23.
6. DeWitt J, DiMaio CJ, Brugge WR. Long-term follow-up of pancreatic cysts that resolve radiologically after EUS-guided ethanol ablation. Gastrointest Endosc. 2010;72(4):862–6.
7. Oh HC, Seo DW, Song TJ, et al. Endoscopic ultrasonography-guided ethanol lavage with paclitaxel injection treats patients with pancreatic cysts. Gastroenterology. 2011;140(1):172–9.
8. Oh HC, Seo DW, Kim SC, et al. Septated cystic tumors of the pancreas: is it possible to treat them by endoscopic ultrasonography-guided intervention? Scand J Gastroenterol. 2009;44(2):242–7.
9. Oh HC, Brugge WR. EUS-guided pancreatic cyst ablation: a critical review (with video). Gastrointest Endosc. 2013;77(4):526–33.

14 How to Manage Cystic Tumors of the Pancreas in High-Risk Individuals

Ingrid C.A.W. Konings, Djuna L. Cahen, and Marco J. Bruno

14.1 Introduction

With the widespread use of high-resolution cross-sectional imaging, (asymptomatic) cystic tumors of the pancreas are being detected with increasing frequency [1–4]. While most pancreatic cysts are benign, some have malignant potential or even harbor invasive cancer. Differentiating these cysts is crucial to provide optimal patient care, but presents clinicians with a challenge. In individuals at increased risk to develop pancreatic cancer, cyst management poses an even greater challenge, as already little is known about the natural behavior of cystic lesions in general, but even less in high-risk individuals.

I.C.A.W. Konings, MD (✉)
M.J. Bruno, MD, PhD • D.L. Cahen, MD, PhD
Department of Gastroenterology and Hepatology, Erasmus MC, University Medical Center, Rotterdam, The Netherlands
e-mail: i.konings@erasmusmc.nl; m.bruno@erasmusmc.nl; d.cahen@erasmusmc.nl

14.2 Pathophysiology of Pancreatic Lesions

In the past years, significant progress has been made in our understanding of the (molecular) biology of pancreatic tumor growth. We have learned that infiltrating pancreatic cancer results from the accumulation of inherited and acquired mutations and arises from histologically well-defined precursor lesions: pancreatic intraepithelial neoplasia (PanIN), intraductal papillary mucinous neoplasms (IPMNs), and mucinous cystic neoplasms (MCNs) [5–7]. Two of these appear as cystic lesions on imaging: IPMNs and MCNs.

IPMNs are epithelial neoplasms that arise from the main pancreatic duct or its side branches and produce mucin. They are divided into three subtypes: those that involve the main duct (main-branch IPMNs), those involving side ducts (side-branch IPMNs), and those involving both (mixed- or combined-type IPMNs). IPMNs are also classified into low-, intermediate-, and high-grade dysplasia, based on the degree of atypia. Some IPMNs are multifocal and, importantly, up to one-third of IPMNs have an invasive component [8, 9]. The molecular alterations in IPMNs are heterogeneous and include loss of *SMAD4*, loss of *STK11* gene expression, activating mutations in the *PIK3CA* gene, and *KRAS* gene mutations [10–12].

Mucinous cystic neoplasms (MCNs) are also mucin-producing cystic lesions, but, in contrast

M. Del Chiaro et al. (eds.), *Cystic Tumors of the Pancreas*, DOI 10.1007/978-3-319-31882-0_14

to IPMNs, they do not involve the ductal system and have a distinctive ovarian-type stroma on pathological examination. MCNs are also classified according to degree of dysplasia, and up to one-third shows an invasive component [13]. At DNA level, activating mutations in the *KRAS2* gene occurs early, and inactivation of *TP53* and *MADH4* occurs in invasive MCNs [14, 15]. Unraveling the molecular pathology of MCNs, however, poses a challenge, partly due to their rare nature.

The further differential diagnosis of pancreatic cysts includes pseudocysts, serous cystic neoplasms (SCNs), solid pseudopapillary neoplasms (SPNs), and even cystic degenerated neuroendocrine tumors or pancreatic adenocarcinomas. Pseudocysts require a history of pancreatitis or abdominal trauma and are therefore generally well distinguishable. SCNs are mixed solid/cystic tumors, composed of numerous small cysts that are conjoined in a honeycomb-like formation. They contain serous fluid and may have a central scar with calcifications. SCNs do not communicate with the pancreatic ductal system and typically occur in young females. Their potential for malignancy is extremely low, so that surveillance is generally not recommended. Although rare, neuroendocrine tumors and pancreatic adenocarcinoma can undergo cystic degeneration and thus present as cystic lesions as well.

Recent observations on the natural course of precursor lesions of the pancreas suggest a significant time period for progression. Patients with noninvasive IPMNs and MCNs are 5–10 years younger than patients with an invasive lesion [16, 17]. A precursor of a neoplastic clone takes approximately 12 years to evolve into a malignant clone, with an additional 7 years to develop metastatic subclones [18]. This, at least in theory, provides a significant window of opportunity for the early recognition of dysplastic lesions and the timely resection of advanced lesions, before they can transform into malignancy. The clinical challenge is to develop diagnostic strategies, i.e., imaging modalities and/or biomolecular tests that can reliably identify and differentiate these lesions.

14.3 Individuals at High Risk of Developing Pancreatic Cancer

Well-known risk factors for pancreatic cancer are older age and cigarette smoking. Smoking doubles the risk, and as many as one in four cases of pancreatic cancer might be attributable to smoking [19, 20]. Heavy alcohol consumption (i.e., three or more drinks per day) also increases the risk of pancreatic cancer by approximately 20 % [21]. Furthermore, an increased risk was demonstrated for long-standing type 1 and type 2 diabetes [22–24], as well as for obesity [25].

A family history of pancreatic cancer is a strong risk factor for developing pancreatic cancer. For decades, case reports have been suggesting that pancreatic cancer aggregates in families, and multiple studies have shown inheritance in an autosomal dominant pattern [26–30]. Although most cases of pancreatic cancer are likely to be sporadic, it is estimated that in 5–10 % of cases, genetic factors are involved [31, 32]. Several genes have been discovered that are responsible for the familial clustering of pancreatic cancer, which can also cause significant morbidity in other organs. At present, in less than 20 % of the familial pancreatic cancers, a known genetic syndrome is identified [31, 32]. With new whole genome sequencing technologies, discovery of additional familial pancreatic cancer genes in the near future is likely.

Thus far, two groups of individuals with a hereditary risk of pancreatic cancer have been identified. First, individuals with a well-defined cancer susceptibility syndrome, of which the gene mutations, are listed in Table 14.1. Germline mutations in the *BRCA1* or *BRCA2* gene increase the risk of pancreatic cancer, independently from the risk for breast and ovarian cancer, the predominant cancer types in the hereditary breast and ovarian cancer (HBOC) susceptibility syndrome. The risk of pancreatic cancer in patients with a *BRCA2* mutation is three- to tenfold increased, as compared to the general population [33, 34]. Male *BRCA2* mutation carriers are at higher risk for pancreatic cancer than females, and the relative risk for pancreatic cancer

Table 14.1 Cancer susceptibility syndromes or inherited disease with a known elevated risk of developing pancreatic cancer

Syndrome	Gene(s)	Risk of pancreatic cancer
Hereditary breast and ovarian cancer (HBOC)	BRCA1 BRCA2 PALB2	RR 2–4 RR 3–10 RR unknown
Familial cutaneous malignant melanoma (familial CMM)	CDKN2A (p16)	RR 8–45
Chronic (hereditary) pancreatitis	PRSS1/SPINK1	RR 60–90
Peutz-Jeghers syndrome	STK11/LKB1	RR 75–135
Familial adenomatous polyposis (FAP)	APC	RR 4.5
Li-Fraumeni syndrome	p53	RR 7.5
Hereditary nonpolyposis colorectal cancer (Lynch syndrome)	MLH1/MSH2/MSH6	RR 9

RR relative risk

increases with age [34]. It is important to realize that the absence of breast cancer in a family with aggregation of pancreatic cancer does not exclude a *BRCA2* mutation, since pancreatic cancer can run in *BRCA2* mutation-carrying families, without associated breast cancer [35, 36]. *BRCA1* mutation carriers have a slightly lower risk of pancreatic cancer than *BRCA2* mutation carriers (relative risk 2–4 [37]). More recently, *PALB2* gene mutations, a gene that codes for a protein that binds to the BRCA2 protein, have also been proven to increase the risk for pancreatic cancer, albeit still unclear to what extent [38–40].

Patients with familial cutaneous malignant melanoma (familial CMM, formerly known as familial atypical multiple mole melanoma (FAMMM)), which is caused by mutations in the *p16/CDKN2A* gene, are at an 8- to 45-fold increased risk of developing pancreatic cancer [41, 42], which is independent from their increased risk of developing melanomas. Patients with hereditary chronic pancreatitis are also at high risk to develop pancreatic cancer (60- to 90-fold increased risk [43]). Hereditary pancreatitis is caused by germline mutations in the *PRSS1* and *SPINK1* genes and is characterized by recurrent episodes of acute or chronic pancreatitis, starting at a young age.

At highest risk for developing pancreatic cancer, with a 75–135-fold increase, are individuals with the Peutz-Jeghers syndrome [44, 45]. This cancer susceptibility syndrome is caused by mutations in the *STK11* or *LKB1* genes that also increase the risk for gastrointestinal, lung, ovarian, and breast cancer. Patients with familial adenomatous polyposis (FAP) and Li-Fraumeni syndrome also have a slightly increased risk of developing pancreatic cancer (4.5- and 7.5-fold, respectively [46, 47]). The risk is comparable to that of patients with Lynch syndrome, caused by mutations in one of the DNA mismatch repair genes, including *MLH1*, *MSH2*, and *MSH6*, and who are at a ninefold increased risk for developing pancreatic cancer [48].

The second and largest hereditary high-risk group consists of individuals with a strong family history of pancreatic cancer, but in whom no mutation was found in any of the known cancer susceptibility genes. This condition is referred to as familial pancreatic cancer (FPC). Depending on the number of affected relatives, the risk increases dramatically: individuals with one first-degree relative with pancreatic cancer have a 4.5–7-fold increased risk, those with two a four- to sixfold increased risk, and those with three or more an up to 32-fold increased risk, as compared to the general population [49, 50]. When at least one family member was diagnosed below the age of 50, the relative risk increases even further (hazard ratio of 1.6 per year of decreased age of the family member) [50].

For FPC families, it is important to realize that at least half of the members are not affected, assuming a dominant inheritance pattern. Unfortunately, because the causative mutation is unknown, it is not possible to test carrier ship and hence increased risk of developing pancreatic cancer. Furthermore, in FPC families, the phenomenon of genetic anticipation has been observed; compared to sporadic cases, pancreatic cancer seems to occur at an earlier age (mean 72 versus 62, respectively) and within affected families; subsequent generations seem to die at an earlier age, compared to the preceding generations [51].

14.4 Prevalence of Cystic Tumors of the Pancreas

In the general population, cystic tumors of the pancreas are being detected with increasing frequency, due to the widespread use of high-resolution imaging modalities [1–4]. The prevalence of asymptomatic cysts is estimated to be approximately 2.5 %, based on two large studies [52, 53]. This prevalence increases with age; below 50, only 1.3 % of individuals had pancreatic cysts, whereas in the category 70–79, cysts were found in 10.6 % [53]. Interestingly, in individuals at increased risk for pancreatic cancer, the prevalence of cystic tumors is also high, up to 39 % [54–64].

14.5 Surveillance in High-Risk Individuals

Because of the poor prognosis of pancreatic cancer, there is great interest in preventive strategies, especially in high-risk individuals. To detect and treat advanced precursor lesions or early-stage cancer may improve the prospects and life expectancy. Therefore, numerous studies on the feasibility of pancreatic cancer surveillance programs are being performed worldwide.

The International Cancer of the Pancreas Screening (CAPS) Consortium provided recommendations concerning surveillance for pancreatic cancer in high-risk individuals [65]. Only individuals with a tenfold increased risk for developing pancreatic cancer (see Table 14.2) and fit for surgery are recommended to participate in surveillance programs for pancreatic cancer. As there is no recommendation given on the starting or finishing age of surveillance, the screening principles for colorectal cancer are mostly used. These advise to initiate surveillance at the age of 50 or at an age 10 years younger than the youngest affected family member, whichever age occurs first, and to end surveillance at age 75. Specific targets for surveillance of the pancreas are the detection and treatment of early and premalignant stages: early invasive pancreatic cancer (T1N0M0), multifocal PanIN3, and IPMN with high-grade dysplasia. For both screening and surveillance, both endoscopic ultrasonography (EUS) and MRI/MRCP are recommended, since both techniques are widely available, have low morbidity rates, and, in particular, are good at detecting early-stage pancreatic cancer and its (cystic) precursor lesions. In the absence of abnormalities, a 12-month interval is suggested, but not agreed upon. Individuals with a non-suspicious cyst are recommended to undergo repeated surveillance after 6–12 months; individuals with a newly detected indeterminate solid lesion or main pancreatic duct stricture are recommended for follow-up after 3 months.

Over the past decade, multiple centers have initiated surveillance programs for pancreatic cancer, to evaluate the diagnostic yield and ultimately improve survival. Results of these studies are summarized in Table 14.3. In the 15 studies listed in Table 14.3, a total of 1085 high-risk individuals underwent annual surveillance of the pancreas. All studies combined, 94 relevant

Table 14.2 Candidates for pancreatic cancer surveillance due to a >10-fold increased risk of developing pancreatic cancer

Individuals with ≥2 relatives affected with pancreatic cancer, of which at least one in the first degree
Individuals with ≥2 first-degree relatives affected with pancreatic cancer
Individuals with Peutz-Jeghers syndrome
BRCA2 mutation carriers with at least one first-degree relative affected with pancreatic cancer or ≥2 affected family members with pancreatic cancer
PALB2 or CDKN2A mutation carriers and individuals with Lynch syndrome with at least one first-degree relative affected with pancreatic cancer

Table 14.3 Overview of results of pancreatic cancer surveillance programs for high-risk individuals

Study	*N*	High-risk individuals	Imaging modalities	Diagnostic yield[a], *N* (%)
Brentnall (1999) [66]	14	FPC	EUS+CT+ERCP	7 (50)
Rulyak (2001)[b] [67]	35	FPC	EUS; ERCP[d]	12 (34)
Kimmey (2002)[b] [68]	46	FPC	EUS; ERCP[d]	12 (26)
Canto (2004) [54]	38	FPC, PJS	EUS; CT[d], EUS-FNA[d], ERCP[d]	2 (5)
Canto (2006) [55]	78	FPC, PJS	EUS+CT; EUS-FNA[d], ERCP[d]	8 (10)
Kluijt (2009) [56]	3	CDKN2A	EUS+MRI; CT[d]	2 (67)
Poley (2009) [57][c]	44	FPC, PJS, CDKN2A, HP, BRCA, p53	EUS; CT[d], MRI[d]	10 (23)
Langer (2009) [69]	76	FPC, CDKN2A, BRCA	EUS+MRI; EUS-FNA[d]	1 (1)
Verna (2010) [58]	51	FPC, PJS, CDKN2A, HP, BRCA, Lynch	EUS and/or MRI; EUS-FNA[d], ERCP[d]	6 (12)
Ludwig (2011) [59]	109	FPC, BRCA	MRI; EUS[d], EUS-FNA[d]	9 (8)
Vasen (2011) [60]	79	CDKN2A	MRI	16 (20)
Scheider (2011)[e] [61]	72	FPC, BRCA, PALB2	EUS+MRI	9 (13)
Al-Sukhni (2012) [62]	262	FPC, PJS, CDKN2A, HP, BRCA	MRI; CT[d], EUS[d], ERCP[d]	19 (7)
Canto (2012) [63]	216	FPC, PJS, BRCA	EUS+CT+MRI; EUS-FNA[d]	5–92 (2–43)
Potjer (2012)[f] [64]	241	FPC, CDKN2A	MRI; EUS[d]	15 (6)

FPC familial pancreatic cancer, *PJS* Peutz-Jeghers syndrome, *HP* hereditary pancreatitis, *EUS* endoscopic ultrasonography, *CT* computed tomography, *MRI* magnetic resonance imaging, *ERCP* endoscopic retrograde cholangiopancreatography, *EUS-FNA* endoscopic ultrasonography-guided fine needle aspiration

[a]Yield is defined as the detection of (pre)malignant lesions (early invasive cancer T1N0M0, PanIN ≥2, or IPMN)

[b]Continuation of Brentnall (1999)

[c]Continuation of Kluijt (2009)

[d]Test performed only as an additional test for detected abnormalities

[e]Continuation of Langer (2009)

[f]Continuation and combination of both data from Langer (2009) and Vasen (2011)

high-grade dysplastic lesions were diagnosed, an overall diagnostic yield of 9 %. Seventy-one of these individuals underwent resection.

Histopathology of the resected pancreatic specimens revealed pancreatic cancer in 15 of the 71 specimens (21 %), of which nine had been detected at the first screening visit and six during follow-up (of which one patient missed the 1-year surveillance visit). Only one of the cancers had risen from an IPMN. IPMNs were found in 25 of 71 specimens (35 %), of which nine were detected at the first screening visit and four during follow-up (three of these had been present at baseline, but showed growth after 1 year). Two IPMNs showed high-grade dysplasia, six moderate-grade dysplasia, and eight low-grade dysplasia. Serous cystadenomas were identified in 3 of the 71 specimens (4 %), and a neuroendocrine tumor was discovered in one (1 %). Six of the 1085 individuals (0.6 %) already had metastatic disease at diagnosis (two were detected at baseline, two after 1 year, and one after 4 years of surveillance).

14.6 Management of Cystic Tumors in High-Risk Individuals

At present, there is no evidence to suggest that the natural behavior of pancreatic cystic neoplasms in individuals with a hereditary pancreatic cancer risk differs from the general

Table 14.4 The revised Sendai criteria for cyst management

Finding	Management
Cystic tumors with any of the following high-risk stigmata of malignancy: Obstructive jaundice in a patient with a cystic lesion in the head of the pancreas Enhancing solid component within cyst Main pancreatic duct ≥10 mm in size	Consider surgery, if clinically appropriate
Cystic tumors with any of the following worrisome features: Clinical: pancreatitis Imaging: cyst ≥3 cm; thickened/enhanced cyst walls; main duct size 5–9 mm; non-enhancing mural nodule; abrupt change in caliber of pancreatic duct with distal pancreatic atrophy AND any of the following features on endoscopic ultrasound: Definite mural nodule Main duct features suspicious for involvement (the presence of any one of thickened walls, intraductal mucin, or mural nodules) Cytology: suspicious or positive for malignancy	Consider surgery, if clinically appropriate
Cystic tumors ≥3 cm and/or inconclusive EUS results on mural nodules, main duct features, or cytology	Close surveillance, alternating MRI and EUS every 3–6 months (or strongly consider surgery in young, fit patients)
Cystic tumors 2–3 cm	EUS in 3–6 months and then lengthen interval, alternating MRI with EUS (or consider surgery in young, fit patients)
Cystic tumors 1–2 cm	MRI annually during 2 years and then lengthen interval if no change
Cystic tumors <1 cm	MRI in 2–3 years

MRI magnetic resonance imaging, *EUS* endoscopic ultrasonography

population. Therefore, the revised Sendai criteria for cyst management (see Table 14.4, [70]) can be applied in this group, but with some modification: the Sendai criteria suggest a longer than 1-year interval for cysts smaller than 2 cm, but in patients with a hereditary risk, annual follow-up is always recommended, according to the CAPS guideline [65].

In the general population, EUS-guided fine needle aspiration (EUS-FNA) is widely used. Although cyst fluid cytology has a high specificity for malignancy (almost 100 %), the sensitivity is low [71]. Cytology, combined with tumor-marker analysis (amylase, CEA, and CA 19–9), can be helpful in differentiating mucinous from non-mucinous pancreatic cysts [1], but is still non-accurate in predicting malignancy. In high-risk individuals, the role of EUS-FNA is limited, as the pretest likelihood of malignancy is so high that clinical decision-making is less dependent on cyst fluid analysis. A lesion with morphological features suspicious for malignancy will be resected, regardless of normal FNA results. Clearly, EUS-FNA should be reserved for those individuals in whom the results will have a direct impact on the decision to operate.

Every pancreatic cyst, suspect of advanced dysplasia or malignancy, should be resected. Limited resections or focal nonanatomic resections (excision, enucleation) may be considered for MCN or side-duct IPMN without suspicion of malignancy. Resection should aim to achieve complete removal of the tumor, with negative margins. Intraoperative frozen sections can help to achieve negative margins. In case of low-grade or moderate-grade dysplasia on the resection margin, further resection is controversial. However, when positive margins for high-grade dysplasia are present, reoperation and additional resection should be performed.

For multifocal side-branch IPMNs, the same surgical approach holds as for unifocal disease: a segmental pancreatectomy to remove the IPMNs at highest oncological risk and close monitoring of the remaining lesions. According to the revised Sendai criteria, however, in patients with a strong family history of pancreatic cancer, one should consider a total pancreatectomy, because of the increased prevalence of high-grade dysplasia elsewhere in the pancreas [72].

It is important to realize that, after partial pancreatectomy, the pancreatic remnant is still prone to develop dysplastic lesions. Therefore, continued surveillance should be performed in these patients at least annually, regardless of pathologic findings in the surgical specimen, as is continued surveillance after IPMN resection.

14.7 Challenges in the Management of Cystic Tumors of the Pancreas in High-Risk Individuals

The true challenge in pancreatic cancer surveillance is to adequately identify both cystic (IPMN) and solid (PanIN) preneoplastic lesions. This means to avoid resection of early-stage lesions (i.e., low- or medium-grade dysplastic IPMN, PanIN1, or PanIN2 lesions) and to timely resect advanced lesions, before cancer develops. Based on present studies, it is not possible to draw a definite conclusion about the (potential) merits of surveillance to prevent pancreatic cancer death. In this regard, it is important to have realistic expectations. For instance, it has taken many years to prove that colon cancer screening is effective. To answer pivotal questions pertaining the yield of pancreatic cancer surveillance and the management of cysts in a high-risk population, large and long-term follow-up studies are required. Moreover, such studies should not merely focus on imaging techniques, but should also include the application of biomarkers.

In summary, the incidence of cystic tumors of the pancreas is high in individuals with a hereditary increased risk for developing pancreatic cancer. At least annual screening of these individuals by EUS and MRI/MRCP is recommended, regardless of the presence of cysts. The management of cysts in these individuals presents a challenge, as little is known about their natural behavior. Large and long-term follow-up studies are required to answer pivotal questions pertaining the yield of surveillance and the management of detected cysts.

References

1. Brugge WR, et al. Diagnosis of pancreatic cystic neoplasms: a report of the cooperative pancreatic cyst study. Gastroenterology. 2004;126(5):1330–6.
2. Lee KS, et al. Prevalence of incidental pancreatic cysts in the adult population on MR imaging. Am J Gastroenterol. 2010;105(9):2079–84.
3. Fernandez-del Castillo C, et al. Incidental pancreatic cysts: clinicopathologic characteristics and comparison with symptomatic patients. Arch Surg. 2003;138(4):427–3; discussion 433–4.
4. Winter JM, et al. Periampullary and pancreatic incidentaloma: a single institution's experience with an increasingly common diagnosis. Ann Surg. 2006;243(5):673–80; discussion 680–3.
5. Matthaei H, et al. Cystic precursors to invasive pancreatic cancer. Nat Rev Gastroenterol Hepatol. 2011;8(3):141–50.
6. Maitra A, et al. Precursors to invasive pancreatic cancer. Adv Anat Pathol. 2005;12(2):81–91.
7. Hruban RH, Wilentz RE, Maitra A. Identification and analysis of precursors to invasive pancreatic cancer. Methods Mol Med. 2005;103:1–13.
8. Schmidt CM, et al. Intraductal papillary mucinous neoplasms: predictors of malignant and invasive pathology. Ann Surg. 2007;246(4):644–51; discussion 651–4.
9. Sohn TA, et al. Intraductal papillary mucinous neoplasms of the pancreas: an updated experience. Ann Surg. 2004;239(6):788–97; discussion 797–9.
10. Iacobuzio-Donahue CA, et al. Dpc-4 protein is expressed in virtually all human intraductal papillary mucinous neoplasms of the pancreas: comparison with conventional ductal adenocarcinomas. Am J Pathol. 2000;157(3):755–61.
11. Sahin F, et al. Loss of Stk11/Lkb1 expression in pancreatic and biliary neoplasms. Mod Pathol. 2003;16(7):686–91.
12. Schonleben F, et al. PIK3CA, KRAS, and BRAF mutations in intraductal papillary mucinous neoplasm/carcinoma (IPMN/C) of the pancreas. Langenbecks Arch Surg. 2008;393(3):289–96.
13. Crippa S, et al. Mucin-producing neoplasms of the pancreas: an analysis of distinguishing clinical and epidemiologic characteristics. Clin Gastroenterol Hepatol. 2010;8(2):213–9.
14. Jimenez RE, et al. Sequential accumulation of K-ras mutations and p53 overexpression in the progression of pancreatic mucinous cystic neoplasms to malignancy. Ann Surg. 1999;230(4):501–9; discussion 509–11.

15. Kim SG, et al. Comparison of epigenetic and genetic alterations in mucinous cystic neoplasm and serous microcystic adenoma of pancreas. Mod Pathol. 2003;16(11):1086–94.
16. Salvia R, et al. Main-duct intraductal papillary mucinous neoplasms of the pancreas: clinical predictors of malignancy and long-term survival following resection. Ann Surg. 2004;239(5):678–85; discussion 685–7.
17. Sarr MG, et al. Clinical and pathologic correlation of 84 mucinous cystic neoplasms of the pancreas: can one reliably differentiate benign from malignant (or premalignant) neoplasms? Ann Surg. 2000;231(2):205–12.
18. Yachida S, et al. Distant metastasis occurs late during the genetic evolution of pancreatic cancer. Nature. 2010;467(7319):1114–7.
19. Gandini S, et al. Tobacco smoking and cancer: a meta-analysis. Int J Cancer. 2008;122(1):155–64.
20. Vrieling A, et al. Cigarette smoking, environmental tobacco smoke exposure and pancreatic cancer risk in the European Prospective Investigation into Cancer and Nutrition. Int J Cancer. 2010;126(10):2394–403.
21. Tramacere I, et al. Alcohol drinking and pancreatic cancer risk: a meta-analysis of the dose-risk relation. Int J Cancer. 2010;126(6):1474–86.
22. Huxley R, et al. Type-II diabetes and pancreatic cancer: a meta-analysis of 36 studies. Br J Cancer. 2005;92(11):2076–83.
23. Stevens RJ, Roddam AW, Beral V. Pancreatic cancer in type 1 and young-onset diabetes: systematic review and meta-analysis. Br J Cancer. 2007;96(3):507–9.
24. Gapstur SM, et al. Abnormal glucose metabolism and pancreatic cancer mortality. JAMA. 2000;283(19):2552–8.
25. Li D, et al. Body mass index and risk, age of onset, and survival in patients with pancreatic cancer. JAMA. 2009;301(24):2553–62.
26. Dat NM, Sontag SJ. Pancreatic carcinoma in brothers. Ann Intern Med. 1982;97(2):282.
27. Friedman JM, Fialkow PJ. Familial carcinoma of the pancreas. Clin Genet. 1976;9(5):463–9.
28. Ehrenthal D, et al. Familial pancreatic adenocarcinoma in three generations. A case report and a review of the literature. Cancer. 1987;59(9):1661–4.
29. Lynch HT, Fusaro L, Lynch JF. Familial pancreatic cancer: a family study. Pancreas. 1992;7(5):511–5.
30. Lynch HT, et al. Familial pancreatic cancer: a review. Semin Oncol. 1996;23(2):251–75.
31. Permuth-Wey J, Egan KM. Family history is a significant risk factor for pancreatic cancer: results from a systematic review and meta-analysis. Fam Cancer. 2009;8(2):109–17.
32. Shi C, Hruban RH, Klein AP. Familial pancreatic cancer. Arch Pathol Lab Med. 2009;133(3):365–74.
33. Iqbal J, et al. The incidence of pancreatic cancer in BRCA1 and BRCA2 mutation carriers. Br J Cancer. 2012;107(12):2005–9.
34. van Asperen CJ, et al. Cancer risks in BRCA2 families: estimates for sites other than breast and ovary. J Med Genet. 2005;42(9):711–9.
35. Goggins M, et al. Germline BRCA2 gene mutations in patients with apparently sporadic pancreatic carcinomas. Cancer Res. 1996;56(23):5360–4.
36. Lucas AL, et al. BRCA1 and BRCA2 germline mutations are frequently demonstrated in both high-risk pancreatic cancer screening and pancreatic cancer cohorts. Cancer. 2014;120(13):1960–7.
37. Mocci E, et al. Risk of pancreatic cancer in breast cancer families from the breast cancer family registry. Cancer Epidemiol Biomarkers Prev. 2013;22(5):803–11.
38. Harinck F, et al. Routine testing for PALB2 mutations in familial pancreatic cancer families and breast cancer families with pancreatic cancer is not indicated. Eur J Hum Genet. 2012;20(5):577–9.
39. Jones S, et al. Exomic sequencing identifies PALB2 as a pancreatic cancer susceptibility gene. Science. 2009;324(5924):217.
40. Tischkowitz MD, et al. Analysis of the gene coding for the BRCA2-interacting protein PALB2 in familial and sporadic pancreatic cancer. Gastroenterology. 2009;137(3):1183–6.
41. Lynch HT, Fusaro RM. Pancreatic cancer and the familial atypical multiple mole melanoma (FAMMM) syndrome. Pancreas. 1991;6(2):127–31.
42. de Snoo FA, et al. Increased risk of cancer other than melanoma in CDKN2A founder mutation (p16-Leiden)-positive melanoma families. Clin Cancer Res. 2008;14(21):7151–7.
43. Rebours V, et al. Risk of pancreatic adenocarcinoma in patients with hereditary pancreatitis: a national exhaustive series. Am J Gastroenterol. 2008;103(1):111–9.
44. Korsse SE, et al. Pancreatic cancer risk in Peutz-Jeghers syndrome patients: a large cohort study and implications for surveillance. J Med Genet. 2013;50(1):59–64.
45. Giardiello FM, et al. Very high risk of cancer in familial Peutz-Jeghers syndrome. Gastroenterology. 2000;119(6):1447–53.
46. Giardiello FM, et al. Increased risk of thyroid and pancreatic carcinoma in familial adenomatous polyposis. Gut. 1993;34(10):1394–6.
47. Ruijs MW, et al. TP53 germline mutation testing in 180 families suspected of Li-Fraumeni syndrome: mutation detection rate and relative frequency of cancers in different familial phenotypes. J Med Genet. 2010;47(6):421–8.
48. Kastrinos F, et al. Risk of pancreatic cancer in families with Lynch syndrome. JAMA. 2009;302(16):1790–5.
49. Klein AP, et al. Prospective risk of pancreatic cancer in familial pancreatic cancer kindreds. Cancer Res. 2004;64(7):2634–8.
50. Brune KA, et al. Importance of age of onset in pancreatic cancer kindreds. J Natl Cancer Inst. 2010;102(2):119–26.
51. McFaul CD, et al. Anticipation in familial pancreatic cancer. Gut. 2006;55(2):252–8.

52. Laffan TA, et al. Prevalence of unsuspected pancreatic cysts on MDCT. AJR Am J Roentgenol. 2008;191(3): 802–7.
53. de Jong K, et al. High prevalence of pancreatic cysts detected by screening magnetic resonance imaging examinations. Clin Gastroenterol Hepatol. 2010;8(9): 806–11.
54. Canto MI, et al. Screening for pancreatic neoplasia in high-risk individuals: an EUS-based approach. Clin Gastroenterol Hepatol. 2004;2(7):606–21.
55. Canto MI, et al. Screening for early pancreatic neoplasia in high-risk individuals: a prospective controlled study. Clin Gastroenterol Hepatol. 2006;4(6): 766–81.
56. Kluijt I, et al. Atypical familial presentation of FAMMM syndrome with a high incidence of pancreatic cancer: case finding of asymptomatic individuals by EUS surveillance. J Clin Gastroenterol. 2009;43(9): 853–7.
57. Poley JW, et al. The yield of first-time endoscopic ultrasonography in screening individuals at a high risk of developing pancreatic cancer. Am J Gastroenterol. 2009;104(9):2175–81.
58. Verna EC, et al. Pancreatic cancer screening in a prospective cohort of high-risk patients: a comprehensive strategy of imaging and genetics. Clin Cancer Res. 2010;16(20):5028–37.
59. Ludwig E, et al. Feasibility and yield of screening in relatives from familial pancreatic cancer families. Am J Gastroenterol. 2011;106(5):946–54.
60. Vasen HF, et al. Magnetic resonance imaging surveillance detects early-stage pancreatic cancer in carriers of a p16-Leiden mutation. Gastroenterology. 2011; 140(3):850–6.
61. Schneider R, et al. German national case collection for familial pancreatic cancer (FaPaCa): ten years experience. Fam Cancer. 2011;10(2):323–30.
62. Al-Sukhni W, et al. Screening for pancreatic cancer in a high-risk cohort: an eight-year experience. J Gastrointest Surg. 2012;16(4):771–83.
63. Canto MI, et al. Frequent detection of pancreatic lesions in asymptomatic high-risk individuals. Gastroenterology. 2012;142(4):796–804; quiz e14-5.
64. Potjer TP, et al. Variation in precursor lesions of pancreatic cancer among high-risk groups. Clin Cancer Res. 2013;19(2):442–9.
65. Canto MI, et al. International Cancer of the Pancreas Screening (CAPS) Consortium summit on the management of patients with increased risk for familial pancreatic cancer. Gut. 2013;62(3):339–47.
66. Brentnall TA, et al. Early diagnosis and treatment of pancreatic dysplasia in patients with a family history of pancreatic cancer. Ann Intern Med. 1999;131(4): 247–55.
67. Rulyak SJ, Brentnall TA. Inherited pancreatic cancer: surveillance and treatment strategies for affected families. Pancreatology. 2001;1(5):477–85.
68. Kimmey MB, et al. Screening and surveillance for hereditary pancreatic cancer. Gastrointest Endosc. 2002;56(4 Suppl):S82–6.
69. Langer P, et al. Five years of prospective screening of high-risk individuals from families with familial pancreatic cancer. Gut. 2009;58(10):1410–8.
70. Tanaka M, et al. International consensus guidelines 2012 for the management of IPMN and MCN of the pancreas. Pancreatology. 2012;12(3):183–97.
71. Khalid A, Brugge W. ACG practice guidelines for the diagnosis and management of neoplastic pancreatic cysts. Am J Gastroenterol. 2007;102(10):2339–49.
72. Bartsch DK, et al. Multiple small "imaging" branch-duct type intraductal papillary mucinous neoplasms (IPMNs) in familial pancreatic cancer: indicator for concomitant high grade pancreatic intraepithelial neoplasia? Fam Cancer. 2013;12(1):89–96.

How to Follow Patients with Resected Cystic Tumors of the Pancreas

15

Katherine E. Poruk and Christopher L. Wolfgang

Intraductal papillary mucinous neoplasm (IPMN) is a mucin-producing cystic lesion of the main pancreatic ducts and its branches. IPMNs were first uniquely described in the literature by Ohashi in 1982, who wrote of patients with pancreatic intraductal neoplasms with cystically dilated ducts containing large amounts of mucin [1]. However, it was not until 1996 that the World Health Organization (WHO) created separate diagnostic criteria to distinguish IPMNs from other cystic lesions of the pancreas [2]. Since that time, increasing focus has been shed on these lesions as precursors to pancreatic adenocarcinomas and, therefore, as a focus for early detection. Recent studies have shown that the risk of recurrence of IPMNs, even benign, is not insignificant. While criteria have been established for the surveillance and resection of IPMNs, very little is known about how to best follow patients who have undergone resection of an IPMN. Therefore, a thorough knowledge of the risk of malignancy and recurrence for IPMNs is needed for clinicians to properly follow these patients after surgical resection.

K.E. Poruk, MD • C.L. Wolfgang, MD, PhD (✉)
Department of Surgery, The Johns Hopkins Hospital, Baltimore, MD, USA
e-mail: kporuk1@jhmi.edu; cwolfga2@jhmi.edu

15.1 Histological Characteristics of IPMN

IPMNs are pancreatic neoplasms characterized by intraductal papillary proliferation of mucin-producing cells and cystic dilatation with the potential to develop into a pancreatic adenocarcinoma. The first distinct report of an IPMN was in 1982, leading to an increased clinical awareness of these cystic lesions. In the following years, numerous reports were published on mucin-producing pancreatic neoplasms under a variety of names, each often focusing on a different histopathological aspect of the tumor [3–7]. In 1989, the term "intraductal papillary neoplasm" was first coined and was later used to define one disease unifying all of the specific histopathological and clinical aspects each previously and individually reported [7, 8]. In 1996, IPMN was defined as a distinct disease with specific diagnostic criteria by the World Health Organization, although these guidelines further categorized IPMNs into three groups based on the presence of benign disease, moderate dysplasia, or carcinoma [2]. IPMNs were further categorized in 2000 by the WHO, and the first set of consensus guidelines on IPMN diagnosis and treatment were published in 2006 [9].

Research on IPMNs has further defined three separate subgroups based on location by imaging studies and/or histology: main duct, branch duct, and mixed duct [9, 10]. Main-duct IPMNs have diffuse or segmental dilatation of the main

M. Del Chiaro et al. (eds.), *Cystic Tumors of the Pancreas*, DOI 10.1007/978-3-319-31882-0_15

pancreatic duct to greater than 10 mm without another cause of obstruction. Branch-duct IPMNs are cysts greater than 5 mm in diameter that are limited to the smaller branches off of but communicate with the main pancreatic duct. A mixed-type IPMN meets the criteria for both main and branch-duct IPMNs, although it is felt to behave more like a main-duct IPMN. The relative frequency and risk of invasive carcinoma vary for each, although all three types have malignant potential [10].

Furthermore, IPMNs can be classified into five subtypes based upon mucin expression and morphology: gastric, intestinal, pancreatobiliary, oncocytic, and tubular or tubulopapillary [1]. The most common type of IPMN is the gastric subtype, which is usually found in the periphery of the pancreas and thus is usually found in branch-duct IPMNs [11]. Of main-duct IPMNs, the most common type is intestinal which tends to occur in the head of the pancreas with cells that resemble villous adenomas of the colon [11, 12]. The pancreatobiliary type also typically involves the main duct, but can be differentiated from intestinal type IPMNs due to its lower expression of mucin and its resemblance of pancreatic and biliary cells. In addition, while all subtypes can lead to invasive cancer, the pancreatobiliary type is the most likely to form classic ductal adenocarcinomas [12]. Both the oncocytic and tubular subtypes are rare. The oncocytic-type IPMNs contain cells with abundant eosinophilic cytoplasm due to the accumulation of mitochondria, but produces very little mucin. The tubular or tubulopapillary type is the most controversial in that it has more solid growth without visible mucin, resulting in little mucin production [12]. However, it is often included in the classification as it is an intraductal lesion [11]. While all types have the potential to form invasive carcinoma, the individual risk varies based on the subtype present [11].

Evaluation of an IPMN's pathology after resection can further distinguish IPMNs based on the presence and grade of dysplasia [12]. IPMNs with low-grade dysplasia contain uniform cells with abundant mucin and little to no nuclear atypia. Intermediate-grade dysplasia involves cells with some nuclear atypia such as nuclear enlargement or increased nuclear-to-cytoplasmic ratio. IPMNs with high-grade dysplasia are composed of atypical cells with nuclear pleomorphism and complex architecture [12]. These are often described as "carcinoma in situ," a term which has been discouraged in recent years [10]. Because a lesion can have more than one grade of dysplasia, IPMNs are graded based on the highest type of dysplasia present [12].

15.2 Clinical Presentation and Diagnosis of IPMN

The clinical presentation of an IPMN varies for each individual patient. The usual age of presentation is generally between 60 and 70 years of age with a slightly higher predominance in males [13–15]. On average, patients with an associated invasive carcinoma tend to present several years older than those with a benign IPMN [13, 14]. The most common symptoms at the time of presentation are often abdominal pain, weight loss, and jaundice, although a substantial group of patients are often asymptomatic at the time of diagnosis [13, 16]. In addition, some patients will first present with pancreatitis, often related to obstruction of the duct by the neoplasm [15, 16]. Generally, main-duct IPMNs are more likely to present with symptoms, while branch-duct IPMNs are asymptomatic and are found incidentally.

Improvements in imaging over the last decade have increased the number of incidentally discovered pancreatic cysts in asymptomatic patients. A review of 2,832 asymptomatic patients undergoing multidetector computed tomography (CT) discovered previously undiagnosed pancreatic cysts in 2.6 %, believed to likely be IPMNs [17]. A review of 118 patients who underwent resection of an incidental periampullary or pancreatic mass found 30 % of operations were for IPMN without an invasive cancer [18]. A similar study of incidentally discovered pancreatic cysts in asymptomatic patients discovered IPMN in 21 patients (27 %), although nine of these were associated with invasive cancer [19].

With imaging increasing the number of incidentally discovered IPMNs, focus shifts to best managing these premalignant lesions in otherwise asymptomatic patients.

15.3 Risk of Malignancy with IPMN

The primary concern with IPMNs is the presence of an associated invasive cancer, found to be the most important factor in determining overall prognosis [20]. The frequency of malignancy found in an IPMN varies according to the specific morphologic type. In addition, differences in observed rates are seen due to variations in the definition and diagnostic criteria for "malignancy" by the different studies. Some define "malignancy" only as the presence of invasive carcinoma, while others will include "carcinoma in situ," high-grade dysplasia, or simply aggressive clinical behavior of the lesion in this category [10]. While this leads to a large variability in the frequency of malignancy reported by various studies, the presence of invasive carcinoma in some IPMNs cannot be disregarded.

Current guidelines define malignant IPMNs as those containing invasive carcinoma [10]. Main-duct IPMNs have been consistently shown to have the highest frequency of malignancy in IPMNs. Malignancy in these lesions ranges anywhere from 36 to 100 % based on classification in published reports, with an average frequency of >62.2 % [10, 21–23]. Looking only at those patients recognized to have invasive carcinoma, this range drops from 11 to 81 % [22, 24]. The frequency of malignancy in branch-duct IPMN ranges from 6.3 to 51 %, with invasive carcinoma specifically noted in 1–36.7 % [21, 22, 25]. The malignancy potential of mixed-type IPMN is unsurprisingly between the two, ranging from 34 to 79 % [22, 26]. Accounting only for invasive disease, however, this range drops from 19 to 68 % [22, 26]. Despite the differences in classification, these studies demonstrate that IPMNs pose a substantial malignant potential.

The presence of an invasive carcinoma associated with the IPMN has been shown to be a significant predictor of survival. Patients with an invasive IPMN have been shown to have similar 5-year survival compared to patients with pancreatic ductal adenocarcinoma (31 % vs. 24 %) and lower survival overall compared to noninvasive IPMNs [13]. A five-year survival in one study for patients with an invasive IPMN was found to be only 36 % compared to 84.5 % in patients with a noninvasive IPMN [14]. Another institution reported 5- and 10-year disease-specific survival of 100 % in patients with noninvasive IPMNs compared to 60 % and 50 %, respectively, for those with IPMNs associated with invasive carcinoma [27]. Studies have shown that the median age for presentation in patients with invasive IPMNs is several years older than those with noninvasive IPMNs, indicating a several-year window between benign disease and the development of an invasive component [12–14]. Thus, resection of an IPMN before the progression to invasive carcinoma is preferable.

15.4 Resection Criteria for IPMN

Resection of IPMNs is usually encouraged based on the location and characteristics in conjunction with the risk of malignancy. In 2006, an international panel published consensus guidelines on the management of IPMNs, commonly referred to as the "Sendai Consensus Guidelines [9]." These guidelines strongly encouraged the resection of all main-duct and mixed variant IPMNs in all patients given the risk of malignancy, provided that the patient was a good surgical candidate. Given the lower incidence of malignancy in branch-duct IPMNs, recommendations mainly varied in relation to symptoms. Resection was encouraged in symptomatic patients not only to relieve their symptoms but also given the higher likelihood of malignancy. Asymptomatic patients had the potential for management with careful observation, provided they were willing to undergo close follow-up [9].

The international consensus guidelines for IPMN management were updated in 2012 based on an increased understanding of these lesions [10]. These guidelines continued to strongly recommend resection in all surgically fit patients with a main-duct or mixed IPMN due to the high frequency of malignancy. In addition, surgery was recommended in patients whose IPMNs contained any "high-risk stigmata" of malignancy, including a main duct at least 10 mm in size, an enhancing solid component within a cyst, and a cystic lesion in the head of the pancreas causing obstructive jaundice. The guidelines were also updated to recommend resection in patients with a branch-duct IPMN with "worrisome features," such as lymphadenopathy, a cyst greater than 3 cm, or a main duct size 5–9 mm. However, in patients who did not have risk factors predicting malignancy or were not good surgical candidates, conservative management was still supported provided the patient was able to undergo close follow-up.

15.5 Risk of IPMN Recurrence after Resection

Concern exists regarding the risk of a new IPMN recurring in the pancreatic remnant after resection of a noninvasive IPMN. This risk was not well understood until recently, when several studies evaluated the recurrence of IPMN in their respective populations of resected patients. Chari et al. looked at the outcomes of 113 patients with resected IPMNs and compared patients based upon the presence of an invasive carcinoma and type of pancreatic resection [14]. Of patients who underwent a partial pancreatectomy, recurrence was noted in 18 of 27 (67 %) patients with an invasive IPMN and in 5 of 60 (8 %) patients with noninvasive IPMNs. Thirteen patients with an IPMN and associated invasive carcinoma underwent a total pancreatectomy; 8 (62 %) had recurrence, primarily due to distant metastases. In patients with a noninvasive IPMN, recurrence occurred between 23 and 75 months (median, 40 months), and 5-year survival was shown to be 84.5 %. This study demonstrated that while invasive IPMNs are associated with high recurrence and poor survival, there is a lower rate of recurrence for noninvasive IPMNs with high survival rates.

White et al. retrospectively reviewed 78 patients who underwent resection for a noninvasive IPMN to evaluate local recurrence [28]. Based on radiographic findings, six patients (7.7 %) were shown to have a local recurrence; four patients had carcinoma in situ, while two had borderline IPMN. The median time to recurrence was 22 months, although all recurred within approximately 5 years. Three patients underwent resection of the recurrent IPMN, while the other three were not surgical candidates due to the extent of their disease. Patients who did not undergo resection all died of recurrent disease, while all patients who had re-resection were alive with no evidence of disease at the last follow-up. Of the factors looked at, a positive margin was associated with recurrence of the IPMN. A five-year recurrence-free survival was 87 %. Based on these results, the authors suggest that indefinite close surveillance is needed for patients who undergo pancreatic resection of a noninvasive IPMN based on the risk of recurrence.

Miller et al. evaluated the risk of recurrence of IPMN after resection based on margin status [29]. Of the 191 who underwent partial pancreatectomy for a noninvasive IPMN, 38 (20 %) had residual disease remaining either at the margin or elsewhere in the pancreas based on radiographic imaging. The 5-year progression-free survival of patients with residual disease was similar to those without remaining disease (88 % vs. 83 %). In addition, only one of the 38 (3 %) patients with residual disease had recurrence of an IPMN with invasive carcinoma. Comparatively, 31 of the 153 patients (20 %) without residual disease after surgery had recurrence of a new IPMN, three of which were associated with an invasive cancer. The median time to recurrence of a noninvasive IPMN was 33 months (range, 7–145 months) compared to 60 months (20–99 months) for an invasive IPMN. Unlike White et al., the authors of this study did not demonstrate an increased risk of developing a new IPMN or invasive disease with disease remaining after a segmental pancreatectomy.

In a recent study, He et al. retrospectively evaluated 130 patients who underwent resection of a noninvasive IPMN [30]. Of the 130 patients, 22 (17 %) developed radiographic evidence of a new or progressive IPMN. Eleven patients underwent resection of the new IPMN by completion pancreatectomy; three were found to have pancreatic ductal adenocarcinoma and three were found to have high-grade dysplasia. Two of the six patients that did not undergo repeated resection had metastatic pancreatic cancer at presentation. The only factor significantly associated with recurrence was a family history of pancreatic cancer. This study calculated the risk of developing a new IPMN to be 42 % at 5 years and 62 % at 10 years, with the estimated chance of developing pancreatic adenocarcinoma 38 % at 10 years. This study also recommended the indefinite close surveillance for patients after resection of a noninvasive IPMN given the high risk of recurrence and risk of cancer development.

15.6 Surveillance After Resection

Based on the studies of IPMN recurrence, long-term surveillance is recommended after resection of a noninvasive IPMN. While there is a lower risk of recurrence and better survival for noninvasive IPMNs compared to those with an invasive carcinoma, this risk is not negligible. Difficulty remains in the lack of specific factors associated with an increased risk of recurrence. Even a positive surgical margin, often a predictor of recurrence in malignancies, has conflicting data on its impact on recurrence. Furthermore, studies have shown a wide range of time to recurrence. Of those studies reporting on recurrence, the median time to recurrence ranged from 22 to 40 months, with individual recurrences seen anywhere between 7 months and 145 months [27–29]. This makes it difficult to identify the best postoperative surveillance regimen or a specific time point at which postoperative surveillance can be safely stopped.

Current guidelines are mixed on surveillance after pancreatic resection for IPMN. For patients without remnant disease after resection and negative surgical margins, the international consensus guidelines suggest to repeat imaging at 2 and 5 years to assess for any new recurrences; however, this is not evidence based [10]. Given the risk of developing pancreatic adenocarcinoma, even after resection of branch-duct IPMNs, others suggest CT or MRCP at 3–6-month intervals [31–33]. In patients with dysplasia at the resection margin, more frequent follow-up is suggested every 6 months by MRCP, with more frequent follow-up based on clinical and radiological findings [10]. In patients with known IPMN remaining due to positive margins or multifocal IPMNs, it is suggested that patients be followed similarly to those with non-resected IPMNs. This typically involves imaging every 3–6 months by pancreatic MRI or CT for those without features worrisome for malignancy [10]. However, there is no conclusive data at this time as to whether surveillance can be spaced out or discontinued based on stability of the lesion. In patients whose IPMN progresses toward findings suggestive of malignancy or who have IPMNs with "high-risk stigmata," shorter interval surveillance of 3–9 months is suggested by international consensus guidelines, especially in those whom resection is not an option [10]. While close follow-up is recommended after surgery, further data is needed to determine the best method for surveillance.

Conclusion

Much has been learned about IPMNs since they were described by Ohashi in 1982. Although a generally benign disease, increasing focus has been shed on these lesions as precursors to pancreatic adenocarcinoma. Survival for patients with noninvasive IPMN is high but drops significantly when invasive carcinoma is found after resection, demonstrating the importance of close preoperative surveillance and resection if worrisome features are discovered. Even after resection of a noninvasive IPMN, risk remains for recurrence of an IPMN or development of an invasive carcinoma necessitating close postoperative follow-up. Currently, no specific guidelines exist for the best method of surveillance, and further research is needed to identify those most at risk of recurrence and how to best follow patients. Until then, close postoperative surveillance involving clinical follow-up and imaging is recommended, especially for the first 5 years, to best identify any recurrence and prolong survival.

References

1. Ohashi K, Murakami Y, Takekoshi T, et al. Four cases of mucin producing cancer of the pancreas on specific findings of the papilla of Vater. Prog Dig Endosc. 1982;20:348–51.
2. Kloppel G, Solcia E, Longnecker DS, et al. Histological typing of tumours of the exocrine pancreas. In: World health organization international classification of tumors. 2nd ed. Berlin: Springer; 1996. p. 11–20.
3. Bastid C, Bernard JP, Sarles H, et al. Mucinous ductal ectasia of the pancreas: a premalignant disease and a cause of obstructive pancreatitis. Pancreas. 1991;6:15–22.
4. Ferrari BT, O'Halloran RL, Longmire Jr WP, et al. Atypical papillary hyperplasia of the pancreatic duct mimicking obstructive pancreatic carcinoma. N Engl J Med. 1979;301:531–2.
5. Warshaw AL, Berry J, Gang DL. Villous adenoma of the duct of Wirsung. Dig Dis Sci. 1987;32(11):1311–3.
6. Yamada M, Kozuka S, Yamao K, et al. Mucin-producing tumor of the pancreas. Cancer. 1991;68(1):159–68.
7. Morohoshi T, Kanda M, Asanuma K, et al. Intraductal papillary neoplasms of the pancreas: a clinicopathologic study of six patients. Cancer. 1989;64(6):1329–35.
8. Sessa F, Solcia E, Capella C, et al. Intraductal papillary-mucinous tumours represent a distinct group of pancreatic neoplasms: an investigation of tumour cell differentiation and K-ras, p53, and c-erbB-2 abnormalities in 26 patients. Virchows Arch. 1994;425:357–67.
9. Tanaka M, Chari S, Adsay V, et al. International consensus guidelines for management of intraductal papillary mucinous neoplasms and mucinous cystic neoplasms of the pancreas. Pancreatology. 2006;6:17–32.
10. Tanaka M, Fernandez-del Castillo C, Adsay V, et al. International consensus guidelines 2012 for the management of IPMN and MCN of the pancreas. Pancreatology. 2012;12:183–97.
11. Grutzmann R, Niedergethmann M, Pilarsky C, et al. Intraductal papillary mucinous tumors of the pancreas: biology, diagnosis, and treatment. Oncologist. 2010;15(12):1294.
12. Shi C, Hruban RH. Intraductal papillary mucinous neoplasm. Hum Pathol. 2012;43:1–16.
13. Schnelldorfer T, Sarr MG, Nagorney DM, et al. Experience with 208 resections for intraductal papillary mucinous neoplasm of the pancreas. Arch Surg. 2008;143(7):639–46.
14. Chari ST, Yadav D, Smyrk TC, et al. Study of recurrence after surgical resection of intraductal papillary mucinous neoplasm of the pancreas. Gastroenterology. 2002;123:1500–7.
15. Hwang DW, Jang JY, Lee SE, et al. Clinicopathologic analysis of surgically proven intraductal papillary mucinous neoplasms of the pancreas in SNUH: a 15-year experience at a single academic institution. Langenbecks Arch Surg. 2010;397:93–102.
16. Lubezky N, Ben-Haim M, Nakache R, et al. Clinical presentation can predict disease course in patients with intraductal papillary mucinous neoplasm of the pancreas. World J Surg. 2010;34:126–32.
17. Laffan TA, Horton KM, Klein AP, et al. Prevalence of unsuspected pancreatic cysts on MDCT. AJR Am J Roentgenol. 2008;191:802–7.
18. Winter JM, Cameron JL, Lillemoe KD, et al. Periampullary and pancreatic incidentaloma: a single institution's experience with an increasingly common diagnosis. Ann Surg. 2006;243(5):673–83.
19. Fernandez-del Castillo C, Targorona J, Thayer SP, et al. Incidental pancreatic cysts: clinicopathologic characteristics and comparison with symptomatic patients. Arch Surg. 2003;138(4):427–34.
20. Hruban RH, Takaori K, Klimstra DS, et al. An illustrated consensus on the classification of pancreatic intraepithelial neoplasia and intraductal papillary mucinous neoplasms. Am J Surg Pathol. 2004;28(8):977–87.
21. Kim SC, Park KT, Lee YJ, Lee SS, et al. Intraductal papillary mucinous neoplasm of the pancreas: clinical characteristics and treatment outcomes in 118 consecutive patients from a single center. J Hepatobiliary Pancreat Surg. 2008;15:183–8.
22. Nara S, Onaya H, Hiraoka N, Shimada K, et al. Preoperative evaluation of invasive and noninvasive intraductal papillary mucinous neoplasms of the pancreas: clinical, radiological, and pathological analysis of 123 cases. Pancreas. 2009;38:8–16.
23. Nagai K, Doi R, Kida A, Kami K, et al. Intraductal papillary mucinous neoplasms of the pancreas: clinicopathologic characteristics and long-term follow-up after resection. World J Surg. 2008;32:271–8.
24. Lee SY, Lee KT, Lee JK, Jeon YH, et al. Long-term follow up results of intraductal papillary mucinous tumors of the pancreas. J Gastroenterol Hepatol. 2005;20:1379–84.
25. Sadakari Y, Ienaga J, Kobayashi K, Miyasaka Y, et al. Cyst size indicates malignant transformation in branch duct intraductal papillary mucinous neoplasm of the pancreas without mural nodules. Pancreas. 2010;39:232–6.
26. Bournet B, Kirzin S, Carrere N, Portier G, et al. Clinical fate of branch duct and mixed forms of intraductal papillary mucinous neoplasia of the pancreas. J Gastroenterol Hepatol. 2009;24:1211–7.
27. Salvia R, Fernandez-del Castillo C, Bassi C, et al. Main-duct intraductal papillary mucinous neoplasms of the pancreas: clinical predictors of malignancy and

long-term survival following resection. Ann Surg. 2004;239(5):678–85.

28. White R, D'Angelica M, Katabi N, et al. Fate of the remnant pancreas after resection of noninvasive intraductal papillary mucinous neoplasm. J Am Coll Surg. 2007;204:987–95.
29. Miller JR, Meyer JE, Waters JA, et al. Outcome of the pancreatic remnant following segmental pancreatectomy for non-invasive intraductal papillary mucinous neoplasm. HPB. 2011;13(11):759–66.
30. He J, Cameron JL, Ahuja N, Makary MA, et al. Is it necessary to follow patients after resection of a benign pancreatic intraductal papillary mucinous neoplasm? J Am Coll Surg. 2013;216:657–67.
31. Tanno S, Nakano Y, Koizumi K, et al. Pancreatic ductal adenocarcinomas in long-term follow-up patients with branch duct intraductal papillary mucinous neoplasms. Pancreas. 2010;39(1):36–40.
32. Tamura K, Ohtsuka T, Ideno N, et al. Unresectable pancreatic ductal adenocarcinoma in the remnant pancreas diagnosed during every 6-month surveillance after resection of branch duct intraductal papillary mucinous neoplasm: a case report. JOP. 2013;14(4):450–3.
33. Ohtsuka T, Kono H, Tanabe R, et al. Follow-up study after resection of intraductal papillary mucinous neoplasm of the pancreas: special references to the multifocal lesions and development of ductal carcinoma in the remnant pancreas. Am J Surg. 2012;204(1):44–8.

16 Oncological Treatment of Cystic Tumors of the Pancreas

Roberto Valente and J.-Matthias Löhr

16.1 Introduction

The mainstay of treatment for cystic lesions with malignant or potentially malignant behavior is surgery [1].

Solid data regarding a possible role of systemic chemoradiotherapy (CRT) either in neoadjuvant, adjuvant, or palliative setting are still largely lacking for both cystic lesions other than IPMN and for IPMNs themselves. For the latter, most commonly clinicians base their clinical decision algorithm extending results from trials regarding pancreatic ductal adenocarcinoma to the management of IPMNs. This approach may not be still completely applicable since, at least for lymph node-negative disease, it is not clear whether they can be considered as two similar entities. Complicating the discussion, there are few data comparing head to head by stage PDAC arising from PanIN from the ones arising from IPMNs [2]. An analysis of SEER registry (1999–2005) compared the outcome of stage-matched 729 IPMNs and 8082 PDAC showing a possible overlap between the two diseases in advanced stages, such as in positive nodes spreading. The survival analysis showed that, in patients with node-negative disease, the 5-year survival was statistically significant ($p<0.001$) in IPMNs than in PDAC (35 % vs 17 %), while this survival benefit was not seen anymore in patients with lymph node-positive disease (7 % vs 9 %, $p=0.54$) [3]. Interestingly such latter cases seem to be the ones having a better response to adjuvant treatment. Anyway the pancreatic cystic lesion spectrum is quite broad, and then, when considering possible medical therapies, a simplifying distinction should be done, at least between IPMNs and cystic lesions other than IPMNs.

16.2 Systemic Adjuvant Chemotherapy for IPMNs

The use of a systemic adjuvant CRT in the treatment of IPMNs has been investigated in four small retrospective series so far (Table 16.1). All of them suffered from inevitable selection biases due to the fact that clinicians in analogy to the treatment of PDAC addressed patients to undergo a CRT in case of advanced disease or in case of clinical/histological more aggressive behavior. All except one [4] suggested a possible benefit from CRT in the setting of adjuvant treatment for invasive IPMNs undergoing surgery especially in the presence of node metastases according to the current European Consensus Conference's indications. In detail, in 2010 Swartz et al. retrospectively reviewed a series of 70 patients from Johns Hopkins who had undergone surgery for pancreatic intrapapillary mucinous tumor of the

R. Valente, MD (✉) • J.-M. Löhr, MD
Department of Gastrocentrum, Karolinska University Hospital & Karolinska Institutet, Stockholm, Sweden
e-mail: robbie.valente@gmail.com; Matthias.lohr@ki.se

M. Del Chiaro et al. (eds.), *Cystic Tumors of the Pancreas*, DOI 10.1007/978-3-319-31882-0_16

Table 16.1 Overview of the four studies analyzing the role of systemic adjuvant CRT in the treatment of IPMNs

Study	Year	Pts undergoing adjuvant treatment	CHT	RT	Aggressive/advanced disease in adjuvant treated patients[a]	Median survival (T/UT)	OS (T/UT)	CSS (T/UT)	Relative Risk/Hazard Ratio (T/UT)
Swartz et al.	2010	70 invasive IPMNs (1999–2004)	5FU together and after RT	Median 50.4 Gy	++++	25.8 months (56 %)/91.9 months (59 %)	–	–	Node-positive-treated pts displayed an RR = 0.43 $p = 0.047$ Overall, CRT was associated with improved survival (RR = 0.43; 95 % CI 0.19–0.95, $p = 0.044$)
Alexander et al.	2010	17 invasive IPMNs (1990–2005)	Infusional 5FU + RT (65 %) Bolus 5FU (24 %) Capecitabine (6 %) 5FU/GEM (6 %) GEM (6 %)[b]	Median 50.4 Gy	++	–	–	Median CSS of node-positive-treated vs untreated was 20 vs 3.3 months	Node-positive-treated pts displayed CSS HR = 0.10 and OS HR = 0.13
Turrini et al.	2010	37 invasive IPMNs (1989–2006)	5 pts GEM 2 pts 5FU 26 pts 5FU + RT 4 pts GEM + RT	Median 45 Gy	+++	–	All pts 5-year OS T/UT was 22 % vs 36 % Pts IIA or lower, negative margins T/UT showed no differences (63 vs 48 months $p = 0.98$) Pts IIB or higher and/or positive margins T/UT showed no differences (17 vs 22 months $p = 0.67$)	–	–

Caponi et al.	2013	33 invasive IPMNs (2005–2011)	23 pts GEM 10 pts GEM+RT	–	+	Disease-free survival in T/UT was 30 vs 44 months $p=0.05$ in N0 pts and 7.5 vs 16.5 months $p=0.04$ in N1 pts	–	–	Disease-free survival HR in treated pts was HR=0.40 (95 % CI 0.19–0.86, $p=0.02$) OS HR in treated pts was HR=0.37 (95 % CI 0.15–0.92, $p=0.03$)

CHT chemotherapy, *RT* radiotherapy, *CRT* chemoradiotherapy, *LN* lymph nodes, *T/UT* treated/untreated, *OS* overall survival, *CSS* cancer-specific survival, *5FU* 5-fluorouracil, *RR* relative risk, *GEM* gemcitabine, *Pts* patients

[a]Criteria for aggressive/advanced disease were vascular invasion, neural invasion, advanced T status/lymph nodes metastasis, undifferentiated disease (+/++/+++/++++)

[b]Five patients in the CRT group also received 4–6 additional months of adjuvant chemotherapy (3 with 5FU and 2 with GEM)

pancreas with associated invasive carcinoma. In this series, 40 patients underwent chemoradiotherapy (CRT) with both concomitant 5FU- and computer tomography-based radiotherapies (median 50.4 Gy) followed by subsequent 5FU administration. Many factors affected the quality of the study such as the small number of patients, the retrospective nature of the study, and significant selection bias due to the fact that a higher proportion of patients undergoing CRT had worse prognostic factors such as positive node ratio (65 % vs 30 %), stage II or III (80 % vs 47 %), perineural (63 % vs 27 %) and vascular invasion, and ductal phenotype. Due to these worse prognostic factors, the median 2 years survival rate after surgery with or without CRT was 28.8 and 91.9 months. Nevertheless margin-positive patients undergoing CRT had improved survival ($p=0.04$), and on multivariate analysis adjuvant treatment was associated to improved survival (RR = 0.43 95 % C.I. 0.19–0.95, $p=0.04$) when considering nodal and margin status, tumor location and grade, and histological type. The overall conclusion was that in patients with IPMN associated with an invasive component, particularly when lymph node metastases or positive postsurgical margins were positives, CRT could offer an adjunctive benefit in terms of survival [5].

After that in 2010 another paper retrospectively analyzed a cohort of 44 patients from Harvard University collected from 1990 and 2005. Within this group, 17 patients (39 %) underwent adjuvant concurrent CRT which consisted of radiotherapy (median dose 50.4 Gy) administrated concurrently with infusional 5FU in 65 %, bolus 5FU (24 %), capecitabine (1 %), and a combination of 5FU/gemcitabine (6 %) for IPMN with an invasive component. The median follow-up for all patients was 19 months and 26 months for survivors. Even in this series, patients treated with CRT showed a statistically significant higher stage ($p=0.035$) and positive node ($p=0.024$). Patients with positive nodes had a significant shorter survival compared to node-negative ones (16 vs 78 months). Patients with nodal disease undergoing CRT displayed a significant better cancer-specific survival (HR = 0.10, 95% C.I. 0.018–0.59) and overall survival (HR = 0.13, 95% CI 0.029–0.56). The median cancer-specific survival in node-positive receiving adjuvant CRT was 20 months compared to 3.3 months in the group who did not receive therapy. The conclusion of the study was that a clear prognostic benefit can be achieved in node-positive invasive IPMNs, while there is not a survival improvement in node-negative IPMNs in which probably a major role is played by a more indolent course of disease itself. It has also to be underlined the difficulty in interpreting the data about the short (3.3 months) survival of patients with positive node status not undergoing CRT, since it could be either the cause or the consequence itself of a missed opportunity for CRT [6].

In 2010 another paper analyzed a double-center experience on 412 resected IPMNs at Indiana University Hospital and at Mayo Clinic, Rochester. 98 (24 %) patients received a diagnosis of invasive IPMNs, the majority of which were main duct or mixed-type IPMNs (89 %). 37 patients (37 %) underwent an adjuvant treatment which consisted of 5FU chemotherapy in 2 cases, gemcitabine chemotherapy in 5 cases, gemcitabine CRT in 4 cases, and 5FU CRT in 26 cases. No patient underwent a neoadjuvant treatment [4].

Overall, the 37 patients who received adjuvant treatment showed a lower 5-year overall survival (22 % vs 36 %; $p=0.002$) and a median lower survival (23 vs 38 months) compared with patients who did not receive adjuvant treatment.

When stage-stratified in two groups (early or advanced), both of them did not show any difference in survival between treated and untreated patients. Particularly, the group of patients lower or equal to IIA stage with negative operative margin and the group equal/higher to IIB stage with positive margins showed no difference in terms of median survival when receiving or not receiving adjuvant treatment (respectively, 63 vs 48 149 months; $p=0.98$ and 17 vs 22 months; $p=0.67$), suggesting that the overall poorer survival with adjuvant treatment mirrored an intrinsic study selection bias. No differences in median survival were noted within patients who experienced a postsurgical recurrence of the disease when comparing adjuvant treated to non-adjuvant treated. A statistically significant survival advantage was anyway noted for the three patients who underwent re-resection for the recurrence of the disease ($p<0.02$) [4].

The conclusion of the study was that a clear prognostic benefit could not be added with adjuvant treatments. The only possible survival advantage regarded operated patients undergoing a reoperation for disease recurrence.

In 2013 also a retrospective series of IPMNs undergoing surgical resection from the University Hospital of Pisa, Italy, was described. Within 64 patients considered in the analysis, 33 received adjuvant treatments: 10 of which RCT (gemcitabine plus radiotherapy) while 23 chemotherapy alone (gemcitabine). Patients with lymph node-negative disease displayed a better median disease-free survival (DFS) when compared to patients with nodal involvement (32.7 vs 14.6, $p<0.01$). The same trend was seen in patients with G1 or G2 tumors when compared to G3 ones (18.4 vs 7.6 months, $p<0.001$). The median OS of the entire study population was 41.8 months (25.1–58.6) with a better OS observed for patients with lymph node-negative tumors compared to node-positive ones (57.4 vs 25.3 months, $p<0.03$) and for patients with differentiated tumors when compared to patients with undifferentiated ones (44.8 vs 9.7 months), $p<0.02$) [7].

When considering the entire population, patients receiving adjuvant treatment did not display significant difference from the ones that did not, in terms of DFS. However when considering both the node-positive and node-negative subgroups, adjuvant treatment seemed to produce a significant benefit 30 vs 44 months in treated versus untreated N0 patients ($p<0.05$) and 7.5 vs 16.5 months in treated versus untreated N1 patients ($p<0.04$), respectively. No survival advantages were seen for radiotherapy use.

In multivariate analysis of the entire cohort, several factors were identified as positive prognostic factors in terms of DFS such as negative lymph nodes (HR = 0.23, $p<0.001$), low tumor grade ((HR = 0.34, $p<0.03$), and adjuvant treatment 203 (HR = 0.40, $p<0.02$).

Negative lymph nodes and adjuvant therapy emerged also as positive prognostic factors for OS after surgery (respectively, HR = 0.22 $p<0.01$ and HR = 0.37 $p<0.03$) [7].

Although there are limits due to the intrinsic biases of the studies, these data taken together seem to underline a possible benefit of adjuvant chemotherapeutic treatment, especially in patients with a more aggressive/advanced disease, like the ones with positive nodes or postsurgical margins.

The possible advantages of radiotherapy are still less clear. While on one hand CRT improved survival in node-positive patients, on the other hand data on pure radiotherapy seems not to support any role of it in the management of invasive IPMNs [4].

Another paper tried to shed light on this aspect by retrospectively analyzing SEER registry and taking into account a cohort of 972 patients with diagnosis of invasive IPMN. Postoperative radiotherapy was administered to 309 patients (31.8 %). Within this subgroup T3 stage, node involvement and absence of metastasis were more common (59.9 % vs 37.1 %, 58.6 % vs 38 %, and 92.6 % vs 74.2 %).

Cancer-specific survival (CSS) in T3–T4-stage patients with positive nodes receiving RT was 20 months (CI 15–25 months) compared to the 12-month survival of patients not receiving RT (CI 10–14 months, $p<0.001$).

In T3–T4-stage patients with positive nodes, adjuvant RT was associated with improved CSS (HR = 0.71, CI 0.52–0.96, $p=0.022$), though there was no difference in overall survival (OS) (HR = 238 0.76, CI 0.56–1.02, $p=0.06$). No differences were noted among T1/T2 tumors and positive nodes or among patients with negative nodes irrespectively for the T status in terms of CCS or OS.

In conclusion the study demonstrated that the survival benefit associated with adjuvant RT was limited to T3–T4-stage patients, with positive regional lymph nodes. Anyway these results should be carefully interpreted because of the possible selection biases related to intrinsic nature of the SEER registry, like the lack of data regarding applied RT protocols, regarding possible concomitant chemotherapies, and regarding many patients, tumor, and hospital characteristics which potentially could influence the survival rate [8].

16.3 Systemic Adjuvant Treatments in IPMNs: Future Directions

A phase II trial tested erlotinib (oral inhibitor of EGFR) in pancreatic IPMNs by measuring the activity of the MUC5AC as a biomarker of the pathway, but the study did not reach definitive conclusions.

At the moment there is a Phase II-R and a Phase III Trial Evaluating Both Erlotinib (PH II-R) and Chemoradiation (PH III) as Adjuvant Treatment for Patients with resected head of pancreas adenocarcinoma including invasive IPMNs. The study, available at clinicaltrial.gov, is still ongoing and is validating the possible effect that gemcitabine with or without erlotinib followed by the same chemotherapy regimen with or without radiotherapy and capecitabine or 5FU may have in treating surgical resected pancreatic cancer patients (NCT01013649).

16.4 Systemic Neoadjuvant and Palliative Chemotherapy in IPMNs

At the moment there are no studies about the possible role of neoadjuvant chemotherapy in malignant IPMNs.

The role of palliative chemotherapy has also been poorly investigated in large series. In a retrospective series of 128 patients with IPMNs and 548 patients with invasive PDAC, 12 patients with invasive IPMN and 73 patients with invasive PDAC experienced a recurrence of the disease and were treated with gemcitabine-based chemotherapy as a palliative approach. The study, even if retrospective and on a small series, did not prove any statistically significant difference in the outcome of the two groups in terms of median survival (9.3 vs 8.8 months $p=0.09$) [9].

The possible role of a palliative systemic chemotherapeutic approach has then finally been suggested by two case reports treating, respectively, a peritoneum metastatic patient that has been treated with palliative peritoneal cytoreduction and intraperitoneal hyperthermic chemotherapy and a patient with a simultaneous occurrence of biliary and pancreatic IPMNs who had refused to undergo a surgical treatment [10, 11].

At the moment it is almost impossible to draw a conclusion stating whether an oncological palliative approach should be proposed to patients with invasive IPMNs, and further studies are strongly needed in order to clarify a possible role of a systemic chemotherapy approach in the setting of palliation for inoperable, metastatic patients and for those who refuse or cannot undergo a surgical resection due to comorbidity and high anesthesiological risk.

16.5 Systemic Chemotherapy in Pancreatic Cystic Lesions Other than IPMNs

The standard therapy for malignant or potentially malignant pancreatic cystic lesion other than IPMNs such as mucinous cystadenoma, serous cystadenocarcinoma, and solid pseudopapillary tumor is surgery. The role of medical therapy has not achieved yet any grade of evidence. Many, different, anecdotal case reports have been described with varying therapeutic protocols and results without having proved any standard of care.

In solid pseudopapillary tumor, even due to the young age of occurrence, the role of surgery has been particularly stressed, being extended to the resection of metastasis and anecdotally to liver transplant [12, 13]. Chemotherapy and radiotherapy should be considered in the management of patients with recurrent disease or with unresectable tumors. Adjuvant protocols, including gemcitabine, epirubicin, docetaxel, paclitaxel, and mitomycin C, have been used in few patients, due to the general resectability of the tumor. Some of these protocols were based on gel droplet-embedded culture drug sensitivity test [14]. Neoadjuvant treatments aiming at causing tumor regression have been anecdotally described using cisplatin, 5FU, gemcitabine with or without RT, or combinations of many drugs (VP-16, cisplatin, cyclophosphamide, doxorubicin, and vincristine), whereas others found no response to multiple agents [15–17].

Intensity-modulated radiation therapy and selective internal radiotherapy (SIRT) have infrequently been used in a neoadjuvant or adjuvant setting [14, 18, 19].

A single case report described the use of chemotherapy with gemcitabine as palliative treatment of mucinous cystadenocarcinoma, while other two reports described the use of gemcitabine and oxaliplatin (GEMOX) as neoadjuvant treatment, to obtain a downstaging and to finally allow surgical resection. In one of them, a subsequent adjuvant protocol with gemcitabine was used [20 22].

In another paper palliative, chemotherapy with gemcitabine was administered to five patients with partial remission and stability in one patient, stability in another patient, and progression in three patients with mucinous cystadenocarcinoma. In that series the median overall survival was 10.5 months [23].

These data taken together do not show any clear indication to the use of chemotherapy in the setting of solid pseudopapillary tumor and mucinous or serous cystadenocarcinoma either in neoadjuvant, adjuvant, or palliative setting. So far in this setting, the choice of undergoing medical treatment should be discussed and weighted with the patient considering his performance status, the possible surgical options, the local expertise, and finally patient's will and the possible gain in quality of life.

Conclusions

In the setting of IPMNs, the use of conventional chemotherapy might have a rationale in the treatment of invasive diseases displaying more aggressive features or in advanced stages such as the ones with positive nodes and positive postsurgical margins. So far new oral chemotherapeutic drugs, such the inhibitors of EGFR, are under evaluation in clinical trials. Possible benefits of radiotherapy are less clear but, as for chemotherapy, they seem either to be limited to the treatment of diseases in advanced stages (T3–T4 stages with positive regional lymph nodes). No evidence-based recommendations can be provided on both neoadjuvant and palliative chemotherapies.

No definitive indications can also be provided for the use of chemotherapy in the setting of solid pseudopapillary tumor and mucinous or serous cystadenocarcinoma either in neoadjuvant, adjuvant, or palliative setting.

References

1. Del Chiaro M, et al. European experts consensus statement on cystic tumours of the pancreas. Dig Liver Dis. 2013;45(9):703–11.
2. Chin JY, Pitman MB, Hong TS. Intraductal papillary mucinous neoplasm: clinical surveillance and management decisions. Semin Radiat Oncol. 2014;24(2):77–84.
3. Wasif N, et al. Invasive intraductal papillary mucinous neoplasm versus sporadic pancreatic adenocarcinoma: a stage-matched comparison of outcomes. Cancer. 2010;116(14):3369–77.
4. Turrini O, et al. Invasive intraductal papillary mucinous neoplasm: predictors of survival and role of adjuvant therapy. HPB (Oxford). 2010;12(7):447–55.
5. Swartz MJ, et al. Adjuvant chemoradiotherapy after pancreatic resection for invasive carcinoma associated with intraductal papillary mucinous neoplasm of the pancreas. Int J Radiat Oncol Biol Phys. 2010;76(3):839–44.
6. Alexander BM, et al. Intraductal papillary mucinous adenocarcinoma of the pancreas: clinical outcomes, prognostic factors, and the role of adjuvant therapy. Gastrointest Cancer Res. 2011;4(4):116–21.
7. Caponi S, et al. Adjuvant chemotherapy seems beneficial for invasive intraductal papillary mucinous neoplasms. Eur J Surg Oncol. 2013;39(4):396–403.
8. Worni M, et al. Adjuvant radiotherapy in the treatment of invasive intraductal papillary mucinous neoplasm of the pancreas: an analysis of the surveillance, epidemiology, and end results registry. Ann Surg Oncol. 2012;19(4):1316–23.
9. Otsuka T, et al. Gemcitabine in patients with intraductal papillary mucinous neoplasm with an associated invasive carcinoma of the pancreas. Pancreas. 2013;42(5):889–92.
10. Arjona-Sanchez A, et al. Long-term survival with peritoneal mucinous carcinomatosis from intraductal

mucinous papillary pancreatic carcinoma treated with complete cytoreduction and hyperthermic intraperitoneal chemotherapy. Int J Hyperthermia. 2014; 30(6):408–11.
11. Valente R, et al. Simultaneous intraductal papillary neoplasms of the bile duct and pancreas treated with chemoradiotherapy. World J Gastrointest Oncol. 2012;4(2):22–5.
12. Dovigo AG, et al. Liver transplantation as treatment in a massive metastasis from Gruber-Frantz pancreatic tumor: a case report. Transplant Proc. 2011;43(6):2272–3.
13. Sumida W, et al. Liver transplantation for multiple liver metastases from solid pseudopapillary tumor of the pancreas. J Pediatr Surg. 2007;42(12):e27–31.
14. Ji S, et al. Management of a malignant case of solid pseudopapillary tumor of pancreas: a case report and literature review. Pancreas. 2012;41(8):1336–40.
15. Romics Jr L, et al. Solid pseudopapillary neoplasm of the pancreas--proposed algorithms for diagnosis and surgical treatment. Langenbecks Arch Surg. 2010;395(6):747–55.
16. Kanter J, Wilson DB, Strasberg S. Downsizing to resectability of a large solid and cystic papillary tumor of the pancreas by single-agent chemotherapy. J Pediatr Surg. 2009;44(10):e23–5.
17. Maffuz A, et al. Preoperative gemcitabine for unresectable, solid pseudopapillary tumour of the pancreas. Lancet Oncol. 2005;6(3):185–6.
18. Zauls JA, Dragun AE, Sharma AK. Intensity-modulated radiation therapy for unresectable solid pseudopapillary tumor of the pancreas. Am J Clin Oncol. 2006;29(6):639–40.
19. Krug S, et al. Successful selective internal radiotherapy (SIRT) in a patient with a malignant solid pseudopapillary pancreatic neoplasm (SPN). Pancreatology. 2012;12(5):423–7.
20. Shimada K, et al. A case of advanced mucinous cystadenocarcinoma of the pancreas with peritoneal dissemination responding to gemcitabine. Gan To Kagaku Ryoho. 2009;36(6):995–8.
21. Obayashi K, et al. Remarkable effect of gemcitabine-oxaliplatin (GEMOX) therapy in a patient with advanced metastatic mucinous cystic neoplasm of the pancreas. Gan To Kagaku Ryoho. 2008;35(11):1915–7.
22. Di Marco M, et al. Preoperative gemcitabine and oxaliplatin in a patient with ovarian metastasis from pancreatic cystadenocarcinoma. Case Rep Gastroenterol. 2012;6(2):530–7.
23. Bjork Werner J, et al. Mucinous cystadenocarcinoma of the pancreas - outcome following different modes of treatment. Ann Gastroenterol. 2011;24(3):213–7.

Comparison Between the IAP and European Guidelines for the Management of Cystic Lesions of the Pancreas

17

Ralf Segersvärd, Takao Ohtsuka, Elena Rangelova, and Masao Tanaka

17.1 Introduction

At the moment, the management of the cystic tumors of the pancreas is regulated by two major guidelines: the one adopted by the International Association of Pancreatology (IAP) [1] and the European expert consensus statement (Euro) [2]. The IAP guidelines are created by the collaboration of 14 pancreatic experts in the field from mainly the USA and Japan even though one author is from South Korea and two authors are from Europe. This makes IAP rather broadly represented, however, with a clear weight toward general practice in the USA and Japan. The Euro guidelines are created by the European Study Group on Cystic Tumors of the Pancreas including about 40 European experts with one representative from the USA. Thus, these guidelines represent mostly the workup and therapeutic strategy of pancreatic cystic lesions conveyed in Europe.

A substantial premise for a guideline is to be widely applied and raise interest to be followed even by nonexpert centers before referral is needed. This is crucial for the equal patient accessibility and inclusion irrespective of where patients live. For preventive guidelines it is also of ultimate importance to aim to recruit all patients that might benefit from treatment.

In this chapter we will try to make an objective analysis of the similarities and differences between the IAP and Euro guidelines.

17.2 Common Features in the IAP and Euro Guidelines

17.2.1 Subject

The guidelines for the management of IPMN and MCN of the pancreas, published by the International Association of Pancreatology (IAP) in 2012 and the European expert consensus statement on cystic tumor of the pancreas (Euro) in 2013, are both consensus guidelines that are based on recognized leading experts' opinion in addition to review of the available literature and the highest level of evidence available. Although the Euro guidelines cover a broader spectrum of cystic lesions representing 90% of all known pancreatic cystic lesions, both guidelines rest

R. Segersvärd, MD, PhD (✉) • E. Rangelova, MD
Division of Surgery, CLINTEC, Karolinska Institutet at Center of Digestive Diseases, Karolinska University Hospital, Stockholm, Sweden
e-mail: ralf.segersvard@ki.se; Elena.rangelova@ki.se

T. Ohtsuka, MD, PhD • M. Tanaka, MD, PhD, FACS
Department of Surgery and Oncology, Graduate School of Medical Sciences, Kyushu University, Fukuoka, Japan
e-mail: takao-o@surg1.med.kyushu-u.ac.jp; masaotan@med.kyushu-u.ac.jp

M. Del Chiaro et al. (eds.), *Cystic Tumors of the Pancreas*, DOI 10.1007/978-3-319-31882-0_17

their major focus on the diagnosis and treatment approaches on the mucinous neoplasms of the pancreas.

17.2.2 Diagnosis

Both the IAP and the Euro guidelines recognize primarily MRI, but also CT, as useful modalities for the initial assessment of all cystic lesions. EUS with FNA, having a reasonable diagnostic value in experienced centers, is considered a complementary method in cases where the initial assessment has not been able to confirm clear indications for resection of a suspected mucinous cystic lesion.

Both guidelines agree upon the histological subdivision of the mucinous cystic lesions into gastric, intestinal, pancreatobiliary, and oncocytic type and on the definition of minimally invasive cancer, as well as on their clinicopathologic significance that might play a role for determining the follow-up strategy of the patient. The distinction whether the main pancreatic duct is involved or the disease is limited to the side branches is substantial, as well as the thorough examination of the specimen for a concomitant PDAC that may coexist.

17.2.3 Clinical Workup

Both the IAP and the Euro guidelines rely on a set of descriptive morphological criteria from the imaging studies to grade the risk for malignant transformation of the diagnosed mucinous cystic lesions that would strongly motivate surgical resection (regarded as "high-risk stigmata" or "absolute indications"). Both guidelines agree upon the two major structural features that should be addressed, that is, the size of the main pancreatic duct and the presence of a solid mass in the cystic lesions. The first one suggests involvement of the main duct by the disease, carrying much higher risk for malignant transformation, and the second feature suggests architectonical changes in the epithelial lining of the cysts with loss of respective layer organization typical for cancer. The only nonimaging criterion that both guidelines point out as a strong predictor of invasive behavior that requires surgery is the clinical symptom suggestive of malignant transformation in the area – obstructive jaundice.

Neither of the guidelines requires cytological or histological verification of existing malignant transformation, as guidance to surgical intervention, which reflects the current limitations with more thorough and specific assessment of the diagnosed cystic pancreatic lesions.

17.2.4 Surgical Intervention

Both the IAP and the Euro guidelines agree that MCNs represent an indication for surgical resection. Whenever the lesions are less than 4 cm in size and without clear signs of malignancy, parenchyma-sparing and spleen-preserving procedures may be used. Both guidelines make some reservations when a more conservative approach could be undertaken, which is smaller MCNs without clear malignant signs, considering the uncertainty for estimating the risk for invasive transformation and the undefined time perspective for that. Both guidelines suggest preventive resections only in surgically fit patients. The Euro group specifies further that particularly with smaller lesions, where diagnosis is uncertain, minding the often very difficult differentiation with BD-IPMN and oligocystic SCN, a similar observational follow-up approach as for BD-IPMN can be undertaken. For the rest of the cases of MCN, where invasive cancer development cannot be excluded, oncologic resections are recommended.

Regarding the surgical strategy toward IPMNs, both IAP and Euro guidelines agree that oncological resections should be considered whenever there is a suspicion of malignant transformation, i.e., whenever the risk factors are present. Both favor partial resection, depending on the localization of the lesion and not total pancreatectomy. Mini-invasive and organ-preserving procedures should be considered when there are no definitive signs of malignancy, but when relative indications, particularly in young or high-risk individuals, are present.

17.2.5 Follow-Up

Both guidelines present a clear algorithm for the continuous follow-up of the mucinous cystic lesions in patients without features meriting resection. Interestingly, neither of the guidelines engages with giving a reasonable time-limited cutoff for the follow-up. It is however not a surprise when there is a lack of knowledge and certainty about the natural history of the mucinous cystic lesions. The only way out of the surveillance program is surgery, even though follow-up of IPMN after surgery is still needed. The Euro group determines the deadline for follow-up of non-resected IPMN to be until the patients are fit for surgery, yet this recommendation does not convey a clearly determined time limit. Yet, becoming increasingly aware of the prevalence of pancreatic cystic lesions in the general population, and particularly the high incidence in the elderly, both guidelines carry a similar risk for excessive accumulation of examinations in the long run which might hamper the use of the available health-care resources. Hence, agreeing on limitations of follow-up is important and an issue that updated guidelines should be addressed.

17.3 Differences Between the IAP and Euro Guidelines

17.3.1 Focus

The IAP guidelines are focused selectively on the treatment and surveillance of IPMN and MCN – the most problematic cystic lesions that carry the high risk for malignant transformation. The Euro guidelines take into consideration also SCN and SPN as these two entities represent often the differential diagnostic challenge. By including these the Euro guidelines encompass recommendations for the clinical workup of about 90 % of all pancreatic cystic neoplasms and give a firm base for the general clinical practice. Clear hallmarks of treatment strategy are given.

17.3.2 Frequency of Follow-Up and Preferred Methods

The IAP guidelines provide a safe way of monitoring all mucinous cystic lesions in terms of not missing potential changes in their characteristics raising the suspicion for malignant transformation and, thus, surgical resection. The guidelines recognize follow-up of cysts of different dimensions, distinguishing between those less than 1, 1–2, 2–3 cm, and >3 cm. In lesion ≥2 cm surveillance is done by EUS or MRI every 3–6 months and surgery is considered in young, fit patients. EUS is the preferred method of surveillance in these lesions, despite being highly investigator dependent, having relatively low sensitivity and specificity, and is not readily available in many centers. This would imply the need for follow-up in high-volume specialized centers. Fine-needle aspiration (FNA) poses a further risk of complications that needs to be considered, particularly if the patient should undergo repeated examinations. In lesions <2 cm noninvasive methods are recommended, and the follow-up periods might be prolonged if no change of the measured criteria has occurred. However, the guideline does not state criteria for when follow-up may be prolonged. Ranges of time rather than exact timing of follow-up are given.

The Euro guidelines are somewhat less complex taking into consideration the differences in cyst size of <3, 3–4, and ≥4 cm, the latter being a relative indication for surgery. The Euro group recommends MRI as a major surveillance method in terms of avoiding radiation and invasiveness. The shortest recommended period of surveillance is 6 months and cyst growth rate is, besides morphological characteristics, taken into consideration for the timing of follow-up. Notably, the frequency of the repeated examinations increases after 5 years, reflecting the natural history of increasing risk for accumulation of neoplastic changes and an accelerated oncogenesis, however, so far only shown in experimental models.

Which guideline – the IAP or the Euro one – carries a psychological advantage for the patient and a premise for better compliance can only be a matter of debate. The somewhat tighter follow-up proposed by IAP might provide a feeling of safety and enhance the patients' compliance; on the other hand, the less invasive Euro approach might be perceived as a more tolerable one. This matter will remain unanswered, as long as no data from patient questionnaires to support one or the other is available.

17.3.3 Cyst Size Cutoff for Follow-Up and Intervention for BD-IPMN

The two guidelines differ in the relative criteria for a more aggressive approach, where IAP guidelines rely on morphology and cytology obtained by EUS ± FNA, whereas Euro guidelines act on MRI appearance, clinical behavior, and recognition of the value of CA 19–9. The size of the cyst itself has no correlation to the incidence of invasive cancer, but the increasing surface of the covering epithelium increases chance for neoplastic changes to occur on this terrain.

The IAP guidelines set the strongest emphasis on the presence of high-risk stigmata or worrisome features to justify the need for intervention. In cases when neither of these features is present, the guidelines stratify the recommended intervals of follow-up strictly dependent on the size of the cysts. No transition period to consider the speed of the cyst growth is recommended.

The Euro guidelines on the other hand consider clinical symptoms attributable to the mucinous cyst of great importance as well as the presence of risk factors. If none of these are present, follow-up at determined periods is recommended irrespective of the cyst size; however a rapidly increasing cyst size (>2 mm/year) is an indication to shorten surveillance intervals. Both guidelines recognize that malignant transformation may exist even in smaller lesions without worrisome features. The IAP guidelines advocate a surgical resection of a cyst to be strongly considered if it is >3 cm and considered if it is 2–3 cm. The Euro guidelines set the border at ≥4 cm but recognize rapidly increasing cyst size as a relative, but objective, indication for surgery.

17.3.4 Grade of Dysplasia at the Resection Margins

Moderate-grade dysplasia at the resection margin is not a recommendation for further pancreatectomy according to the IAP guidelines. The Euro guidelines, however, advise to at least consider further resection when moderate-grade dysplasia is present, in case the patient is fit for extended surgery. This consideration is made due to the fact that clear-cut differentiation between moderate and high-grade dysplasia, particularly on a frozen section, is very difficult to assess and there is no complete agreement on its estimation even among expert pathologists.

17.3.5 Use of EUS and CEA in Cystic Fluid

The IAP guidelines put more emphasis on the use of EUS (and FNA) as a method to evaluate the presence of worrisome features in cystic lesions, whereas the Euro guidelines are less hearted to utilize these as primary methods, rather only as a part of a multimodality diagnostic evaluation. The difference in methodology may reflect the differences in availability of EUS in Europe compared to the USA and Japan.

17.3.6 Risk Factors, High-Risk Stigmata, and Worrisome Features

Both the IAP and the Euro guidelines generally agree that malignant cyst-related symptoms, mural nodules, and dilatation of the main pancreatic duct are the key features that might predict invasive transformation and thus are strong indications for intervention. However, whereas IAP guidelines distinguish the presence of obstructive jaundice as a high-risk stigma and pancreatitis as a worrisome feature, the Euro guidelines do not make such a differentiation, but rather summarizes all symptoms that are known to be associated with cancer development (obstructive jaundice, newly diagnosed diabetes, acute idiopathic pancreatitis, etc.), as equally important to advocate further intervention. The same pattern regarding the assessment of the size of the main pancreatic duct may be observed. The IAP guidelines consider a dilatation of the main pancreatic duct above 10 mm as a high-risk sign, while a size of 5–9 mm is a worrisome feature. The Euro guidelines regard a size of the duct above 6 mm as uniformly requiring attention. Furthermore, while the Euro guidelines regard a rapid increase in size as worrisome, the IAP guidelines do not include this parameter, rather put weight on the results of further investigations with EUS with or without FNA.

Thus, the consequences following the Euro guidelines would be a somewhat more aggressive interventional strategy, maybe reflecting a difference in clinical attitude between Europe and the USA/Japan.

17.4 Strengths of the IAP Recommendations

The IAP guidelines are very thorough, describe in detail all aspects of the diagnosis of the mucinous cystic lesions, and clarify all the definitions, concepts, and reasoning behind the recommendations suggested. They dissect into smaller subcategories all of the morphological features of the cysts and present modified attitude in all the different scenarios, leaving space for the different physicians to adapt them to their practice without being very strict in neither the timing nor the absolute decisiveness of their recommendations. A premise, though, is that the consumers of the IAP guidelines need to be somewhat of an expert themselves in order to safely navigate through the possibilities of interpretation that is at hand. Finally, the IAP guidelines open the opportunity for new treatment modalities such as EUS-guided cyst ablation, e.g., in patients with comorbidities making them poor candidates for surgery. Even though clearly stated that more research is needed before this treatment can be recommended, it is important to emphasize possible future alternatives when intervention is required, but surgery is not feasible.

17.5 Strengths of the Euro Recommendations

The Euro guidelines encompass all cystic neoplastic pancreatic lesions that can be encountered and cover the workup aspects of the most often encountered cystic lesions and give clear recommendations for follow-up, including the interval time spans. The guidelines give the grade of recommendation and recommend a treatment or follow-up strategy, with certain reservations, of course, even when the grade of evidence is not high. The latter is substantial to decrease confusion and enhance the compliance in following the guidelines. Thus, the recommendations are practically oriented and can be used by most centers as a first approach, irrespective of volume or expertise. Lastly, Euro guidelines also look forward and points out pancreaticoscopy, today only to be used within research protocols, as a future possibility to enhance the workup of suspected main-duct IPMN.

References

1. Tanaka M, Fernández-del Castillo C, Adsay V, Chari S, Falconi M, Jang JY, Kimura W, Levy P, Pitman MB, Schmidt CM, Shimizu M, Wolfgang CL, Yamaguchi K, Yamao K, International Association of Pancreatology. International consensus guidelines 2012 for the management of IPMN and MCN of the pancreas. Pancreatology. 2012;12(3):183–97. Epub 2012 Apr 16.
2. Del Chiaro M, Verbeke C, Salvia R, Klöppel G, Werner J, McKay C, Friess H, Manfredi R, Van Cutsem E, Löhr M, Segersvärd R, European Study Group on Cystic Tumours of the Pancreas. European experts consensus statement on cystic tumours of the pancreas. Dig Liver Dis. 2013;45(9):703–11. Epub 2013 Feb 14.

Index

M. Del Chiaro et al. (eds.), *Cystic Tumors of the Pancreas*, DOI 10.1007/978-3-319-31882-0

MIX
Papier aus verantwortungsvollen Quellen
Paper from responsible sources
FSC® C105338

If you have any concerns about our products,
you can contact us on
ProductSafety@springernature.com

In case Publisher is established outside the EU,
the EU authorized representative is:
Springer Nature Customer Service Center GmbH
Europaplatz 3, 69115 Heidelberg, Germany

Printed by Libri Plureos GmbH
in Hamburg, Germany